Communication Skills Training for Health Professionals

An instructor's handbook

Communication Skills Training for Health Professionals

An instructor's handbook

D.A. Dickson
Head, Social Skills Training Centre,
University of Ulster, Jordanstown

O.D.W. Hargie
Head, Department of Communication,
University of Ulster, Jordanstown

N.C. Morrow
Director, Continuing Pharmaceutical Education,
The Queen's University, Belfast

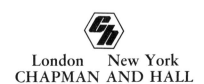

London   New York
CHAPMAN AND HALL

First published in 1989 by
Chapman and Hall Ltd
11 New Fetter Lane, London EC4P 4EE

© 1989 D.A. Dickson, O.D.W. Hargie and N.C. Morrow

Typeset in 10/12 Sabon by
Best-set Typesetter Limited, Hong Kong

Printed in Great Britain by
T.J. Press (Padstow) Ltd, Padstow, Cornwall

ISBN 0 412 32710 4

British Library Cataloguing in Publication Data

Dickson, David, *1930*–
    Communication skills training for health
    professionals: an instructor's handbook.
    1. Health services. Personnel. Communication skills
    I. Title   II. Hargie, Owen   III. Morrow, N. C.
    (Norman C.)
    302.2

ISBN 0-412-32710-4

This book is dedicated to:

Kerri and Shona;
Ernest, Pat and Elizabeth;
and
Michael, Victoria and David.

Contents

Preface

The importance of skilful interpersonal communication to the provision of effective health-care is now widely recognized. In addition to the various other dimensions of expertise which health professionals draw upon they must be able to interact successfully with colleagues and other health workers as well as patients and clients. It would seem, however, that standards of practice, in this respect, frequently fall short of public expectations and levels of professional acceptability. Interpersonal communication is consequently beginning to emerge from the 'hidden curriculum' to form an integral part of the training of, for instance, doctors, dentists, nurses, pharmacists, health visitors, physiotherapists, occupational therapists, speech therapists and dietitians. At present, however, those intent upon implementing such a training initiative often feel ill-prepared to do so having little to direct them in the planning, operation and evaluation of communication skills training (CST) procedures. This handbook has been prepared to meet this need for information and advice by tutors faced with the task of contributing inputs in this area as part of either pre- or in-service education programmes.

The book is essentially concerned with elaborating a structured and systematic instructional procedure for enhancing skilful *face-to-face* communication. (Utilizing representational media e.g. reports, pamphlets, newspapers, etc. and mechanical media e.g. telephone, etc. is excluded). It is organized in four parts. Part One contributes a firm conceptual base for the rest of the text by introducing and examining the notions of communication and communicative competence. The importance of effective interpersonal communication in the health professions is assessed and contrasting approaches to facilitating performance considered. An initial overview of CST is also given. Part Two is devoted to the *content* of training. Here a theoretical model of skilled communication is developed incorporating interpersonal, intrapersonal and situational determinants. A range of skills, commonly documented as being relevant to health-care personnel, are presented and analysed. These include nonverbal communication, questioning, listening, explaining, reinforcement and assertiveness. Furthermore the incorporation and integration of such skills within the strategic contexts of interviewing, counselling and influencing is discussed.

The CST *process* encompassing preparation, training and evaluation stages is the subject of Part Three. Having established the aims and objectives of the training intervention, techniques are presented for isolating and identifying appropriate skills content. Sensitization, practice and feedback phases of training *per se* are expounded and guidelines offered as to their implementation. This section is concluded by focusing upon methods of programme evaluation. The fourth and final part of the book brings a more integrative perspective to bear upon CST. A detailed exposition is given of the major considerations which the tutor must acknowledge in designing and implementing training and the influence of these, at different levels, on the instructional sequence formulated. Finally the impact of CST upon the communicative competence of professionals is discussed from within the institutional and organizational framework of the present Health Service.

It has been our intention to produce a book which is fundamentally practical in orientation, containing not only information and guidance but also material which trainers can directly apply in planning, teaching and evaluating programmes. Practical exercises are inserted throughout, together with suggestions as to how they may best be made use of. Material is also contained which can be utilized in analysing performance, identifying skills and presenting structured feedback to trainees. This can either be accepted in its present form or adapted to more fully meet particular requirements.

In outlining CST procedures and techniques we have, however, avoided a 'cook-book' approach which merely describes a stereotypical sequence of steps to be reflexively followed on each and every occasion. This is not how we see CST. Rather we have resolved to document the underlying rationale for this type of training and illuminate the theoretical, conceptual and empirical underpinnings of the various instructional mechanisms which contribute to it. Trainers who have a firm understanding of *why* they are doing what they are doing are infinitely better prepared to maximize the potential which CST has to offer with different groups in disparate settings. An inevitable consequence of this stance is that the book takes on some of the trappings of an 'academic' publication. Nevertheless, no prior knowledge of CST techniques is assumed on the part of the reader although those with a background in the behavioural sciences, particularly psychology, will be at an advantage.

Perhaps a mention should be made of the nomenclature which we have adopted. In the literature terms including 'interpersonal skills', 'social skills' and 'interactive skills' can sometimes be found to refer to what practitioners do when they relate to others and what we have here called 'communication skills'. Again methods of training in these skills, sharing many fundamental similarities with those presented in this book, have been variously labelled 'Interpersonal skills training', 'Social skills training', etc. (Furnham *et al.* 1980; Rae, 1985). While in practice there is little consistency, with these terms being applied interchangeably, we detect an emerging orthodoxy favouring 'Interpersonal communication skills training', or simply 'Communication skills training' in professional contexts. Throughout the book we have endeavoured to avoid sexist forms of expression. Where this proved difficult we have tried to ensure that gender-specific forms are applied on a reasonably random basis.

This book could not have been completed without the help of a great many people – we owe them all a very real debt of gratitude. We would like to acknowledge the support received from Professor Roger Ellis, Dean of the Faculty of Social and Health Sciences, University of Ulster, and the financial backing of the Faculty's Research Committee. Colleagues, including Christine Saunders, who contributed ideas and suggestions upon which we have developed a number of the exercises included in the book also deserve a word of thanks. We are especially appreciative of the continued encouragement and advice so freely given by all the tutors who have been involved with us, at the University of Ulster, in planning, presenting and assessing CST programmes in various Health Professions including District Nursing, Health Visiting, Occupational Therapy, Physiotherapy and Speech Therapy. Students who undertook such training also deserve to be mentioned – we have learned a lot from them about CST! An expression of gratitude is due to Mrs Audrey Mitchell for her proficient and expeditious typing of the manuscript. Finally we are eternally indebted to our long-suffering wives for their support and forbearance throughout.

David Dickson

Owen Hargie

Norman Morrow

May 1988

PART ONE

Background

The first part of the book introduces the topic of communication, its importance in the health professions, and training approaches to improving its effectiveness. As such, this part is designed to orient the reader to the detailed exposition, in subsequent sections, of the content and process of CST for health-care personnel.

Part One is comprised of two chapters. Chapter 1 provides a firm conceptual base which is built upon and extended throughout the remainder of the text. It begins with an initial examination of the salience of effective face-to-face communication within the health-care context and continues by assessing the present effectiveness of practitioners in this respect. The bulk of the chapter, however, is given over to a detailed analysis of the concepts of communication and communicative competence with knowledge, the ability to use it, and consequent appropriate performance, isolated as the central defining features of the latter. Extending this theme, the notion of communication as an essentially skilful activity is introduced and elaborated.

The manner in which the nature of interpersonal communication is construed will have clearly inescapable implications in respect of training. Three general approaches to instruction in this area are identified and labelled 'On-the-job', 'Model-the-Master' and 'Directed training'. Having established some of the weaknesses of the first two, 'Directed training' procedures are concentrated upon and descriptions given of methods based variously upon 'thinking', 'feeling' and 'doing'. CST goes some way to synthesizing these three methods and the chapter is brought to a close with an overview of the CST process.

Chapter 2 re-introduces the issue of the importance of effective communication in the health professions and examines it more thoroughly. At the outset a skill-based model of professional competence is developed incorporating a significant communicative dimension. The promotion of professional competence must, therefore, include training in interpersonal skills in addition to the more traditional areas of the curriculum. The chapter continues by examining a number of sources of influence which have resulted in the increasing acceptance, of late, of the legitimacy of CST and the contribution which it can make in the training of health workers. The extent to which CST procedures presently form part of professional curricula, is surveyed, particularly in the fields of medicine, dentistry, nursing and pharmacy. The chapter finishes with a brief consideration of the outcomes of such training and conclusions are drawn concerning the efficacy of this type of intervention.

1

Introduction

The young mother waited on her own. She had taken her baby to the hospital that morning, as arranged, to have tests of some sort carried out – her GP had been somewhat vague about it. Deep down she was more concerned than she cared to admit yet she reassured herself that there was really nothing to worry about – everything would be alright. Nevertheless it had to be faced that Emma was decidedly small and underweight for her age. She simply didn't seem able to fend off the constant colds and chest infections to which she was prone. It was on account of these respiratory problems that Dr Brown, her GP, had made the appointment at the hospital. Suddenly the door opened and a ward sister entered.

'Mrs Jones'
'Yes'
'Are you alone? Where is your husband?'
'He's at work. Why?'
'Dr Smythe would like a word with both of you. Could you contact Mr Jones right away and ask him to come here as quickly as possible. We have found out what is wrong with your baby. She has cystic fibrosis!'

With that the sister left letting the door slam behind her. Mrs Jones had heard of cystic fibrosis before but couldn't recall what it was. But she knew that there was something seriously wrong with Emma. Initial confusion quickly gave way to a growing anguish as she stood alone in that room.

It would be comforting to be able to describe the above story as a work of fiction – unfortunately the incident really happened, although the names have, of course, been changed. Nor can we console ourselves in the belief that it is unique. No doubt there are many like Mrs Jones who have been subjected to unnecessary levels of distress under similar circumstances. Other have experienced bewilderment, rejection, shame, guilt or humiliation due to the insensitivity and interpersonal ineptitude of some well-intentioned health professional who probably remained totally oblivious to the effects of her action. The story serves to emphasize the importance of communicating effectively with patients and yet how poor practitioners sometimes are at it.

The major focus of this book is upon how the communicative competence of health-care workers can be best promoted. To this end a systematic instructional framework is elaborated which encompasses, firstly, procedures for identifying aspects of communication which could most usefully be considered by particular trainee groups, secondly, a structured technology for training in these skills and thirdly, a variety of approaches to the evaluation of outcome. Several types of interaction that staff may be involved in and that require specialized knowledge and skill are also examined. These include interviewing, influencing and counselling. In addition, a range of specific skills which facilitate these processes are outlined. In this way it is hoped that the book will, in at least some small measure, contribute to a health service which is 'caring' in the fullest sense of the word.

1.1 THE IMPORTANCE OF EFFECTIVE COMMUNICATION IN THE HEALTH PROFESSIONS

During the past decade there has been an ever increasing appreciation of the importance of the interpersonal dimension of the work undertaken by health-care personnel and its contribution to patient well-being. Indeed the health professions can collectively be regarded as a particular sub-set of what recently has been termed, by Ellis and Whittington (1981), the 'interpersonal professions'. This label is applicable when the major proportion of the professional's working day is spent in face-to-face interaction with a variety of others and where the fundamental objectives of the service offered are largely achieved by this means. Thus Smith and Bass (1982, p.5) point out that, 'Much of health care is communication-centred. As a health professional, you give directions, offer reassurances, provide consolation, commiserate, interpret, receive information, and carry out directions. The more effectively and efficiently you learn to communicate, the more accomplished you become in fulfilling your health service role'. This book is explicitly devoted to improving the health worker's interpersonal proficiency.

The establishment of facilitative levels of communication enabling meaningful and trusting relationships with patients to be developed is now widely accepted as fundamental to effective management and care. There is some evidence to suggest that beneficial outcomes may be physiological as well as psychological and behavioural (Gerrard *et al.*, 1980).

1.2 ARE HEALTH PROFESSIONALS SKILLED COMMUNICATORS?

In the light of what has just been said, it is reasonable to assume that health professionals should manifest particularly high levels of interpersonal skill.

This, unfortunately, would appear not to be the case. Pettegrew (1982) suggests that perhaps it is the very fact that communication plays such a pervasive role in health care that has sadly led, all too often, to, '... neglect and complacency by those who must rely on it so routinely' (p.1). In any case empirical findings have largely corroborated the popular impression of the practitioner as someone who tends to do things rather than say things, being essentially concerned with the functioning of some part of the body rather than the patient as person. Having reviewed a number of studies surveying patient attitudes to the quality of care which they received, Gerrard *et al.* (1980) concluded that in many cases considerable dissatisfaction with the interpersonal dimension was revealed. Indeed patients tended to be more critical of poor communication between themselves and staff than any other facet of their experience in hospital. This is borne out by the NHS Ombudsman's report for 1978 in which it emerged that problems to do with poor communication were evident in most, if not all of the 120 complaints dealt with (HMSO, 1978). Sadly, it would appear that complaints of this type are still increasing (MacLeod Clark, 1985).

This decidedly depressing picture is made worse by those who have investigated the interpersonal competence of health professionals directly. Observation studies of senior medical students conducting history interviews unearthed deficits in certain essential skills. Even experienced hospital doctors were accused of showing a lack of interest in patients and failing to acknowledge their needs. As a consequence psychosocial dimensions of cases were largely neglected (Maguire, 1981). Nurses whose conversations with patients have been studied have fared little better. MacLeod Clark (1985) summarized the findings by saying that: 'The overall picture was one of tactics that discourage communication rather than skills that encourage it' (p.16). Again, in the community the social skills of the district nurse have been called into question by Kratz (1978). Unfortunately there is no good reason to believe that this state of affairs is atypical of the health professions as a whole.

In general it would appear that problems which arise centre around deficiencies in four major areas. The first is in getting information. Badenoch (1986) highlights this deficiency by relating the apocryphal story of the busy physician rapidly writing out the patient's history without looking up and blithely unaware that the patient is deaf and his questions are being answered by the blind patient in the next bed! Practitioners have been found to neglect important areas when interviewing or they collect the detail in such a way that it is likely to be inaccurate or incomplete (Maguire, 1981).

Secondly, the giving of information frequently invites criticism either because the amount provided is inadequate or alternatively is delivered in an insensitive or unintelligible way. This can cause compliance problems (Di Matteo and Di Nicola, 1982). Thirdly, and in a sense related to the last issue, health-care personnel have been accused of taking little time to listen to what the patient wants to say (Freund, 1969). Fourthly, communication which does take place tends to be primarily factual, addressing physical aspects of the condition (Byrne and Long, 1976). As a consequence it is thought to be inappropriate, even abnormal, for patients to have and divulge strong feelings to staff. Their role in offering comfort and emotional support is thereby neglected. Techniques for improving communication in each of these respects will be considered in Chapters 4, 5 and 6.

1.3 CAUSES OF POOR COMMUNICATION

The causes of what would appear to be rather disappointing standards of communication in the health professions are, no doubt, multifarious. Attention, though, has been directed to deficiencies in the basic training received by, for example, pharmacists (Hargie and Morrow, 1987a), nurses (Davies, 1976) and doctors (Pendleton *et al.*, 1984). The interpersonal dimension has all too frequently been ignored, underestimated or misunderstood. Davis (1981) highlights the assumption, held by some, that 'such skills are common-sense, inborn not learnt, and only a matter of conscientious application' (p.44). There is the view that communication cannot be taught. On the one hand it is argued that it is a 'natural attribute' and that 'you either have it or you haven't.' Alternatively it is suggested that it can only be taught in the practice environment and that intelligent individuals have no difficulty picking it up through experience. As a consequence communication has tended to be relegated to the 'hidden curriculum'. Recently there have been encouraging signs of a change of attitude on the part of those bodies with responsibility for monitoring standards of professional preparation and practice. As discussed more fully in Chapter 2, the need for more explicit instruction in this area is increasingly being recognized.

When training has been attempted, inappropriate methods have frequently been implemented leading to largely ineffective outcomes (Hargie and Morrow, 1986a). Many of those tutors who have been given the task of providing formal instruction in interpersonal skills are unfamiliar with training possibilities which exist (MacLeod Clark and Faulkner, 1987). Approaches which define communication skills in more explicit terms and offer a systematic and structured approach are advocated by many (Maguire, 1984a; Eastwood, 1985). The instructional procedure which we present in this book is of this type.

1.4 THE HEALTH PROFESSIONAL'S COMMUNICATION
   NETWORK

So far we have thought of communication involving the patient. But the health-care worker is at the centre of a much wider network of relationships as depicted in Fig. 1.1.

Depending upon the specific profession and the particular role played

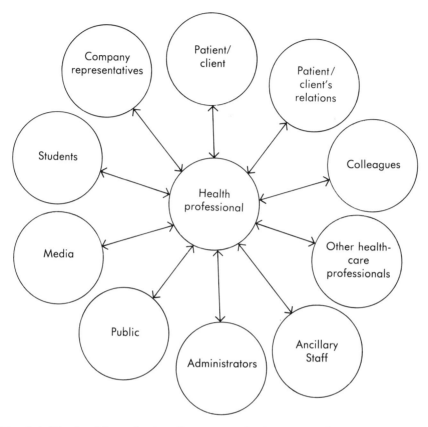

Fig. 1.1 The health professional's communication network.

within it, some of these contacts will be more common and important than others. Taking the example of a GP, consultations with patients, without doubt, are foremost in importance. But the GP may also discuss the patient's progress with members of the family, with colleagues and, indeed, with other caring professionals e.g. district nurse, health visitor, social worker, etc. during a formal case conference. There will also be contacts with administrative staff including receptionists, secretaries, etc. and, perhaps, with representatives from various pharmaceutical companies. The GP could additionally be invited to speak to members of the local womans' group on some aspect of health care; be interviewed on the topic on local radio; or act as a practice tutor to a student undergoing training in General Practice. This network could probably be further extended!

To attempt a comprehensive coverage of each of these various contexts is beyond the scope of this text. We will concentrate, for the most part, on dyadic (two person) interaction in those relationships with, for instance, patients, relatives, colleagues and other professionals which, it could be argued, are more central to the work of the practitioner. However the general instructional mechanism, encompassing preparation, training and evaluation stages, which is detailed in the following chapters has a much wider application.

1.5   WHAT IS COMMUNICATION?

But what exactly is this phenomenon that seems so central to the health professions and yet is often neglected? We have taken the term 'communication' somewhat for granted. It may be useful, therefore, to pause at this point to examine the concept and what it involves.

The first thing that strikes one about communication is its ubiquity – it is widespread throughout the animal kingdom. This has led Ellis and Beattie (1986) to describe it as a 'fuzzy' concept since its boundaries are blurred and uncertain. Yet, in spite of what has been said heretofore, it is something that, in relation to other species, humans excel at, having evolved a system of unequalled sophistication. In the interests of simplicity and relevance, attention will be restricted to human communcation and, essentially, to face-to-face interaction in the dyadic (or small group) situation. At a stroke this eliminates representational media e.g. reports, files, books, etc. and mechanical media e.g. telephones, telexes, TV, etc. What we are left with has been defined as, 'the process by which information, meanings and feelings are shared by persons through the exchange of verbal and non-verbal messages' (Brooks and Heath, 1985, p.8).

Characteristics of interpersonal communication

A number of central features of interpersonal communication have already been intimated in the preceding definition. These, together with several others, will now be examined in some detail.

Communication is a process

According to Fiske (1982) the conceptualization of communication as a systematic process is a common theme in the literature. At its simplest level, the components of this process include communicators, message, channel, noise, feedback and context.

Communicators For interpersonal communication to take place at all, there must be at least two people involved in the exchange of information. In the earlier theoretical accounts of the activity, such as that by Shannon and Weaver (1949), one was designated the *Source*, the other the *Receiver*. The process was held to commence when the source encoded ideas, thoughts, feelings, intentions, etc. or translated them into the form of a message capable of being transmitted to the receiver who then decoded them to reveal the underlying meaning.

More recently it has been stressed that each communicator is both a source and a receiver in the ongoing exchange. The notion of *source-receiver* is, therefore, a more accurate representation of the role played by each participant in the process (Myers and Myers, 1985). More will be said on this point later when the transactional nature of communication is discussed.

Message Messages can be thought of as signals, both verbal and non-verbal (in the form of postures, gestures, facial expressions, tone of voice, etc.), that pass between interactors and convey meaning. They may be auditory, visual, tactile, olfactory or gustatory. Frequently they comprise combinations of these possibilities.

Channel This refers to the physical means by which the message is relayed from one person to another. It can be regarded as the link between source and receiver. Light waves, sound waves and the nervous system, are examples.

In some cases, and in a wider sense, the means of communication in the form of face-to-face interaction, telephone, newspapers, TV and so on, are also referred to as channels (DeVito, 1986). Other writers, including Fiske (1982), label these 'media'.

Noise This is more than sound. It is anything that interferes with the success of the communicative act by distorting the conveyed message so that the meaning received is different from that sent. As such it may originate in the source, how the message is encoded, the channel, or the receiver.

Noise can be essentially psychological in nature. Unintended meanings can easily be attached to messages due to the beliefs and attitudes of the receiver. For example, although the doctor did not tell her, the hypochondriac is convinced, from what was said, that there is something seriously wrong with her state of health. Semantic noise is also possible when the doctor, perhaps, uses medical terminology which the patient either does not understand or misunderstands. In addition, physical noise in the form of intrusive sound, uncomfortable chair, unpleasantly warm room, poor lighting, or the patient having his hand over his mouth, can detract from effective communication.

Feedback By means of feedback, the sender determines the extent to which the message transmitted has been successfully received and its impact. Monitoring 'return messages' given by the receiver enables subsequent communications to be adapted and regulated to achieve a desired outcome.

Context All communication takes place within a context and is influenced, in an important way, by it. Context encompasses the physical location of the interaction – whether it is the health clinic or the patient's home; psychosocial factors such as the status relationships between the participants; the affective 'climate' of the meeting and the rules which govern it; and a temporal dimension in that the point at which a particular message is sent in an ongoing conversation can be highly significant (DeVito, 1986). Argyle (1983) discusses how participants must succeed in synchronizing their contributions in order to enjoy a properly organized conversation.

These various components of the process are represented in the model of interpersonal communication developed in Chapter 3.

Communication is transactional

Communication was viewed by earlier theorists such as Shannon and Weaver (1949) as fundamentally a linear process. The message was determined by the source and sent to the receiver. This opinion has given way to a more transactional conceptualization. The process is now generally regarded as characteristically dynamic and changing. Both participants are at the same time sources and receivers of messages. Each affects, and is affected by, the other in a system of reciprocal influence (Mortensen, 1972). Indeed each of the elements, previously identified, that form part of communication share an interdependent relationship. Changes in one will have implications for each of the others.

Communication is purposeful

Those who engage in communication do so, for the most part, with the achievement of some end state in mind. In broadest terms these goals may be instrumental or consummatory (Ruffner and Burgoon, 1981). Instrumental communication leads to some specific outcome e.g. asking the patient to 'open wide' enables the dentist to inspect for dental decay. Consummatory communication, on the other hand, satisfies the communicator without the active mediation of the other. In a sense the goal is achieved by the act of communicating e.g. feelings of relief having disclosed some guilty secret. Both types of outcome may be achieved by the same piece of interaction.

A more fine-grained functional analysis is offered by Dimbleby and Burton (1985). Communication may be used to:

1. give, get or exchange information
2. persuade and influence
3. form and maintain relationships
4. regulate power

5. reach decisions and solve problems
6. make sense of the world and our experiences of it
7. express ourselves.

This list can be extended by including some additional functions noted by Stevens (1975) which have relevance for the health professions. These are to:

8. alleviate anxiety and distress
9. provide physical, emotional and intellectual stimulation
10. facilitate further contact.

Commenting more single-mindedly upon the aims of communication entered into by the nurse when interacting with a patient, French (1983) identified the following. To:

1. establish and maintain a relationship
2. promote the equality of the relationship
3. collect information
4. give information
5. facilitate self-expression on the part of the patient
6. promote recovery
7. provide reassurance
8. control behaviour.

It should not be assumed, however, that communicating is inevitably a conscious activity. On occasion we may be completely unaware of having sent a particular message e.g. a look of disappointment when a patient regresses. Indeed, DeVito (1986) goes further by suggesting that messages may be conveyed unintentionally e.g. disgust on the face of a nurse dealing with an incontinent patient.

Communication is multi-dimensional

The complex nature of the phenomenon has already been alluded to. Messages exchanged are seldom single or discrete. Watzlawick *et al.* (1967) point out that human communication takes place at two separate but, nevertheless, inter-related levels. One has to do with substantive issues, with 'the words, language, and information in a message ...' (Northouse and Northouse, 1985, pp.8–9). The other concerns relationship matters and determines how participants define their association. Messages characteristically have elements of both. The directive, 'Nurse Smith, get on duty immediately', delivered brusquely by the ward sister serves to illustrate this. The informational message is contained in the verbal content, while the choice of expression and particularly the way in which it is delivered (i.e. nonverbal behaviour) serve to confirm the relationship which they share. There can be no doubt, for instance, who enjoys the higher status!

Elaborating upon these notions, Wilmot (1979) proposed that not only has every statement a relational meaning but that relationships cannot be orchestrated solely by relational talk.

In addition to addressing relationship issues, nonverbal behaviour seems to be centrally involved in conveying information about affective state (Argyle, 1975). Patients may be reluctant to discuss their emotions openly for fear of being thought 'weak' perhaps, but an astute practitioner will be able to detect anxiety or disappointment, for example, through such cues as the voice and facial expressions.

The nonverbal dimension has a further contribution to make. Messages of this sort may confirm, negate or modify the meaning attached to the substantive content (Myers and Myers, 1985). The nonverbal accompaniment can indicate how what is said is intended to be interpreted, for instance. 'Mr Brown, you are the worst patient on the ward', can be either a stern rebuke by a churlish member of staff or a friendly tease, depending upon *how* it is said. Furthermore the choice of medium together with the channel used to carry the information can contribute to the global meaning.

Communication is inevitable

Those who stress this facet adopt a broad view of what constitutes communication. In situations where two people are present and one is aware of the other, communication is taking place. The observed individual need not speak, indeed may be sitting quite passively, nevertheless the observer is able to form judgements as to sex, age, occupation, emotional state, etc. based upon the cues available. (There is no guarantee, of course, as to the accuracy of these opinions and they may be revised in the light of subsequent evidence.) Such observations led Freud to conclude that it is impossible for any individual to keep a secret, arguing that although a person's lips may remain silent he will betray himself in a profusion of nonverbal ways. Essentially the same belief was expressed by Watzlawick *et al.* (1967, p.48) in the statement: '. . . no matter how one may try, one cannot *not* communicate. Activity or inactivity, words or silences all have message value: they influence others and these others, in turn, cannot *not* respond to these communications and are thus themselves communicating.'

But not all who have written on the topic would agree with the above sentiment. Some have a much more restricted view of what constitutes communication. Gahagan (1984) distinguishes between *information* and *communication* on the grounds that the latter is an *intentional* act involving the *deliberate* encoding, transmission and decoding of messages in accordance with common codes of meaning. Other actions, such as blushing, are expressive rather than communicative. This conceptual distinction makes informing, but not necessarily communicating, inevitable. The implications are significant. As we shall see, intentionality and control are entailed when referring to communication as a skilled activity.

The most important practical point is that the accomplished health professional must be alert to the totality of the detail being provided: to what is said, how it is said, what else is happening while it is being said, to what is not being said, etc.

Communication competence

Communication that is consistently effective invokes the idea of competence. There must be some enduring and underlying predisposition to say and do things in ways acknowledged to be successful. The exact specification of what this 'predisposition' is, however, is more problematic.

Definitions of communicative competence abound. While Wiemann (1977, p.198) construed it as, 'the ability of an interactant to choose among available communicative behaviours in order that he (she) may successfully accomplish his (her) own interpersonal goals during an encounter while maintaining the face and line of his (her) fellow interactants within the constraints of the situation', as many alternatives can be found as there are authors. Part of the inconsistency resides in how the relationship between competence and performance is held. Following the distinction drawn by Chomsky (1965) between these constructs, competence can be thought of narrowly as knowledge; the knowledge which an individual has of his language and the rules which govern it. More broadly this knowledge-base incorporates characteristics of the psychosociological context within which it is embedded. For such knowledge to be of any practical significance the individual must also possess the ability to make use of it. This has spawned further differentiations between, as Fillmore (1979) puts it, 'knowing that' and 'knowing how' or 'knowledge' and 'the ability to use it' (Cooley and Roach, 1984). According to Hymes (1972) both knowledge and the capacity of the individual to utilize it are essential determinants of communicative competence. A consequence of this extended conceptualization is that 'competence' is not solely determined by cognitive factors but must also accommodate both motivational and affective concerns. (For example, a medical student may know how to conduct a history interview but anxiety may interfere with his ability to do it.) Performance is restricted to the implementation of such knowledge and ability – to 'actual use and actual events' (Hymes, 1972, p.283) – and distinguished from competence on this basis.

Communicative competence may accordingly be confined to knowledge about people and communication or to this knowledge together with the ability to behave in accordance with it. Some theorists go even further to include performance considerations (Spitzberg and Cupach, 1984). The construct will be used in this broad way in this book following Hymes.

Several additional features of communication competence are worth highlighting. The first is that it is very much culturally determined. Thus what constitutes competent behaviour in one context may not do so in another. In many parts of India an interactor of lower status will avert eye-contact by looking at the ground when interacting with another of higher position. Such behaviour, in the Western world, would commonly signal a lack of competence. More generally, Backlund, (1977, p.15) stipulated that, 'Appropriateness, then, appears to be the single criterion with the power to discriminate the phenomenon of communication competence from other communicative phenomena'.

Communicative competence is circumstantially determined in another sense. The values, beliefs, attitudes and standards of *the observer* reflected in *his* customary ways of relating must not be overlooked in establishing which performances warrant this label. Roloff and Kellermann (1984) stress this phenomenological dimension of the construct. Regardless of knowledge and its implementation, a communicator is only competent when he is judged to be so by another. Such a judgement entails that the interactor's performance conformed to a certain standard of acceptability; that it has been positively evaluated according to particular criteria.

One criterion upon which such a judgement may be made involves the outcome which results (Spitzberg and Cupach, 1984). Performances which lead to the desired outcome are more likely to attract this accolade than those which fail in this respect. More will be said on outcome considerations in the following sub-section on communication skill.

According to McCroskey (1984), communicative competence depends upon four constituent elements. In addition to the appropriate knowledge base and cognitive understanding, certain behavioural skills are essential. Without a repertoire of such skills, effective performance is impossible. Thirdly, the competent individual should manifest a positive affective predisposition towards communicating. Without it, cognitive and behavioural elements may be inhibited. Finally, there must be an opportunity for communicative competence to be operationalized. If not used, performance will atrophy.

The significance of this analysis of communicative competence should not be overlooked. The way in which the construct is defined will largely determine the approach adopted when faced with the task of training and evaluating health workers in this respect. Training implications will be returned to later in the chapter.

Communication apprehension

When the sort of positive affective predisposition towards interacting with others, mentioned above, doesn't exist, communication apprehension may be experienced and competence suffer as a result. Communication apprehension is a fear or anxiety associated with real or anticipated communication with another person or persons (McCroskey, 1977). It has to do with the way a person feels about communication rather than how they communicate.

It is likely that this condition is multi-causative (Daly and McCroskey, 1984). In some instances the negative effect associated with it may stem from an unfamiliarity with, and inability to successfully handle, certain encounters. Appropriate ways of coping may never have been acquired, perhaps inappropriate techniques learned in their stead. In any case anxiety is a reaction to the primary problem of skill deficit. The type of training procedure with which this book is concerned has been found to be an effective approach to overcoming difficulties of this type, especially when the anxiety is mild (Kelly, 1984). Nevertheless the trainer must be ever aware of the emotional demands being made on such a trainee and take steps to ensure that the tasks presented are capable of being undertaken without causing distress.

When performance suffers from the inhibiting influences of an anxiety which is more deep-seated and etiologically distinct – when anxiety *per se* is the essential problem – CST is unlikely to work and could indeed even exacerbate the condition. Here specialist clinical help may be required.

Communication as skill

The word 'skill' tends to conjure up images of manipulative procedures with various objects in the environment. In an artistic sense we may think of an acclaimed pianist playing a difficult piece of music; in sport, a top golfer driving the ball long and straight; in craft, a cabinet-maker turning a piece of wood; in medicine, a surgeon performing some delicate operation. If pushed we may even begin to consider some of the more mundane activities that form part of the workaday world of many, such as cooking a meal or driving a car. In other words, we tend to focus primarily upon perceptual-motor skills – that is 'activities involved in moving the body or body parts to accomplish a specified objective (Marteniuk, 1976). The scientific study of such skills has a long and illustrious pedigree within psychology.

The possibility of 'skill' being applicable to what takes place during an interpersonal exchange is less immediately evident. Crossman (1960) is generally credited with having first drawn parallels between perceptual-motor skill performance and the processes underpinning social interaction. In a report on the effects of automation on management and social relations in industry he noted that a crucial feature of the work of the operator of an automatic plant was his ability to communicate easily with his fellows, understand their points of view and put his own across. If 'skill' was an appropriate term to use in relation to the technical facets of the operator's job then why, it was reasoned, could it not apply to his communicative performance. The analogous nature of social and motor skills was further elucidated by Argyle and Kendon (1967). Both types of activity, it was argued, are carried out with the intention of achieving some end-state; both rely upon a complex system of perceptual, central and motor mechanisms;

and in both cases purposive actions are associated with commensurate environmental changes the careful monitoring of which enables decisions to be taken as to goal achievement. Limitations of the analogy were also recognized. These are taken up in Chapter 3.

But what exactly is communication skill? Again there is no single, commonly accepted answer to this question. Dimbleby and Burton (1985, p.58) define it as, '. . . an ability to use means of communication effectively, with regard to the needs of those involved'. It is therefore accomplished within the parameters of communicative competence already identified. Acknowledging the needs and rights of all concerned is a feature strongly endorsed by Phillips (1978). Accordingly, the degree of skill evinced depends upon 'The extent to which he or she can communicate with others, in a manner that fulfils one's rights, requirements, satisfactions, or obligations to a reasonable degree without damaging the other person's similar rights, satisfactions or obligations, and hopefully shares these rights etc. with others in free and open exchange' (p.13). Skilled communication, therefore, involves much more than the mere encoding, transmission and decoding of a message in such a way that it is understood.

But the main defining feature of communication skill offered by Dimbleby and Burton would appear to be the effective use of available means. Argyle (1983) also regards the extent to which the desired outcomes of communicators are accomplished as a key consideration in attributing 'skill'. This criterion is encompassed within the comprehensive definition given by Hargie *et al.* (1987). Thus by skilled behaviour we mean 'a set of goal-directed, inter-related, situationally appropriate social behaviours which can be learned and which are under the control of the individual' (p.3) Here six separate components of skilled performance are stressed:

1. Goal-directed. The purposive nature of communication has already been highlighted. Communication which, other things being equal, succeeds in accomplishing some preordained goal tends to be regarded as more highly skilled than that which fails. But 'skill' implies not only that acceptable intentions have been actualized but that they have been actualized in a particular way. There is a connotation of efficiency in the manner in which the goal state is attained. It has sometimes been described as obtaining the maximum effect from the minimum of effort. As with 'communicative competence' there is the further implication that skilful behaviour has been adjudged to conform to acceptable standards of propriety.
2. Inter-related. Elements of communication, both verbal and nonverbal, must be closely synchronized in order to bring about a desired consequence.
3. Appropriate. It has already been mentioned that appropriateness of use is a prerequisite of communicative competence. This applies both to the

goals striven for and the manner in which they are sought. Behaviour must not violate accepted situational rules and conventions. The skilled individual must, therefore, be aware of these matters and be sufficiently flexible to adapt to meet the demands of particular individuals in different social contexts.

4. Behaviours. Skills involve identifiable units of behaviour which the individual displays. These may take the form of questions, reflections, explanations or reinforcing utterances as outlined in Chapters 4 and 5. But this does not mean that such activities have a mystically inherent quality by dint of which they are skilful in some absolute sense. What makes them 'skilled' is their use within the framework of characteristics of skilful performance already identified. When we refer to a particular behaviour as a skill, this should be taken as read.

   Neither should it be assumed that skills are exclusively behavioural phenomena. While they undoubtedly have an indispensible behavioural dimension, performance, as outlined in the preceding sub-section, draws inescapably upon a body of knowledge, attitudes and abilities. Further perceptual, affective and cognitive complexities of the process will be introduced in Chapter 3.

5. Learned. It is widely accepted that most forms of behaviour displayed in social contexts, apart from basic reflexes, are learned by the individual. Verbal communication is a very obvious case-in-point. This fact, of course, makes CST a viable proposition and strongly counters the naive assumption, sometimes voiced, that 'good communicators are born, not made', with the implication that nothing much can be done to improve those who are weak.

6. Control. To be considered as skilful, communicators must have a measure of control over their behaviour. An important dimension of interpersonal competence relates to the timing of certain elements of performance. Learning *when* to communicate is just as crucial as learning what techniques to use (Tomlinson, 1985; Hargie and Morrow, 1987). Further characteristics of communication skill pertinent to the task of skill identification will be elaborated in Chapter 7.

1.6 APPROACHES TO TRAINING

Since communication and skill are essentially learned entities they must be amenable to training. Several broad approaches which can be contemplated have been identified and discussed by Hargie and Saunders (1983a).

'On-the-job' training

The 'logic' behind this strategy is that, having been successful in obtaining a certain job, one then beings to train oneself to do it, while doing it! Yet this approach is the one that has traditionally been employed in the health professions in respect of the interpersonal parameters of the work undertaken. It is still invoked by those who view communicative competence as something that will 'come with experience' being essentially 'caught rather than taught'. The available empirical evidence would seem to offer scant support for the comfortable assumption that this aspect of the professional role is gradually but inevitably acquired through increased experience (MacLeod Clark, 1985; Maguire, 1986). More generally, Argyle (1983), in reviewing research conducted into learning-on-the-job concluded that, '. . . this seems to be a very unreliable form of training. A person can do a job for years and never discover the right social skills . . .' (p.273).

Among the inherent weaknesses of this method can be mentioned:

1. Learning is predominantly by trial and error;
2. The learner may develop habits of 'survival' rather than situationally appropriate strategies and skills;
3. The learner may be unable to cope in certain situations or cope at the expense of the patient;
4. It raises profound ethical issues.

'Model-the-master' training

This technique consists of a learner being assigned to an experienced professional. The rationale would appear to be that through observation of 'the master' at work the skills displayed will be grasped by the novice. This, of course, is the philosophy underpinning the apprenticeship system of vocational training. Indeed elements of it can be found in most courses incorporating periods of practical placement or clinical experience. Many medical schools and postgraduate training programmes continue to rely upon it. But when exclusive reliance is placed upon this technique, training can be limited as Maguire *et al.* (1978) discovered in relation to the history-taking skills of medical students.

Some of the problems of this mode of instruction are:

1. The notion of the 'master practitioner'. Even experts have bad habits and can make mistakes.
2. No guarantee that the neophyte will identify the subtleties of effective performance and discriminate between that and inappropriate ways of relating.
3. Particular difficulties may occur in modelling when there are marked differences between the experienced professional and the student in, for instance, cultural background, attitude, personality, age, sex and behavioural style.
4. It promotes conservatism and militates against innovation, given that few 'experts appear to be aware of the considerable literature on factors

that enhance patient comprehension, recall, satisfaction and compliance' (Maguire, 1981, p.64).

Directed training procedures

This rubric encompasses disparate techniques for providing instruction prior to job experience. They are all classroom-based and explicitly directed to the furtherance of interpersonal functioning. While sharing this general aim, marked differences exist in relation to the formulation of specific training objectives and, more evidently, the procedures implemented in order to achieve them. Following the system of classification suggested by Phillips and Fraser (1982) we can regard them, on a methodological basis, as being either 'thinking', 'feeling' or 'doing' oriented.

'Thinking' based methods of training

This approach tends to favour more traditional, didactic techniques. The emphasis is upon providing information and effecting conceptual learning by means of, for example, readings, formal lectures, seminars, group discussions, films and case studies. Throughout, trainees are expected to be essentially passive and receptive. They are required to assimilate content and thus further their knowledge and understanding of interpersonal communication and its various facets, but to do little else. In relation to the different dimensions of competence it is, therefore, *knowledge* about communication which is, primarily, targeted.

While this approach is non-threatening and safe, familiar and, if well done, intellectually satisfying, Phillips and Fraser (1982) highlight some of its weaknesses. It:

1. Provides little opportunity for skills to be developed;
2. Trainees may fail to personalize the knowledge;
3. Fosters too great a dependence upon the trainer;
4. Fails to adequately address the complementary dimensions of communicative competence.

'Feeling' based methods of training

Here training concentrates upon the affective component of social functioning and the illumination of interpersonal operation is achieved by this means. Approaches which can be grouped under this heading rely upon experiential learning afforded by some sort of small group participation. Perhaps the best known of these is the T-group, but there are others such as Encounter groups, Tavistock groups or, more generally, Sensitivity training groups. Broadly speaking the aim of this type of training is to increase awareness and sensitivity. At the end of the experience members should be more aware of themselves, their needs and feelings, and the impact that they have on others. They should also be more sensitive to those with whom they may come in contact. This is achieved through the process of group involvement – the group itself is the learning resource. The group studies itself and what is happening within it. Participants, therefore, share perceptions of each other and what is taking place and by so doing exchange feedback. A corollary of this is that the group is responsible for its own learning making it much more difficult for the trainer to specify pre-determined learning objectives.

In addition to utilizing the group as a vehicle for learning, T-groups share several other features. They tend to have a 'here-and-now' orientation: discussion is based upon what is being experienced at that time in the group. They are less structured than many of the 'thinking' and 'doing' approaches; are typically process-directed; and the internal and external bases of various behaviour in the group are explored (Cooper, 1981).

Advantages of this method are in providing trainees with total involvement in, and responsibility for, training; increasing awareness of self and others; and heightening appreciation of the role of the affective domain in interpersonal relationships. Among the disadvantages, on the other hand, can be included:

1. May be threatening especially for the more shy, introverted, timid and serious participant;
2. Can prove damaging for some trainees;
3. Little conceptual framework given for what takes place;
4. Difficulty in setting precise training objectives;
5. Relevance of what takes place to the job may be unclear;
6. Places more emphasis upon increasing interpersonal awareness than on the various other parameters of communicative competence.

'Doing' based methods of training

These techniques rely upon action as a means of bringing about learning. Trainees undertake practical tasks of different kinds necessitating interpersonal communication with one or more others. The task may be a simulated exercise or could involve roleplay e.g. counselling a 'patient'. Throughout, the theme of training is closely related to what takes place during the task – with the performative aspects of the encounter. Practice opportunities can be built in to enable trainees to identify and implement various ways of dealing with the situation. Encouragement is often given by the trainer to try out different interpersonal skills and strategies. Based upon feedback provided decisions can be reached as to those which are most comfortable and seem to work best. This is undertaken within the context of a tightly structured and controlled programme derived from clearly articulated learning objectives (Phillips and Fraser, 1982).

A positive feature of this approach is that it focuses directly upon what individuals actually do when they communicate – upon the contribution of performance considerations to communicative competence. There are drawbacks nevertheless:

1. Little insight may be gained into *why* what took place happened if exclusive emphasis is placed upon behaviour;
2. Feelings may be neglected;
3. Trainees may be more concerned with performing well and not making mistakes, than with learning.

A summary reflection on these three orientations to improving communication reveals not only that each has attendant strengths and weaknesses but that the strengths of one frequently mark the weaknesses of another. Rather than being thought of as inherently diverse and incompatible a more fruitful framing may therefore countenance their unique contributions complementing each other in a comprehensive training framework. Such a framework is reflected in the instructional procedure outlined in this book which utilizes a variety of techniques including lectures, readings, group discussions, videotape displays, roleplay, simulation exercises and games, *in vivo* practice and focused feedback. Again the focus of training acknowledges communication as a complex and multi-faceted phenomenon. While it must, accordingly, be concerned with behaviour it must not be so to the exclusion of, for instance, the underlying needs and motives, feelings and emotions, perceptions and sensitivities of the individual. Consonant with the conception of communicative competence and skill already presented, effective instruction must provide knowledge, enable that knowledge to be used appropriately and ultimately make possible successful performance.

Communication Skills Training (CST)

Thinking of communication in terms of skill has profound implications for training. In keeping with other examples of skill, what transpires when two (or more) people interact can be reduced to a set of sub-processes and constituent elements. Just as playing golf may be thought of as involving driving, chipping and putting so an encounter with a patient may comprise greeting, getting information, giving information and parting. But analysis can take place at different levels within a hierarchical structure of performance (French, 1983). At the broad level of strategy the health worker could, perhaps, be interviewing, counselling or indeed influencing the patient to follow some course of action (Chapter 6). Each of these procedures is, in turn, capable of further analysis. At a more fine-grained level we can view the process as comprising molecular elements such as questioning, listening, explaining, asserting, and so on. Each of these skills is amenable to further reduction (Chapters 4 and 5).

A corollary of this reductionist philosophy is that the resulting sub-skills can usefully form the content of training. Allen and Ryan (1969) draw attention to the fact that similar procedures have featured for some time in training medical personnel in the technical aspects of the job. Similarly, actors don't learn 'a part' as an undifferentiated whole but rather break it down into scenes and indeed interjections within scenes. In like manner trainees undergoing CST are not expected to attempt a full-blown display of the performance, be it interviewing or counselling, from the outset. Instead the programme is organized in such a way that, in the early stages, isolated components are concentrated upon. A session, for instance, may be given over to questioning, another to nonverbal behaviour, the next to explaining, etc. Due to the progressive and systematic nature of instruction, by the end of the programme the repertoire of skills practised should be synthesized into a complete and effective performance of the communicative task. This is brought about in a number of ways and alternatives for structuring training will be presented in Chapter 12.

Regarding communication as skill implies not only that instruction can be planned, executed and evaluated but points the way to the sorts of training methods which may prove suitable. CST, as elaborated in the chapters to follow, is procedurally based upon fundamental concepts of learning theory including modelling, practice and feedback. Its origins reside in 'micro-counselling', a technique pioneered by Allen Ivey to offer training in the skills of interviewing and, more particularly, counselling (Ivey and Authier, 1978). Microcounselling in turn, grew out of the 'microteaching' methods used by Allen and Ryan (1969) to provide student teachers with classroom skills. 'Microtraining' is a more generic label for this type of instruction and has been reported to be 'an effective method for improving the communicative competence of trainees . . . and . . . well received by both trainers and trainees alike' (Hargie and Saunders, 1983a, p.163).

The three key phases of the CST process have been identified and labelled Preparation, Training, and Evaluation, by Hargie and Saunders.

Preparation   An initial starting point with any training endeavour lies in identifying the needs of the trainees. The objectives of the devised intervention accrue from these. This entails establishing the specific skill requirements of the group. Some of the techniques available for unearthing precisely what health professionals do when they relate to others in particular situations will be outlined in Chapter 7. The outcome of such inquiry furnishes the content of training.

Training   The training process combines *sensitization*, *practice* and *feedback* components. During the sensitization stage, the student is presented with an analysis of the skill under consideration by means of a lecture together, perhaps, with group discussion and readings. This, it will be recalled, is very much a 'thinking'-oriented facet of the procedure designed to contribute the necessary knowledge-base. Skill discrimination also forms part of sensitization training. Practical examples of the skill in use, typically presented on video- or audio-tape, facilitate a more concrete appreciation of what is involved and promote modelling. The emphasis here is with fostering the ability to make appropriate use of the knowledge acquired as a result of skill analysis (see Chapter 8).

The next stage of training requires that ability to be put to use. Trainees are given the opportunity to practice the skill in an interactive context. Chapter 9 examines this part and outlines some of the modes of practice available together with their advantages and disadvantages. The reader will recognize this as very much a 'doing' form of training which addresses the performative dimension of communicative competence.

Following on from practice is feedback. Here participants are made more fully aware of what they did during practice in relation to what they were striving to achieve and the effects which it had on the other party. This is a particularly important stage for promoting greater awareness of self and others, if properly handled by a skilful trainer. It forms the content of Chapter 10.

The rationale underlying this sequence has been characterized as, 'telling them what to do, having them do it and telling them how well they did it'. While this is a crude oversimplification and mistakenly depicts an extremely trainer-centred operation, it does reflect the three essential training components outlined above.

Evaluation The final phase of CST has to do with evaluation. This can be contemplated on a more or less formal basis and may be instituted for a number of reasons including student assessment and programme evaluation. At the very least it should ensure a more successful intervention 'next time around'. Chapter 11 is devoted to these issues.

In sketching this operational framework, we may have unintentionally created the impression of CST as an extremely fixed and inflexible procedure, uncompromisingly adhered to on each and every occasion. Nothing could be further from the truth. While accepting the basic tenets of this approach (namely that communication can rightly be construed as skilful, that analysis can reveal constituent elements and that these skills can be systematically taught), trainers have modified and adapted the *modus operandi* of instruction just outlined, to more fully meet the needs of specific groups of trainees and/or accommodate exiguous resources and limiting circumstances (See Chapter 12 for more detail.)

This reflective strategy is strongly recommended. It has, nevertheless, spawned a plethora of idiosyncratic programmes, each representing something of a 'variation on a theme'. Inconsistencies in nomenclature also abound. Some programmes can be located bearing titles such as 'Social Skills Training' or 'Interpersonal Skills Training'. While not wishing to deny that subtle conceptual distinctions can be drawn between social, interpersonal and communication skills, in practice, these terms tend to be used interchangeably (Hewitt, 1984), with essentially similar training procedures masquerading under different labels (Furnham *et al.*, 1980; Rae, 1985). This confusion is compounded by the fact that skills training of this genre has been implemented in remedial and developmental contexts in addition to that of professional education (Ellis and Whittington, 1981). As far as the latter application is concerned though, there would seem to be an emerging orthodoxy favouring the adoption of the term, 'Communication Skills Training'. Our choice of title was made essentially on this basis.

1.7 OVERVIEW

In this chapter the concepts of communiction and communicative competence were introduced and examined. Furthermore communication was presented as skilled activity and its associated characteristics expounded upon. One significant implication countenances the possibility of improvement in this respect through training and contrasting approaches to training were considered. The particular training procedure featured in this book – Communication Skills Training (CST) – was identified and briefly outlined.

The importance of effective communication in the health professions and the extent to which practitioners manifest it were further issues which were introduced. It is to these fundamental matters that we return in the following chapter.

2

The importance of effective communication in the health professions

2.1 INTRODUCTION

The foundations of a case advocating a place for CST in the training of health professionals were laid in Chapter 1. Some of the issues introduced there are taken up again in this chapter and developed. The notion of professional competence is examined in accordance with a model depicting the integration of several sets of sub-skills. Communication skills are identified together with those of a technical and cognitive nature which have more commonly been associated with effective health care. A corollary of this extended view of professional competence is the acknowledgement of the necessity for instruction to be targeted on all its facets. Continuing this theme, several major sources of influence are revealed which have resulted in the increasing acceptance of CST procedures as part of training courses for health workers. These influences include a growing realization, in many quarters, of the traditional neglect of the social and behavioural sciences in the preparation of health professionals and the contribution of these disciplines to health care. Secondly, bodies within the different professions charged with the responsibility of maintaining standards of training and practice have begun to recognize a need for improvements in practitioner communication. Thirdly, this need has been underscored by research outcomes into what takes place at the patient/practitioner interface and its potential ramifications for patient satisfaction and well-being.

The extent to which CST currently features in the professional curriculum is surveyed, particularly in respect of medicine, dentistry, nursing and pharmacy. Some of the empirical work which has been conducted into the assessment of training outcomes is examined and conclusions reached as to the efficacy of this type of intervention.

For the present, though, we continue with a more fundamental considera- tion of the concepts of health and health need.

2.2 HEALTH AND HEALTH NEEDS

At the receiving end of any therapeutic intervention is a person. The concept of a person rather than a patient is not often fully appreciated by health-care personnel, and is an issue largely neglected in professional training. Thus, the delivery of care is frequently conducted at an impersonal or functional level, reminiscent of a production line approach, with little attention being devoted to the interpersonal dimensions of practice, or indeed to the indivi- dual's behaviour and attitudes towards health and illness. It is, therefore, often a salutary lesson in interpersonal communication for the health pro- fessional to experience being a patient and thereby subjected to the realities of the health care system.

Moreover, within the health professions the concept of health is often viewed within narrow limits, the focus of attention being on the physical well-being of the individual. However, it is important to understand that being 'healthy' can and does mean different things to different people. Ewles and Simnett (1985) have presented several practical exercises designed to help health practitioners examine their attitudes to, and concepts of health in relation to their own lifestyle and practice, and the reader is referred to this resource material. These authors indicate that health needs to be understood not only in physical terms but also embracing mental, emotional, social and spiritual domains. The physical aspects of health relate to the mechanistic functioning of the body; mental health to the ability to think clearly and coherently; emotional health to the recognition and appropriate expression of emotions and also the ability to cope with stress, tension, anxiety and depression; social health to the initiation and maintenance of relationships with other people, and spiritual health to religious beliefs and ethical and moral codes the keeping of which may be a means of achieving peace of mind.

These five aspects obviously apply at an individual level. However, the concept of health must also be viewed at a societal level in that health is related to society at large. This means that the idea of being truly healthy in a holistic sense must be questioned in societies where there is oppression, violence, famine, racial prejudice and mass unemployment. Thus, at the practitioner-client level it will be important to recognize and perhaps relate across a much broader framework of health needs in order to provide effec- tive health care within the context of a helping relationship. Exercise 2.1 can be used with students to stimulate thought along these lines.

Exercise 2.1 The helping relationship

Instructions

Divide the training group into small sub-groups of three or four people. Give each member a copy of the case study and the questions for discussion. Each group should appoint a secretary and/or a spokesperson to feedback the group's response to the tutor. The responses should be tabulated and the main issues to emerge from the discussion highlighted.

Case study

Jane is a nineteen year old single parent with a six month old baby. She has no family support but is visited regularly by a social worker, whom she views as interfering in her affairs. The baby has been very irritable recently and hard to manage although Jane has not expressed this difficulty to the health visitor. To ease her own tension Jane has taken up smoking again which she had stopped during her pregnancy. She asks a health professional for something to help her stop smoking.

For discussion

- What factors are affecting (a) Jane's health; (b) her baby's health?
- Analyse these factors within a holistic approach to health.
- What communication problems/dilemmas/issues would you envisage in dealing with Jane?
- What actions or strategies would you employ to help Jane?
- What behaviour would be consistent with the helping relationship?

Unfortunately, in communicating with patients the tendency of the health practitioner is to do what has been learned, that is to teach, to sell or to tell. Such behaviours are more likely to serve the professional rather than the patient, to the extent that the patient may be disadvantaged in negotiating his/her own needs.

For example, in a review of the clinical implications of social scientific research allied to doctor-patient communication, Waitzkin (1984) has indicated that in regard to the sociolinguistic structure of communication, doctors often maintain a style of high control, involving many doctor-initiated questions, interruptions and neglect of patients' real 'life world'.

In contrast, the practitioner-patient consultation when conceived as a helping relationship is by definition different. Here a co-operative communication process exists in which the patient's needs and wishes are expressed and responded to by the practitioner. It is the adoption of a holistic approach to patient care which acknowledges and addresses not only physical needs but psychological and social needs, among others, that will result in greater patient satisfaction and more effective and comprehensive health care. Indeed with patients who have undergone surgery, there is some evidence to suggest that frequent contact, the establishment of a caring relationship and full and informative communication can contribute to a shorter recovery period and subsequent discharge from hospital (Ley, 1977a).

2.3 PROFESSIONAL COMPETENCY

This book is premised on the assertion that any conceptualization of professional competence in the health setting, must make reference to the inevitable communicative dimension of the job. Health practitioners are comprised of a number of professional groups who are related not only on the grounds of health as a common focus, but also by the fact that their activities involve pre-eminently face-to-face interaction and whose objectives, in terms of service, are largely effected through this means.

In relation to physiotherapy Caney (1983) formulated a homoeomorphic model of the competent practitioner which featured the integration of skills involved in communication together with those, traditionally recognized, of a more cognitive and technical nature. Applying this model on a wider basis, professional competence involves the ability to execute three main sets of sub-skills, namely cognitive, technical or psychomotor and social or communicative.

Cognitive skills

This represents the knowledge base of the profession, the body of knowledge which characterizes it and makes it unique from other groups of professionals. Obviously within the health-care field there will be some overlap in the knowledge base because of the implications to practice activities. Cognitive skills enable informed judgements to be made and decisions taken in relation to assessing and meeting need.

Technical or psychomotor skills

This relates to the manipulative skills inherent in the profession. This is quite obvious within the physiotherapy discipline but is also exemplified by surgical and palpable techniques, blood pressure measurements, the application of dressings and analytical skills in other health professional domains.

Communication skills

This refers to the ability of the individual to interact effectively with others in the professional context. It represents the aspect of health practice concerned with practitioner-patient relationships, inter- and intra-professional relationships and attitudes and behaviour to the delivery of health care and compliance with therapeutic managements. It is also the area which historically has received least attention in the curricula of the various health professional groups.

2.4 IMPETUS FOR SKILLS TRAINING WITHIN THE HEALTH PROFESSIONS

In relation to communication in the medical context Waitzkin (1984) has stated:

> 'Communicating well is an important part of practising medicine. Previously, practitioners have often paid lip-service to doctor-patient communication, have felt that it is someone else's problem, and have immersed themselves in the technical challenges of practice. The common assumption has been that communication is either too obvious or too mysterious to justify much detailed attention' (p.2446).

Applied to other health disciplines the statement is equally true, for, as has been previously indicated CST has been largely neglected in health professional training. Within the professions themselves there has been the feeling that the interpersonal dimensions of practice are naturally and automatically understood and acted upon, and that socially skilled action is not amenable to training and education. Furthermore, research within this area has been met with a considerable degree of scepticism and resistance by those committed to traditional scientific investigation. Indeed, the viability of some university departments is seen to be dependent upon being able to attract significant amounts of external funding for 'scientific' research. It must also be recognized that part of the justification of this is that the end product from scientific research is also much more easily quantifiable than a 'better' practitioner. Resistance to change is also evidenced by the conservatism that exists in various health disciplines, where the form and structure of education is very similar to that which existed some thirty years ago or more and which produces the attitude, 'what did for me is good enough for you now!'.

In addition and also summary to the above the development of CST within the health professions will be strongly influenced by a number of factors:

1. the need to clearly identify and define interpersonal skills pertinent to particular contexts of practice
2. the lack of training or experience of teaching staff to actually teach communication skills
3. the lack of facilities and resources required to teach communication skills
4. the limited time available in already crowded curricula
5. the hidden curriculum syndrome
6. the lack of commitment from educators to introduce new areas of training

7. the limited cross fertilization of teaching and research by the behavioural sciences to the health disciplines
8. the need for more evidence of benefit of CST courses in terms of patient outcomes
9. the need for a better understanding of the social and psychological contexts of health-care practice
10. the need to ensure an integrated form of CST.

Against this background it is important to highlight what have been the major factors that have contributed to the current upsurge in interest in the behavioural aspects of health care practice and the development of communication skills programmes in particular. Among these can be identified the recognition of the neglect of the social and behavioural sciences in traditional training; the outcomes of reviews of professional practice; and research into patient/practitioner communication. These sources of influence will now be examined in turn.

The contribution of the behavioural and social sciences

There has been a move to redress the imbalance in training through neglect of the behavioural and social sciences in their contribution to health care. It may be argued that the relevance and success of these sciences in the education of health personnel will depend largely upon the multi-disciplinary context in which they are presented, the degree to which they are considered as basic to the delivery of effective health care, their teaching and reinforcement throughout an individual's training both at pre- and post-qualification stages, the extent to which humanization occurs within the learning experiences of these personnel and the degree to which the teaching and learning of the social and behavioural sciences result in improved patient care. On this latter point it must be admitted that the cost benefits of such a programme are unknown, yet to ignore this area is a greater cost. It is, therefore, a path that must be explored if health professionals are to address the complexities of the individual, not only in chemical and biological terms, but emotionally, intellectually and socially.

Professional review of practice

Various reports following reviews of professional practice have strongly endorsed the need for better communication at the practitioner-patient interface.

This is perhaps best exemplified by reference to the pharmaceutical profession both within the USA and UK. In the USA, the Dichter Institute for Motivational Research in 1973 reported that many of the pharmacist's problems could be traced back to his failure to adequately communicate the value of his services to the patient. The pharmacist was stereotyped as the hidden practitioner closeted in his dispensary, typing labels and putting pills in little bottles but who did not see, speak with or touch the patient. Furthermore, the Report indicated that patients expressed the desire that pharmacists should communicate with them. Two years later the Millis Commission (1975) gave strong emphasis to the need for good communicative ability among pharmacy practitioners, and called for increasing the training of pharmacy students in communication skills.

More recently, the Association of Colleges of Pharmacy Study Committee (Chalmers, 1983) on the preparation of students for the realities of contemporary pharmacy practice addressed, among others, the issue of deficiencies in comunication training and abilities. The report stated that '. . . the core and elective courses throughout the curriculum should include instruction, guided experience, and formal evaluation and feedback to students regarding their written and oral communications' (p.398).

In the UK, the Working Party report on pharmaceutical education and training (Pharmaceutical Society of Great Britain, 1984) stressed the importance of developing the interpersonal skills of students and graduates. It was pointed out that without such skills pharmacists would not have an adequate basis for the provision of the full range of professional services which should be available in community practice. Indeed, a satisfactory level of communication skills was suggested as a criterion for graduation and professional registration.

Perhaps more importantly the recent report of the Nuffield Inquiry into Pharmacy (1986) clearly identified 'pharmacy's neglect of its own social context, and social science's neglect of pharmacy' (p.98). The Report advocated that the pharmacy curriculum should be restructured to include the behavioural sciences to involve the teaching of 'social psychology especially in relation to the behaviour of health-care professionals and patients' (p.104). Specific attention was also drawn to the importance and need to develop CST as part of both undergraduate and postgraduate education. Further, the Inquiry Committee recommended that 'research into pharmacy practice in co-operation with social and behavioural scientists should be increased' (p.139).

The importance of these issues was also highlighted by the Government's discussion paper on Primary Health Care (Department of Health and Social Security, 1986) which pointed out that it will be important to ensure that pharmacists' training supplements their scientific training with skills relevant to their wider roles, that is, skill in communication, counselling and behavioural science.

It is possible to trace similar stimuli from within the other health disciplines. For example, in medicine the UK General Medical Council in 1980 issued new guidelines governing the form and content of the undergraduate medical curriculum. Within these recommendations there are twenty stated objectives of undergraduate medical education of which no less than three include explicit reference to the skills of interpersonal communication. Further, the teaching of communication skills to new trainees in general practice is a stated part of the programme of vocational training as laid down by the Joint Committee on Postgraduate Training for General Practice (1982).

Similarly within the nursing domain the General Nursing Council for England and Wales (1977) stressed the need for nurses to learn the skills of communication in association with an understanding of the nurse/patient relationship. More importantly the teaching of these skills is a specific requirement in the General Nursing Syllabus of the National Board for Nursing, Midwifery and Health Visiting for Northern Ireland (1983) as can be seen from Table 2.1.

Practitioner/patient communication

The findings of research into the patient/practitioner interface have had substantial effect on the development of skills training programmes in the health professions. Indeed, Eastwood (1985) has suggested that the need to improve nurse/patient communication is supported from three distinct sources: (1) patient opinion studies which show social need; (2) expressed needs within the profession to improve communication performance; and (3) nursing research into the clinical needs of patients particularly in respect of reducing patients' anxiety. Research evidence from the dental field indicates that the attributes that patients seek in their dentists concern (a) the dentist's ability to perceive and cope with patient anxiety; (b) the dentist's ability to establish and maintain rapport with patients; and (c) the dentist's ability to inform patients and provide explanations (Furnham, 1983a).

More specifically the results of research at the patient/practitioner interface can be summarized under five headings.

Patient dissatisfaction with advice and information received

McGhee (1961) in a survey of 490 patients discharged from hospital reported that 65% of them saw communication with medical personnel as the least satisfactory part of their hospital stay. In a similar study, Cartwright (1964) showed that 60% of 739 patients recently discharged from hospital reported difficulty in getting the information they required about their illness, treatment, progress and tests. Their levels of dissatisfaction were strongly linked to their 'need to know'. Interestingly they expressed difficulty in knowing whom to ask. Only 11% of patients said that the nurse was the main source of information with 70% reporting that they received no information from nurses. Korsch, Gozzi and Francis (1968) in a study of child care referrals showed 40% of mothers highly dissatisfied with the consultation with the doctor as a whole. The overall evidence suggests that on

Table 2.1 Interpersonal skills in nursing*

Interpersonal skills required to meet the social and psychological needs of patients should be developed both in the classroom and clinical situations. The importance of roleplay, simulation and similar teaching methods in the classroom situation, and supervised clinical practice in these skills, is emphasized.

Interpersonal skills, to include:

- verbal and nonverbal communication
- receiving and interpreting social signals
- listening
- empathy, taking the role of the other
- self-presentation
- assertive skills
- reinforcing skills
- modelling skills
- stimulating interaction; commencing, controlling, continuity and meshing, concluding social interaction.

The application of interpersonal skills in nursing, to include:

- observing patients; perceiving and interpreting verbal and nonverbal signals
- establishing rapport with patients
- interviewing patients and relatives
- giving information to patients, relatives and colleagues
- reassuring patients and relatives
- fostering independence and self-respect in patients; involving patients in care
- asserting oneself as a member of the nursing care team and wider inter-disciplinary team.

* Taken from: National Board for Nursing, Midwifery and Health Visiting for Northern Ireland: General Nursing Syllabus for Part 1 of the Register of Nurses, Midwives and Health Visitors, (1983), p.10.

average 35−40% of patients are dissatisfied with communications with their doctors (Ley 1982a) and that the aspect of medical care that gives rise to greatest dissatisfaction is the amount and form of information received (McKinlay, 1972).

Non-compliance with advice

Crichton, Smith and Demanuele (1978) presented three primary factors which influence patient compliance with medication instructions. Firstly, the credibility of the information as viewed by the patient is an integral aspect of compliance. Here the patient must believe that the psychological, financial and physiological costs of taking the prescribed medication are less than the perceived benefits. Secondly, compliance is a feature of behavioural modification in the patient, and as such is a series of trade-offs by the patient between his daily routine and the restrictions imposed upon him by his drug regime. Thirdly, the knowledge of the patient concerning his medications is important, in that if instructions are not understood medication errors and defaulting occurs.

Against this background decisions have to be made regarding what information should be given. Ley (1982b) lists three basic criteria that may be used to establish the information needed by patients, namely behavioural objectives, rationality and empirical criteria. The first is primarily knowledge related, in that it is concerned with information of the disease itself, recognition of drug effects etc. The second criterion demands that a patient is given sufficient information to make rational decisions about treatment (e.g. weigh up the risks-to-benefit ratio). The third depends on having established correlation between the provision of certain information and particular outcomes. Thus, effective explaining skills will be a fundamentally important part of the health practitioner's interpersonal communicative ability.

Patient satisfaction and compliance are related

In his review (Ley, 1982a) showed that almost 50% of patients were non-compliant with not only their medication but with other forms of medical advice. At a more specific level non-compliance was viewed as being related to a number of discrete variables, (a) duration and complexity of regime, (b) patients' levels of dissatisfaction, (c) lack of support or follow-up, (d) patients' perceptions of their vulnerability to the consequences of the illness, (e) the seriousness of the illness, (f) the effectiveness of the treatment, and (g) the problems caused by treatment. Correlations between satisfaction and compliance have also been made with the patient's perceptions of convenience and waiting time before and during appointment (Becker and Maiman, 1975).

In their study of child care referrals Korsch *et al.* (1968) demonstrated the relationship between satisfaction and compliance and the practitioner. These workers showed that compliance was more likely if the doctor was friendly, engaged in some informal discussion, talked with the child and talked for a substantial time during the consultation. Compliance was also enhanced if the doctor inquired about and tried to meet the mother's expectations, took action to alleviate the mother's anxieties and gave information in addition to asking questions. A decade later, despite these observations, Plat and McMath (1979) were able to demonstrate significant deficiencies in doctor-patient consultations. In a study of 300 physician interviews these workers reported several key defects. Patients were not greeted adequately or provided with explanations of what the doctor was doing. Doctors appeared eager to terminate the interview and missed key leads. Their comments were not very supportive or understanding, nor did they ask how the patient was feeling. They were also poor in giving reassurance. Not surprisingly, Becker and Rosenstock (1984) have stated that 'compliance is greatest when patients feel their expectations have been fulfilled, when the physician listens and respects patient concerns and provides responsive information about their condition and progress, and when sincere concern and sympathy are shown' (p.197).

A final aspect of the satisfaction-compliance relationship is the fact that it can be linked to the provision of information by the practitioner. For example, McKenny *et al.* (1973) have shown that in a group of hypertensive patients exposed to medication counselling by pharmacists, their knowledge, regimen compliance and blood pressure control were significantly increased over a control group continued at the usual level of care.

Patients often forget or fail to understand what they are told

Failures of comprehension are related to at least three factors, (a) oral or written material is too difficult in terms of vocabulary, terminology etc. for some patients (Becker and Maiman, 1980); (b) patients often lack elementary technical medical knowledge such as the position of vital organs (Ley, 1977b); and (c) patients are often reluctant to ask their doctor for more information (Maguire, 1984a). As far as recall of medical information is concerned, Ley (1977a) has clearly shown that on average patients forget some 30–50% of what they are told and that this occurs within a short time following the consultation. Furthermore, Cassata (1978) has made a number of other observations in relation to patient distortion and forgetting of medical recommendations:

1. Instructions and advice are more likely to be forgotten than other information;
2. The more a patient is told the more he/she will forget;
3. Patients will remember what they are told first and what they consider most important;
4. Intelligent patients do not remember more than less intelligent patients;
5. Older patients remember just as much as younger ones;
6. Moderately anxious patients recall more of what they are told than highly anxious patients or non-anxious patients; and
7. The more medical knowledge a patient has the more he/she will recall.

This leads to the final aspect of patient/practitioner communication.

Patient understanding and recall can be improved which in turn will enhance patient satisfaction and compliance

A number of factors pertain to this issue. Firstly patients remember best the first instructions presented (Podell, 1975; Cassata, 1978). Secondly, instructions that are emphasized are better recalled. Ley *at al.* (1973) used the term 'explicit categorization' to refer to attempts by the communicator to emphasize and label the message given to the patient. For example, a doctor, nurse or pharmacist may tell the patient that he/she should be aware of three things, the drug dose, how it should be administered and potential side effects, and then go on to give specific information on each point. Thirdly, repetition of instructions aids recall. Fourthly, the fewer the instructions given, the greater the proportion of remembered information (Podell, 1975). Fifthly, simplification of information aids recall (Ley *et al.*, 1972; Bradshaw *et al.*, 1975). Finally instructions should be concrete and specific. An explanation or instruction which employs vague indeterminate words and expressions is not as clear as one which employs concrete and specific information (Hargie, Saunders and Dickson, 1987). This is particularly true of situations where a helper is giving directions to a client (Ivey and Gluckstern, 1976). (See Chapter 5 for further information on the skill of explaining).

Overall then, the patient/practitioner focus provides compelling reasons why CST is and indeed must be incorporated into the education and training of health personnel. Such training will by necessity have to consider not only models of the communication process but the range of social skills required to interact effectively at the practitioner/client interface.

2.5 COMMUNICATION SKILLS TRAINING IN THE HEALTH PROFESSIONS

Within the health professions medicine has had the longest tradition of CST. The refinement and development of interpersonal skills training in dentistry followed that of medicine, certainly within the USA (Jackson and Katz, 1983). Within the last 10–15 years skill-based training has become a more central part of nursing and pharmaceutical training. Individual initiatives within other health disciplines have been described more recently including occupational therapy (Furnham, King and Pendleton, 1980), physiotherapy (Dickson and Maxwell, 1985), health visiting (Crute, 1986), psychiatric nursing (Hargie and McCartan, 1986) and speech therapy (Saunders and Caves, 1986). An analysis of the experiences of these professions in relation to CST is of benefit in directing future developments and for those commencing initial training programmes.

Medicine

In their survey of 111 medical schools in the USA, Kahn *et al.* (1979a) attempted to ascertain the extent to which interpersonal skills were being taught and also which specific skills were addressed within the curriculum. These workers also aimed to identify at what stage of training this teaching was being focused, who taught the courses, what instruction methods were being used and also what evaluation methods were employed.

Results of the survey showed that of the 79 (71%) schools responding, 76 (96%) offered courses in interpersonal communication. The majority of programmes (61%) were directed to preclinical (first and second year) students, with 26% being offered to clinical students. The remaining 13% spanned both stages of the undergraduate course. An average of 2.5 official school-instituted interpersonal skills programmes were reported per school. Over 500 individual medical school faculty members were stated to be involved in such teaching (over 4 per school). Psychiatrists were reported to be the most frequently used teachers followed by psychologists.

A wide range of specific skills were taught within these courses with most courses focusing on the component skills of the interpersonal process, information gathering and psychological intervention. During the clinical years more specialized areas such as sexual counselling, counselling on death and dying and pre-surgery counselling were likely to be addressed. The main teaching method employed was that of video instruction for formal presentation, demonstration and skills practice/feedback. Some form of student evaluation was carried out by 95% of schools. Indirect assessment (e.g. multiple choice examination) was undertaken by 87% of schools while 69% conducted direct assessment through staff observational methods. Programme outcomes were determined by 35% of schools in terms of assessing patient satisfaction or patient compliance.

Two surveys in the UK (General Medical Council, 1977; Fletcher, 1979) have indicated that during the period 1975–1977 approximately one-third of medical schools (9 out of 30) offered no training in communication skills. In the remainder a wide variety of initiatives were made to address students' interpersonal skills. Such programmes were normally provided within general practice or psychiatry disciplines and amounted to one or two hours video-recording and replay. Only one medical school determined the policy that CST should form a defined part of the undergraduate course for all students. The most common teaching method involved CCTV with video feedback. Most of the teaching was directed to developing students' history-taking skills with little or no attention being directed to how to give information to patients. Evaluation of CST programmes was limited. More recently, however, a number of evaluation procedures have been described (Maguire *et al.*, 1978; Irwin and Bamber, 1984; Weinman, 1984; Knox and Bouchier, 1985).

At the practitioner level a number of programmes have been described. Kahn *et al.* (1979b) carried out a parallel survey of family practice residencies parallel to their medical school survey. In this study 88% of respondents indicated formal programmes in interpersonal skills. To a considerable extent the results mirrored the undergraduate situation in terms of the skills addressed, the tutors and the instructional methods used. Pendleton (1981) has described a CST programme as part of a Vocational

Training Scheme for medical practitioners. Similarly, Boulton *et al.* (1984) have described the programme for general practice vocational trainees focused more specifically to the development of skills to help patients achieve a good understanding of what they have been told in the consultation. Further, some of the issues relating to interpersonal skills training allied to general practice consultation have been discussed (Hasler, 1983; Schofield, 1983). Despite these initiatives, Kerr (1986) has suggested that in reality only lip service is paid to CST within postgraduate medical education in the UK and there is little evidence of organized teaching of the subject on a large scale.

The final aspect of the medical situation is the implications for CST arising out of an assessment of the teaching of clinical interviewing. Carroll and Monroe (1980) reviewed 73 studies of the teaching of medical interviewing. They concluded that instruction in clinical interviewing has generally promoted significant gains in students' interview skills. Furthermore, they suggested four principles for designing instructional programmes: (a) the provision of direct observation and feedback on students' interviewing behaviour; (b) the use of standardized presentations of illustrative patient interviews; (c) the explicit stating of the skills to be learned and evaluated; and (d) the provision of sufficient time to undertake small group or individualized instruction.

Dentistry

Dworkin (1981) has traced the development of the application of the behavioural sciences to dental education in the USA. During the 1960s considerable impetus was given to the notion that dental education should not be just concerned with the teaching of technical and clinical skills emanating from a biological science base. There was a need to integrate the behavioural sciences into dental education in order to 'humanize the dental student'. The overall object was to train practitioners who were not only technically capable and biologically orientated but who were socially sensitive. Such was the impact of this movement that in 1970 about 70% of USA dental schools had departments of Social Dentistry teaching diverse subjects such as biostatistics, epidemiology, and patient management.

The patient management aspects of training have been addressed in two main ways. The first is concerned with patient behaviour and how this can be managed or controlled. It is perhaps best exemplified by the efforts made to teach dental students and practitioners how to manage anxiety and fear in the paediatric patient (Chambers, 1970; Weinstein and Getz, 1978). In the second, the focus is on the patient's feelings and emotions as the basis for developing interpersonal skills, and finds its expression in training, for example, counselling skills (Hornsby, Deneen and Heid, 1975; Eijkman *et al.*, 1977; Jackson, 1978; Runyon and Cohen, 1979).

Within the USA it is difficult to estimate the amount of time given to interpersonal skills training. Dworkin (1981) has indicated that behavioural science in its broadest sense comprises from 4–6% of the total dental curriculum in terms of clock hours. To this extent the behavioural science enterprise is not large and is poorly supported. However, the presence of at least one or two 'behavioural/social science type' faculty members in each school is indication that the concept, at least, is well established. More specifically, the results of a curriculum study conducted by the American Dental Association (1977) indicated that, although 92% of schools offered courses in the interpersonal aspects of dental care, these occupied less than 2% of the entire curriculum of the average school.

More recently, a number of initiatives have been described in relation to interpersonal skills training in dentistry (Bader, 1983). These relate to the type of courses that have been implemented, the skills content of the courses and the teaching techniques and materials that have been employed. Videotape technology formed an important element of the instruction methods used and considerable emphasis was placed on experiential learning. Other programmes of training have been described together with evidence of their positive effects on trainees (Brown and Elmore, 1982; Ter Horst, Leeds and Hoogstraten, 1984).

In contrast to the USA situation, CST in the dental discipline in the UK is still largely underdeveloped. Furnham (1983a) has provided compelling reasons why social skills training is important to dentists, in terms of improving patient satisfaction, compliance and attendance, as well as possibly reducing occupational stress and improving job satisfaction. However, despite the fact that dentistry, like the other health professions, is an 'interpersonal profession', social skills training occupies no part of the formal curriculum of training institutions in the UK but is supposed to occur in the 'hidden curriculum'.

Nursing

In the USA Sparks *et al.* (1980) carried out a study of interpersonal skills training in nursing practitioner programmes parallel to that of Kahn *et al.* (1979a) in medicine. At least 78% of the 120 programmes surveyed included courses on interpersonal communication. A wide variety of individual skills were taught including, among others, interpersonal process skills, information gathering skills, information giving/counselling skills and psychological intervention skills. The most frequently cited skill was that of psychosocial history taking. Listening skills were also strongly emphasized within these courses, a skill which Whyte (1980) has drawn particular attention to as being fundamental to good nursing practice.

The majority of courses were taught by academic non-physician clinicians including nurses, psychiatric social workers, clinical psychologists etc.

Behavioural scientists were involved in teaching almost 20% of courses. In terms of instructional methods used lectures predominated in didactic teaching. Videotape exemplars were used by 66% of faculties, and videotape and live observation were employed most frequently for skill practice and feedback. Course evaluation was carried out most often using indirect methods. However, 63% of courses included direct assessment, involving both tutor and peer observation of live and videotaped performance. Several course descriptions have been reported which are illustrative of the teaching initiatives in the USA (Higgins, McCabe and Vanetzian, 1984; Friedrich, Lively and Schacht, 1985; Menikheim and Ryden, 1985).

In the UK, Nurse (1977) surveyed twenty-four schools of nursing in an attempt to establish the extent to which CST was implemented with student nurses undertaking general nurse training. Of the fifteen schools responding only two stated that communication skills were taught in discrete sessions where roleplaying was occasionally involved. Other schools reported that communication was discussed in the context of other areas of nursing practice. More recently, in a survey of all Directors of Nurse Education in England, Wales and Northern Ireland, 32% indicated that 5% or less time was given to planned communication sessions, while 43% thought that less than 10% of time was given to the subject. Furthermore, tutors indicated that they felt generally ill-prepared to teach communication skills (Faulkner *et al.*, 1983). Gott (1984) in a review of three schools of nursing found that interpersonal skill development was not a curricular goal in any of the schools and no formal teaching in communication skill was provided.

Although the evidence suggests that CST for nurses is still in its infancy in the UK some more positive initiatives are emerging. Firstly, as has been previously stated, 'the new syllabus' for nurse education in Northern Ireland places considerable emphasis on developing interpersonal skills such that Smith (1983) has claimed that CST in nursing education in the Province is more established than in the rest of the UK. However, Eastwood (1985) has also indicated that for further improvement in communication skill development to occur there is need to: (a) train the trainers in the teaching of these skills; (b) provide a more structured approach to learning for students; and (c) equip training centres with the modern resources required to teach these skills.

Secondly, an increasing number of practice research reports have been published which focus on the interpersonal dimensions of the nursing process. These are largely directed at examining the context in which interpersonal interactions take place, identifying the skills to be trained appropriate to the practice situation, and the implementation and evaluation of CST for nurses (Kagan, 1985).

Thirdly, and related to the former is the recent proliferation of texts which bring together issues of research and practice related to interpersonal skills in nursing, and which seek to serve researchers, trainers and nurse practitioners in the development and learning of the subject area (Faulkner, 1984; Gott, 1984; Porritt, 1984; Kagan, 1985; Sundeen *et al.*, 1985; Kagan *et al.*, 1986).

Pharmacy

Within the pharmaceutical discipline CST has historically been a neglected part of training. The origins of teaching in this area can be traced to the early 1970s in the USA, where currently the majority of pharmacy schools offer formal classroom instruction in communication skills (Pillow and Schlegel, 1981). The evidence from the USA does however indicate that there is enormous variation in regard to the content of these courses and also the strategies that are employed to develop professional social skills (Morrow, 1986). Experience in the UK of social skills training is more limited. In a recent survey of the eighteen schools of pharmacy in the UK and Ireland (Hargie and Morrow, 1986a) three schools indicated that they did not include a communication component within the undergraduate curriculum. Of the remaining fifteen schools, only four indicated that they devoted twenty hours or more per student to this training. In five schools less than seven hours per student was allocated. Four schools stated that the amount of time given was variable and of the remaining two one devoted ten hours and the other thirteen hours.

In relation to training strategies, twelve schools made use of roleplay, four closed-circuit television and six used exemplar video films. Only four institutions used all three of these teaching methods. Student assessment was carried out by seven departments using written assessment and examinations. An examination of the content of courses revealed eleven distinct areas of teaching of which interviewing, questioning and theoretical perspectives predominated.

Like medicine there is little evidence within the pharmaceutical discipline to indicate that CST is widely conducted at the continuing education level, despite the fact that the majority of practitioners have never been exposed to this form of training. In the USA, Love, Weise and Parker (1978) and Hanson (1981) have described individual programmes to develop the social skills of practising pharmacists. In the UK a major initiative has been mounted in Northern Ireland where the disciplines of pharmacy and applied psychology have been brought together to mount successful endeavours in the interpersonal dimensions of pharmacy practice (Morrow and Hargie, 1985a; 1987a).

2.6 ASSESSMENT

Much has been published to describe what should or should not happen in any patient/practitioner consultation, but there is little empirical evidence to clearly identify the effects of CST among health practitioners. As has been previously stated there is some evidence to indicate that good communicative technique enhances patient satisfaction, aids compliance and improves recovery. However, does training improve performance? What happens to performance over time? Are there any differences in specific outcomes? Do skills become habituated and do they become generalized across different situations? What objective criteria can be established to measure performance and to what extent can reliability and validity be built into evaluation scales?

The need for training

That there is a need for training is clear. For example, Byrne and Long (1976) in a study of over 2000 audio recorded doctor/patient consultations concluded that the preferred focus of attention of the practitioner was an organic illness with a neglect of emotional or social problems. Furthermore, there was little attempt to clarify that they had correctly identified or understood the patient's problems, and little opportunity was given to patients to ask questions.

Maguire (1985) in analysing the key communication deficiencies among nurses described their tendency to use closed or leading questions so biasing the response made by the patient. In addition, reflective questioning skills among nurses have been found to be lacking (Faulkner, 1980) thereby closing down any extension or development of any particular theme. Both authors also cite the poor ability among nurses to pick up cues covertly given off by patients. More recently, Maguire, Fairbairn and Fletcher (1986) in a study of forty young doctors concluded that most of them were extremely incompetent in giving information and advice to patients. In addition, few obtained and took any account of patients' views or expectations of their own predicament. There was also a tendency to avoid social and psychological aspects within the consultation, a factor which has been previously identified within doctor/patient interactions (Rosser and Maguire, 1982).

Improvements in skilled performance

In a comprehensive review of the teaching of clinical interviewing in the health professions, Carroll and Monroe (1980) concluded that 'instruction in clinical interviewing has generally promoted significant gains in students interview skills, as measured by various cognitive tests, affective instruments and observed behaviours' (pp.35–36).

Related to the assessment of CST within the medical domain Maguire (1984a) has indicated that the most promising results would seem to follow training that has involved audio or television feedback. Using these feedback techniques improved skills in empathy, responding to patients' feelings, covering psychosocial aspects and taking clinical histories have been demonstrated. Other evaluative studies within medicine have shown similar improved performance (Boulton *et al.*, 1984; McPherson *et al.*, 1984; Omololu, 1984; Weinman, 1984; Knox and Bouchier, 1985) but it is of interest to note that the majority of published reports relate to students in training.

Part of the reason is obviously that this is a 'captive' group who have no alternative but to participate in evaluative procedures as part of their course assessment. It may also reflect the difficulty of carrying out similar studies in the real practice environment because of a reluctance or fear among practising doctors to submit to an audit of their communication performance. Where it has been carried out the interviewing skills of doctors who had received feedback training were superior to those of doctors who had undergone conventional training in interviewing skills (Maguire, Fairbairn and Fletcher, 1986).

Within the pharmaceutical profession a similar situation exists where the majority of evaluative studies of CST occur in the undergraduate curriculum (Morrow, 1986). Again the findings support the notion that training actually promotes skill performance in both content and process skills. Where assessment of CST among practising pharmacists has occurred it has been limited to self-reported methodologies the results of which suggest changes in attitudes, abilities and actual behaviour at the pharmacist/client interface (Hanson, 1981; Morrow and Hargie, 1987a).

In the nursing situation evaluation of skills based programmes has been carried out during the training and post qualification stages. For example, Menikheim and Ryden (1985) have described a self-reported methodology to assess skill development. Here students expressed a significant increase in their communicative competence following training. Davis and Ternuff-Nyhlin (1982) have described a more controlled study using observer ratings of performance and also patient feedback to assess the impact of CST. The results suggest that in relation to interviewing technique the training produced positive outcomes at attitudinal, intentional and behavioural levels.

Specific outcomes

Maguire *et al.* (1980a) have also demonstrated the ability of nurses to acquire, through training, key social and assessment skills necessary for monitoring patients who had undergone mastectomy. In a further study Maguire *et al.* (1980b) showed that in a follow-up of these patients those who had been seen by the specially trained nursing staff had a more favourable outcome than those continued at the usual level of care.

The relationship between communication skills and specific outcomes, particularly patient outcomes, is as yet largely unclear. However, in the psychiatric context Goldberg *et al.* (1980) have indicated that those doctors who establish good eye contact, pick up verbal leads, clarify key complaints, while at the same time exercising appropriate control in the consultation are more likely to identify problems than doctors who do not have these skills. Moreover surgical patients have been found to rate students who possess good interviewing skills as being more understanding and empathic than those who lack them (Thompson and Anderson, 1982).

Duration of effect and generalization of training

More recently, Maguire *et al.* (1986) have demonstrated the greater clincial competence of doctors who had received feedback training on communication skills than those who had not. Their findings also suggested that the level of skilled performance decreases with time and this fact is also supported by other findings (Poole and Sanson-Fisher, 1981; Kauss *et al.*, 1980; Morrow and Hargie, 1987a).

That the influence of training diminishes with time suggests that generalization of the effects of training have a temporal dimension. However, in relation to the degree to which generalization of effects occurs, other factors such as tasks and persons may play a significant part (Mullan, 1986). Interestingly, Maguire *et al.* (1986) showed that there was some degree of generalization of interview skills training across persons, in that the skills trained in a psychiatric setting were successfully applied to interviews with physically ill patients.Techniques for improving generalization of training effects will be detailed in Chapter 12.

Assessment procedures

In relation to objectivity, reliability and validity of assessment procedures, a wide range of measurement strategies have been employed. These will be considered in Chapter 11.

2.7 OVERVIEW

This chapter has outlined the importance of adopting a holistic approach to patient care. Futhermore, it has identified the communicative competence of the practitioner as a fundamental part of the effective delivery of care. Historically however, CST has been a neglected part of the training of health personnel and to date is still inadequately addressed within training curricula. Yet the evidence suggests that skills training is effective in improving communication performance, clinical practice and patient satisfaction.

PART TWO

Content of communication skills training

A distinction commonly made by curriculum theorists is that between the subject matter to be taught and the methods and techniques utilized in this endeavour (Jarvis, 1983). Part Two, which subsumes three chapters, is concerned with the former: the content of CST.

Chapter 3 extends some of the notions of communication as skill introduced in the first chapter of the book. Here a theoretical model of the communicative process is developed which highlights its transactional nature. What takes place when people interact is mediated by a complex of perceptual, cognitive and affective factors operating within a person-situation framework. The activity is held to be energized by the desire to achieve particular goals and is directed by the ongoing monitoring of both personal and environmental changes, including those represented by the other or others involved in the encounter. It is important for those undergoing CST to be made aware of the nature of communication and the underlying mechanisms by means of which it is effected.

The performative dimension of communication – what practitioners actually *do* when they communicate with patients or significant others – is concentrated upon in Chapters 4 and 5. A pervasive stylistic feature of interaction mentioned by Dickson (1986), would seem to be that of *directness*. This has to do with the degree of constraint imposed by interviewers upon interviewees, and their responses, at each stage of the interaction. Health workers adopting a less direct style tend to make greater use of responding skills such as reflecting, reinforcement, listening and self-disclosure, which form the content of Chapter 4. Chapter 5 outlines a number of initiating skills including questioning, asserting and explaining which suggest a more direct style of relating. There will be occasions, of course, even within the same consultation, when skills of both types are called for. Taken together, these two chapters present a set of what could be regarded as key basic skills of communicating which should be part of the interpersonal skills repertoire of all health workers.

What transpires when two people interact can be analysed at a number of different levels (French, 1983). We can think of the doctor producing phonetic segments, morphemes, saying a word, asking a question, putting the patient at ease or conducting a consultation, depending upon the degree of resolution we bring to the analytical task. The last chapter of Part Two adopts a much more holistic perspective than that which identified the skills detailed in the two preceding chapters, by examining broad strategies which practitioners characteristically employ in order to achieve desired outcomes. These are interviewing, influencing and counselling and their central features and functions form the content of Chapter 6. Furthermore, the responding and initiating skills already examined are re-introduced and synthesized within each of these strategic contexts.

3

Communication as
skilled performance

3.1 INTRODUCTION

This chapter details a theoretical model of interpersonal communication, which provides a conceptual framework for programmes of CST. It develops and extends the analysis of communication skill presented in Chapter 1, where the analogy between social skills and motor skills was introduced.

In noting the similarities between motor and social skills, Argyle and Kendon (1967) put forward a model of motor skill operation, which they claimed could usefully be applied to the analysis of interpersonal behaviour. As outlined in Fig. 3.1, this model has five main components, namely goals, translation, motor responses, feedback and perception. In relation to motor performance, an example of this model in practice would be someone sitting in a room where the temperature has become too cold (*motivation*), and therefore wanting to warm up (*goal*). This can be achieved by considering various alternative plans of action, such as putting on extra clothing, closing a window, turning on a heater etc. (*translation*). Eventually one of these plans will be decided upon and executed. For example, a heater is turned on (*response*). The temperature in the room is thereby increased (*change in outside world*). This change in temperature will be *perceived* by the individual, and the goal deemed to have been achieved.

With regard to social performance, an example of the model in action would be a female at a party seeing a male whom she 'fancies' (*motivation*) and would therefore like to get to know (*goal*). In order to do so, she can *translate* various plans of action (e.g. look at him and smile, move close to him, introduce herself etc.). Eventually, she will decide upon one of these plans and execute it (*motor responses*) by, for example, saying 'Hello, my name is Joan, I don't think we've been introduced'. As she does so she will receive feedback from the male in the form of his reactions to her (*change in*

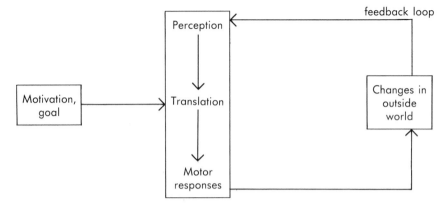

Fig. 3.1 Argyle and Kendon's motor skill model.

the outside world), will *perceive* this feedback and, on the basis of this perception, decide upon her future course of action.

As these examples illustrate, there are clear parallels between motor, and social performance in terms of the main processes involved. However, in exploring this issue Hargie and Marshall (1986) also noted the following important differences between these two sets of skills:

1. Social performance, by definition always involves other people, whereas certain motor skills, such as eating, walking, operating a machine, do not. Since other people are present during interpersonal interaction, it is necessary to consider the goals of all those involved, as well as their actions and reactions towards one another. In this sense, social performance is often more complex than motor performance.
2. The motor skill model does not satisfactorily account for the role of feelings and emotions during interpersonal encounters. Yet, it is clear that the emotional state of the interactor will have an important bearing upon their responses, goals and perceptions. In addition, we often take into account the feelings of other people with whom we interact, whereas in motor skill performance this, typically, is not applicable (e.g when operating a machine we do not need to consider its feelings!)
3. Person perception differs in a number of ways from the perception of objects. Firstly, we perceive the responses of the other person with whom we communicate. Secondly, we perceive our own responses, in that we hear what we say, and can be aware of our nonverbal behaviour. Thirdly, there is the process of metaperception which can be defined as the perception of the perception process itself. Thus, we make judgements about how other people are perceiving us, and also attempt to ascertain how they think we are perceiving them. Such judgements influence our behaviour and our goals during social interaction.

4. The nature of the social situation in which interaction occurs has an important bearing upon the responses of those involved. The roles which people play, the rules governing the situation, the nature of the task and the physical nature of the environment all affect the behaviour of the interactors.
5. Personal factors pertaining to those involved in the interaction also have a significant influence upon their responses. Such factors include age, gender and appearance. Thus a nurse will obviously behave differently towards a 4-year old child and a 40-year old woman!

Having distinguished these important differences between social and motor skills, Hargie and Marshall (1986) put forward a revised model of dyadic interaction to take account of all of these facets. As presented in Fig. 3.2, this extended model takes into consideration the goals of both parties involved in interaction. It also recognizes the more complex nature of person perception as emanating both from one's own responses and from the responses of the other person. The term 'mediating factors' is introduced to encompass the role of feelings and emotions, as well as cognitions, during interpersonal communication. Finally, the importance of both personal and situational characteristics is recognized.

The remainder of this chapter is concerned with an evaluation of each of the processes outlined in Fig. 3.2. This model can usefully be presented to trainees at the outset of the CST programme.

3.2 GOALS

A central feature of the extended interaction model is the goal of the interactors, since behaviour is usually carried out in order to attempt to achieve certain pre-determined objectives. However, the individual may not be consciously aware of these. Thus, just as a skilled car driver does not have to consciously think 'I want to switch on the engine, therefore I must insert the key into the ignition', so a skilled doctor does not consciously think 'I want to obtain an accurate diagnosis, therefore I must question this patient'. Indeed, one of the features of skilled performance is that it is carried out at a sub-conscious level, thereby enabling the individual to act in a smooth, skilled fashion.

A distinction also needs to be made between long-term and short-term goals. Our behaviour is guided by short-term goals, with long-term goals being achieved through a sub-set of short-term ones. For example, a nurse may have the long-term goal of obtaining an accurate medical history from a patient who has been admitted to hospital. In order to do so, however, there are a number of short-term goals which need to be achieved such as establishing rapport, explaining the task, asking appropriate questions, ensuring accurate responses are obtained, and so on. Indeed, these sub-goals

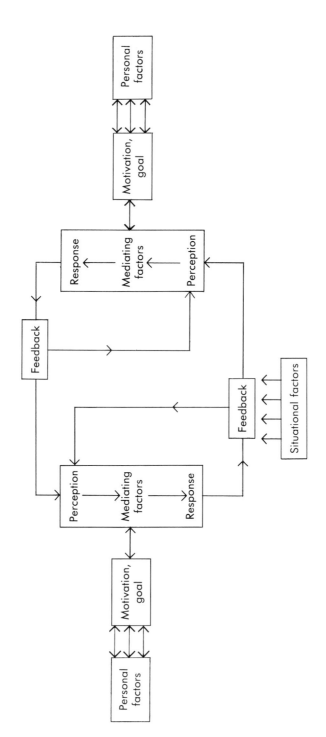

Fig. 3.2 Extended model of interpersonal interaction.

could also be further sub-divided. Thus, in order to establish rapport, the nurse needs to introduce herself, ensure that the patient is comfortable, adopt appropriate nonverbal behaviours, etc. If any of these sub-goals are not achieved, then the long-term one of obtaining an accurate medical history is made much more difficult.

Goals are influenced by our degree of motivation to pursue them, while motivation, in turn, is influenced by needs. There are a large number of human needs which have to be satisfied to enable us to obtain maximum satisfaction from life. Some of these needs are more important than others, and a number of different need hierarchies have been put forward by psychologists. The best known probably remains that proposed by Maslow (1954) as exemplified in Fig. 3.3.

At the bottom of Maslow's hierarchy, and therefore the most important, are the physiological needs, which are concerned with the survival of the individual including the necessity for food, water, heat and pain avoidance. Unless these needs are secured, the individual will not be particularly concerned with those at a higher level. Health professionals often deal with patients who are concerned with physiological needs, and who will therefore have a strong motivation to ensure that these are satisfied. Patients who are in severe pain or who, for example, at the pre-operative stage,

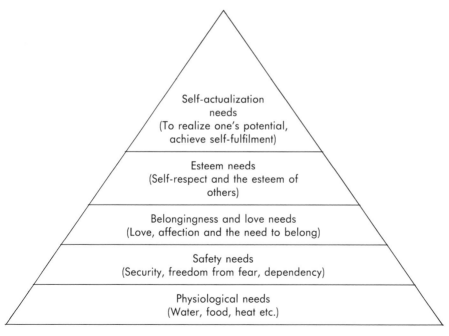

Fig. 3.3 Maslow's hierarchy of human needs.

are worried about survival, will want the professional to deal directly with these concerns.

The second most important needs relate to the safety of the individual and include protection from physical harm, freedom from fear and the need for security. Thus, someone who has developed a serious illness may be worried about whether they will be able to work again and, if not, how they will survive financially, Indeed, it is for this reason that some people take out insurance policies to cover such eventualities. At the next level are belongingness and love needs, including the need for love, affection and the desire to be part of a group. One of the problems with hospitalization, of course, is that the individual is cut off from friends and family who usually meet these needs. As a result, it is important that the health professional should be sensitive to feelings of loneliness or isolation by patients. Nurses, particularly, have an important befriending role to play in this respect. It is also interesting to note that patients often make friends with one another, and this is an important process in itself. In addition, hospital visits by friends and family are crucial in maintaining belongingness and love bonds.

Esteem needs are also important. Maintaining self-respect, dignity and the esteem of others can be difficult, for example, in the case of patients who have become bedridden, are incontinent, or can no longer feed themselves. Equally, an attractive individual who suffers severe facial lacerations, a woman who has a mastectomy, or someone who has a limb amputated, are all likely to suffer from a loss of esteem. Thus, sensitivity, patience and counselling skills are required when dealing with such patients. The final type of need is concerned with higher-order aspects, including the desire to achieve one's true potential.

As French (1983) points out, Maslow's hierarchy raises two important guidelines for health professionals. The first of these is concerned with the principle of meeting the lowest needs first. Severe pain in a patient requires to be dealt with, before belongingness and love needs. Secondly, once lower needs are met, others further up the hierarchy will emerge, and the professional has to monitor such changes and respond accordingly. In this way, the goals of patients will be influenced by their level of needs, and an important goal for the professional should be to recognize, and effectively deal with these.

The goals of the interactors in any situation are important determinants of behaviour. It is for this reason that we attempt to determine what the goals of other people with whom we interact might be. In fact, we are usually fairly accurate in making judgements about these, and this is why we are shocked if we discover that someone, whom we trusted as having honourable goals, turns out to have been deceiving us. In the health context it is important for the professional to explain as fully as possible any actions taken with a patient. Within the hospital setting, where patients are especially vulnerable, it is necessary to answer overt or covert patient questions such as: 'Why is this happening to me?' 'Why is she asking me this?' or 'Why do I need this medication?' In other words, the professional should pay attention to the important goals of the patient.

However, on many occasions there may be goal conflict between practitioner and patient. As Di Matteo and Di Nicola (1982) point out, 'Sometimes this conflict is explicit, such as when the patient wants a prescription and the clinician is unwilling to give it . . . In other cases, however, the conflict and negotiation may be much more subtle and remain unstated. . . . An excellent example of this difference in perspectives is the interaction in the emergency room between a physician and a patient who is complaining of abdominal pain. Until the diagnosis is made, the practitioner must withhold pain-relieving medication in order to chart the course of the pain. The patient does not know this (and the practitioner does not explain it). The patient believes that the physician is withholding medication out of cruelty, and is witholding communication (of diagnosis and prognosis) out of secretiveness' (pp.74–75). Such goal conflicts need to be overcome before effective interpersonal communication can take place.

Goals, therefore, represent an essential starting point in the interaction model. Once appropriate goals have been decided upon, they will have an important bearing upon our perceptions, responses, and on intervening mediating factors.

3.3 MEDIATING FACTORS

Mediating factors are the internal states, activities or processes which mediate between the goal being pursued, the feedback which is perceived and the responses to be made. These factors influence the way in which people and events are perceived, and determine the capacity of the individual to assimilate, process, and respond to, the information received during interpersonal interaction. This process of mediation is important, since it allows individuals to evaluate to what extent their goals can be achieved, or whether new goals need to be adopted and different action plans implemented. In terms of such decision-making the two main mediating factors are cognitions and emotions.

Cognitions

Cognition can be defined as 'all the processes by which the sensory input is transformed, reduced, elaborated, stored, recovered and used' (Neisser, 1967, p.4). From this definition it can be seen that cognition involves a number of important processes. These include *transforming* or decoding the information received from the sensory channels. Since there may be a large volume of such information it is necessary to *reduce* this in order to cope effectively. Paradoxically it is sometimes also necessary to *elaborate* upon minimal information by making interpretations, judgements or evaluations (e.g. she is not speaking to me because she is a shy child, is upset at being in hospital and is missing her mother). It is also necessary to *store* information in memory in order to cope successfully in social interaction. In particular, social information is dependent upon the effective use of a short-term memory store, so that individuals who suffer impairments in this facility find difficulty during social encounters (Antaki and Lewis, 1986). This is quite common among some elderly patients who may have a very good long-term memory and can vividly recall the names of school friends or teachers, yet, due to impairment in short-term memory, forget the professional's name seconds after being told it.

Information that is stored can then be *recovered* and *used* by the individual to facilitate the processes of decision-making and responding. Existing circumstances are compared with previous knowledge and experience in making decisions about action plans. There is evidence to suggest that professionals make use of conceptual 'schemas' to facilitate the process of problem-solving during social encounters (Carroll, 1980; McIntyre, 1983). For example an experienced nurse will have a number of schemas such as: 'patient looks distressed', 'patient getting agitated', each with accompanying action plans – 'spend some time with him and give reassurance where appropriate', 'calm him down to prevent the agitation escalating and upsetting other patients on the ward'. Such schemas are formulated and developed primarily through experience, although one of the advantages of CST is that is can 'short-circuit' the time needed for their development (Crute, 1986). By providing college-based skill learning with related practical experience, in advance of actual clinical practice, it is possible to contribute to the schematic development of trainees.

The development of a wide range of schemas enables the practitioner to respond quickly and confidently in the professional context. This ability to respond rapidly, and appropriately, is in turn a feature of skilled performance (Gellatly, 1986). Thus, the skilled professional has developed a cognitive ability to analyse and evaluate available information and make decisions about how best to respond. He will also have, at the same time, formulated a number of contingency plans which can be implemented immediately should the initial response be ineffective. The skilled individual, in addition, has a greater capacity for what Snyder (1974) terms 'self-monitoring', which is the ability to monitor and regulate one's own responses in relation to the responses of others. This process of regulation necessitates an awareness of the ability level of the person with whom one is interacting and of the 'way they think'. Wessler (1984) maintains that, 'in order to interact successfully and repeatedly with the same persons, one must have the capacity to form cognitive conceptions of the other's cognitive conceptions' (p.112). This process of meta-cognition is therefore also an important component of social skill.

Thus, cognitions play a central role during social encounters. The skilled professional will have developed a wide range of cognitive schemas to facilitate problem-solving and decision-making during interpersonal interaction, together with the ability to make rapid, accurate, judgements about people and situations.

Emotions

As mentioned earlier in this chapter, the role of emotions in social interaction needs to be recognized. Izard (1977) has identified three specific components of emotion. Firstly, the direct conscious experience or feeling of emotion; secondly the physiological processes which accompany emotions; and thirdly the observable behaviours which are used to signal and express emotions. In noting these processes, he further claims that, 'virtually all of the neurophysiological systems and subsystems of the body are involved in greater or lesser degree in emotional states. Such changes inevitably affect the perceptions, thoughts and actions of the person' (Izard, 1977, p.10). The emotional state of the individual therefore influences how he 'sees' the world, thinks about what is happening, and how he responds. Thus, a depressed patient will tend to pick up negative cues and ignore the positive ones, be pessimistic about the future, and typically adopt a slouched posture, lowered head, avoid eye contact, speak in a dull, flat, monotone and generally avoid interacting with others. Conversely, a happy person will focus upon positive cues, be optimistic, and display signs of happiness by smiling, looking at others, adopting an attentive posture and engaging in conversation.

There is, however, debate about the exact nature of the relationship between cognitions and emotions. Some theorists argue that the latter are caused by the former, so that for example, fear or anxiety can be caused by irrational beliefs (e.g. Ellis, 1962). Such a perspective is, however, regarded by others as being an over-simplification of the nature of the relationship between these phenomena. It is argued that rather, there is a reciprocal relationship between cognition and effect. For example, it is pointed out that emotional states can have a direct influence on thought processes, so that someone may be so worried that they can no longer 'think straight'. As Forgas (1983, p.138) points out: 'We not only differentiate between, and represent social episodes in terms of how we feel about them, but mood and emotions also play a crucial role in thinking about and remembering such events'. Thus the way we feel can have a direct bearing on the way we think, and vice versa.

Emotions are therefore very important determinants of behaviour. Furthermore, during social interaction it is important to be aware of the emotional state of others. In many health contexts, patients may be highly emotionally charged. The curve of the relationship between emotional arousal and performance takes the form of an inverted 'U' shape so that high levels of arousal are dysfunctional in that performance is severely impaired. Thus, trainee doctors or nurses, on occasion, faint when observing their first surgical operation. Similarly, health professionals need to be aware of the level of arousal of patients, and take steps to reduce it where necessary (e.g. by providing reassurance, giving careful explanations of what the patient will experience, etc.).

In addition to cognitions and emotions, there are other mediating factors which influence how people are perceived and responded to. These include the values and beliefs of the practitioner. For example, a devout Catholic would find difficulty in advising patients about the procedures for obtaining an abortion. Our political, moral and religious beliefs therefore influence our attitudes towards other people, which in turn affect our thoughts, feelings and behaviour as we interact with them. The attitudes we have towards others are also influenced by our previous experiences of the person with whom we are interacting, or our experiences of similar people. Finally, the disposition of the individual is an important facet in determining responses in social situations. Factors such as whether the practitioner is shy, outgoing, competitive, affiliative, dominant or submissive, influence behaviour.

All of the above mediating factors are operative at the decision-making stage of interpersonal interaction. Thus cognitions, emotions, values, beliefs, attitudes and disposition are important determinants of social responses.

3.4 RESPONSES

When a goal has been decided upon, and a response plan formulated, the next stage is to implement this plan in terms of direct action. It is the function of the response, or 'effector', system to implement the translated strategies, mentioned above, into appropriate behaviours. Social behaviour may by categorized as follows:

1. Verbal – the purely linguistic message. That is, the actual words used;
2. Nonverbal – the use of posture, gestures, facial expressions, and other forms of body language, together with vocal aspects of speech, e.g. pitch, tone, accent, etc.

It is at this level that skills become manifest. Someone who can give a detailed description about how to behave effectively during social interaction, but who cannot put this knowledge into practice, would not be described as socially skilled. In this sense, skilled performance depends upon the ability to *perform* tasks effectively and efficiently. (See Chapters 4, 5 and 6 for further information on skilled responses.)

3.5 FEEDBACK

Following the response stage, feedback will be available to the individual. Such feedback allows the performer to assess the effects of his performance and take corrective action where necessary. Indeed, in order to carry out any task effectively, it is essential to receive such feedback in terms of 'knowledge of results' of performance (Annett, 1969). The crucial role of feedback has been noted by Bilodeau and Bilodeau (1961, p.250) who argue that this is 'the strongest, most important variable controlling performance and learning'.

Thus, it is necessary to receive feedback in order to behave in a skilled, efficient manner. We could not ride a bicycle, play tennis, or perform numerous other tasks if we were unable to perceive the results of our actions. Similarly, in interpersonal interaction we require feedback from others in order to make judgements about the effectiveness of our communications. Such social feedback takes the form of the verbal and nonverbal reactions of others. In situations where we receive little feedback from those with whom we interact, we are generally discontented, since we are unsure about how we are 'being received'.

As illustrated in Fig. 3.2, during social interaction we not only receive feedback from others but also from our own responses. When we interact we hear what we are saying and, if we are highly skilled, may be aware of our nonverbal responses (hand movements, postures etc.). This is part of the process of self-monitoring, mentioned earlier, which includes the ability of the person to monitor his own behaviour and take corrective action based upon this feedback. High self-monitors monitor or control the images of self they project in social interaction (Snyder, 1987). In other words, they control and adjust their behaviour to meet the requirements of particular people, or situations in which they interact. This is clearly an attribute which is important for health professionals, who have to deal with a wide range of patients and other professionals, and need to adapt their skills and strategies to suit the particular context in which they are involved.

Fitts and Posner (1973) have identified three important functions of feedback. Firstly, it provides *knowledge* about the results of behaviour. Secondly, it can provide *motivation* to continue a task, by conveying information concerning the likelihood of goal attainment. Finally, it may act as a *reinforcer*, thereby encouraging the individual to repeat that particular response in the future (see Chapter 10 for further information on feedback). These functions emphasize the importance of this component of social interaction.

During interpersonal encounters a constant stream of feedback impinges upon the individual both from the stimuli received from other people and from the physical environment. As Hargie *et al.*, (1987) point out, in order to avoid overloading the system, the individual must selectively filter this information either into the conscious or the subconscious (Fig. 3.4). As a result, only a certain amount of information will be consciously perceived. Evidence that subconscious perception occurs can be seen during hypnosis, when individuals can recall information which they were not consciously aware of. The extent to which such subconscious information guides

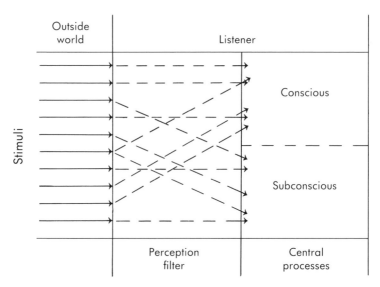

Fig. 3.4 Selective perception process.

behaviour is unclear, although judgements such as 'There was something about him I didn't like', may well be based upon it.

The difference between feedback and perception is that, in many contexts, there will be a huge volume of feedback available, but only a small amount will be consciously perceived. For example, within the physical environment, the ticking of clocks, the pressure of one's feet on the floor, the hum of central heating systems etc. are usually filtered into the subconscious. However, if we are bored during an encounter then these items may intrude into our awareness.

Perception is therefore an active selective process. For this reason it is important for practitioners to be aware of the need to consciously perceive important cues from others, while filtering out only the less essential information. This is especially important in busy environments such as the hospital ward, where the sensory input available to the professional may include visual and auditory stimuli such as the patients, other professionals, visitors, catering staff, beds, magazines, extraneous noises, bright lights and so on. In such contexts, concerted perceptual focus is essential.

3.6 PERCEPTION

Our perceptual system enables us to acquire information about our environment through our five senses: sight, sound, taste, touch and smell. We use these senses to accumulate information both about physical objects and about other people. 'Person perception' is of crucial importance during interpersonal communication since it represents 'the first, crucial stage in any interaction between people. We must first perceive and interpret other people before we can meaningfully relate to them' (Forgas, 1985, p.21). Thus, an awareness of some of the facets which influence the way in which we perceive others is of vital importance in the study of social interaction.

Perceptual accuracy

One important feature of the perceptual process is that our perceptions are frequently inaccurate and our appreciation of many situations can often be distorted. For instance, in Fig. 3.5 the impossible figure seems like three parallel tubes at one end but a magnet-like object at the other. Yet, in reality, it is neither. A similar phenomenon occurs in clinical practice when a patient presents in an apparent state of well-being yet their medical record indicates an emotional or personality disorder. Again, like the impossible figure, the overall picture is difficult to relate to.

Our perceptions are also influenced by the context in which they are received. For example, in Fig. 3.6 the figure 13 will be viewed as the letter B in the upper line, but as the number 13 in the bottom line. Likewise with the hypochondriacal patient who requires 'a pill for every ill' there is the danger of 'seeing' the presenting symptoms in a less serious light, with potentially adverse consequences.

Another form of misperception involves associating physical disability with mental incapacity. Thus, bedridden patients, particularly geriatrics, are often treated as having some degree of senile impairment regardless of their true mental state. Similarly people confined to wheelchairs may be viewed as being somehow less mentally capable.

Misperception may not always be the fault of the practitioner. Our perceptions can be inaccurate because some patients deliberately aim to deceive. Indeed, cases have been documented in terms of clinical conditions, such as

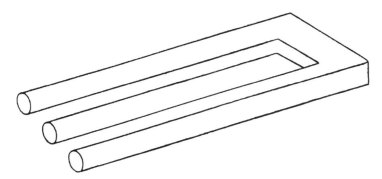

Fig. 3.5 Impossible figure.

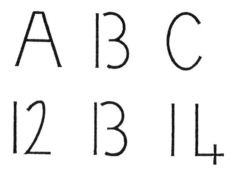

Fig. 3.6 The context of perception.

Munchausen's syndrome. Here the patient describes and enacts textbook symptoms of a disease state, and even undergoes investigation and/or treatment, yet in fact has no such illness.

Interpreting perceptual information

There are a number of related processes which need to be taken into account when considering the role of perception during social interaction:

1. *Attribution* This refers to the process whereby we attribute reasons or motives to the behaviour of others. When attempting to interpret the behaviour of other people we take into consideration situational and dispositional causes. What is known as the 'fundamental attribution error' occurs through 'the tendency to over-estimate the role of dispositional factors and to underestimate the role of situational factors when judging the causes of behaviours' (Kleinke, 1986, p.193). Interestingly, we tend to emphasize dispositional causes when interpreting negative behaviour of others, but highlight the importance of situational factors when explaining our own poor performance (Feldman, 1985). It is likely that such bias is essentially self-serving in that it prevents our sense of self-worth being called into question. Negative self-inferences can be unpleasantly ego-threatening leading, in the longer-term, to poor self-concept and diminished levels of self-esteem. Under such circumstances feelings of self-efficacy may suffer as the individual begins to lose belief in his ability to achieve desired goals (Pennington, 1986). In making judgements about our own, and other people's behaviour, it is therefore important to carefully consider both situational and dispositional factors.

   Kelley (1971) highlighted the importance of three main variables during attribution. Firstly, the *consistency* of the observed behaviour, that is, how often the person displays this behaviour in this situation; secondly its *distinctiveness* which refers to whether or not the behaviour is commonly displayed in different situations; and thirdly the *consensus* in terms of whether the behaviour is typical of how other people behave in this situation. These three variables can best be represented by considering a situation where a nurse bursts into tears when dealing with a particular patient:

Consistency	Distinctiveness	Consensus	Attribution
1. High. She has often cried with this particular patient.	High. She has never cried when dealing with other patients.	High. Other staff on the ward were also very upset.	To this particular patient.
2. High. She has often cried with this particular patient.	Low. She has often cried when dealing with other patients.	Low. No other members of staff on the ward were upset.	To the nurse.
3. Low. She has never cried with this patient before.	High. She has never cried when dealing with other patients.	Low. No other members of staff on the ward were upset.	To the situation, or to prevailing circumstances.

As this example illustrates, when interpreting the behaviour of others in any situation, we make decisions based upon how they have behaved in the past, and how other people behave in the same situation.

2. *Labelling* We use labels to enable us to categorize and deal with people more readily. These labels may be influenced by an individual's age, physical appearance, dress, gender, and other aspects of their verbal and nonverbal behaviour. Such labelling is an intergrated process derived from past experiences, expectations and interpretations of the situation. The function of labelling is to simplify complex information which would otherwise become unmanageable. One type of label is that of the social *stereotype*, which is an attempt to force people into certain categories or 'pigeon-holes' without paying attention to how they actually are (Pennington, 1986). In this way, set patterns of behaviour are anticipated in someone belonging to a specific group (racial, class, religious etc.) and their behaviour interpreted in the light of pre-set expectations about the stereotype. This can often result in a *self-fulfilling prophecy* occurring.

For example, person A may believe that coloured people are aggressive and unfriendly. When A meets a coloured person, B, he then reacts as if B was unfriendly and aggressive, with the result that B is likely to respond in a less friendly manner. In this way, the stereotype is strengthened.

Another example of labelling in the health field is the tendency to refer to patients as illnesses (e.g. 'The hysterectomy in bed 5'). Here, the result is to de-individualize patients, and treat them as medical or technical problems. Other common examples of labels include 'hypochondriac', 'malingerer', 'troublesome patient'. The danger with all such labels is that the professional responds to the label rather than to the person.

3. *Implicit personality theory* People seem to have 'implicit personality theories' (Bruner and Tagiuri, 1954) which they employ to make judgements about others. This refers to the way in which we associate certain characteristics of an individual with a range of other characteristics. For example, in the following instances judge the characteristic in parentheses which best seems to complete the sentence:

   Alan is conscientious, industrious, lively and (fat, thin).
   Patricia is vivacious, attractive, stylish and (young, old).

   In the first instance Alan will be more likely to be judged as 'thin', while in the second case Patricia will be viewed as 'young'. These are two simple examples of how we associate characteristics. This process causes a *halo effect* to occur, in that if someone possesses a number of positive characteristics, we are more likely to infer that they will possess other positive qualities. Likewise, a negative halo effect can occur, with people who display a number of negative characteristics being perceived as possessing a range of other negative qualities.

   Rosenberg *et al.* (1968) found that university students used two major dimensions along which people were differentiated, namely intellectual good – bad, and social good – bad. Certain traits were clearly associated with one another along these two dimensions. Thus, people viewed as warm were also perceived as sociable, popular, happy, good natured and humorous. Interestingly these traits were perceived as good socially, but as indicators of less intellectual individuals. In fact, the traits 'warm' and 'cold' have been found to be of crucial importance, in that once a judgement is made as to whether a person is warm or cold, a large number of other positive or negative judgements respectively are inferred (Wishner, 1960).

4. *Primacy and recency effects* The primacy effect refers to the way in which information we receive initially can affect how we later interpret further information. In person perception, the first impressions we make of others can influence how we respond to them (Gergen and Gergen, 1981). However, a recency effect would also seem to be operative, in that the final information perceived is also influential in making judge-

ments. This suggests that health professionals should pay particular attention to the way in which they greet, and part from, patients. (Chapter 5 has further information on opening and closing interactions.)

5. *Metaperception* This refers to our perception of the perception process itself. When we interact with others we attempt to ascertain how they are perceiving us and try to evaluate how they think we are perceiving them. Both of these facets play an important role in interpersonal interaction.

Person perception is clearly a crucial element of social interaction. Professionals need to develop an ability to perceive accurately the cues being emitted by others, while also being aware of their own responses. They also need to be sensitive to the range of factors which can cause distortion or inaccuracy during the perceptual process.

Perception is the final central process involved in the interaction model presented in Fig. 3.2, and, together with goals, mediating factors, responses and feedback, comprises the core of dyadic interaction. However, in order to gain a fuller understanding of social interaction, it is necessary to consider two related aspects, namely situational and personal factors.

3.7 SITUATIONAL FACTORS

As discussed earlier in this chapter, the behaviour of others is judged upon dispositional and situational factors. For example, someone who gives a large sum of money to a charity collector may be seen as generous (dispositional), or alternatively as showing off in front of those he wishes to impress (situational). It is therefore necessary to be aware of the influence of a range of situational factors in determining the behaviour of people during social encounters. Argyle *et al.* (1981) identified nine main features of social situations:

Goals

The goals that we seek are influenced by the situation in which we are interacting, while conversely, the goals that we seek also influence the situation in which we choose to interact. Thus, the nurse on the ward will have goals directly related to dealing with patients. However, if the nurse is hungry he will seek out situations where food is available. In this way, goals and situations are inter-dependent.

Rules

An analogy is often made between social interaction and games, in that both are governed by rules which must be followed, if a successful outcome is to be achieved (Furnham, 1983b). Rules can be explicit or implicit. For example, there are explicit rules forbidding sexual relationships between doctors and patients. It is an implicit rule that the doctor will provide a chair for patients to sit in. Professionals need to be aware not only of the rules of the situations which they will encounter, but also how to deal with patients who break the rules (e.g. aggressive patients).

Roles

In any social situation, people play a variety of roles. These roles carry with them a set of expectations about the behaviour, attitudes, feelings, beliefs and values of the individuals involved. Indeed, an important aspect of professional training has to do with learning how to effectively play the role of the professional. Thus, a nurse is expected to be concerned about the well-being of patients, to behave in a caring manner, to dress in a certain fashion, and so on. The trainee nurse who fails to learn these role responsibilities will not be allowed to register. As we move from one situation to another, our roles often change, for example from nurse in the hospital, to fiancée on a date, and to daughter at home. Problems can arise, however, where there are conflicting expectations about how a role should be played. Thus, a nurse may expect patients to respond in a certain way, whereas a particular patient may not 'see' his role in that light. In such instances, communication problems are very likely to arise.

Repertoire of elements

In different contexts of professional practice, different responses are appropriate. Thus, when taking a medical history, the skill of questioning is of crucial importance, when giving instructions about how to use medication the skill of explaining is central, and when breaking bad news the use of empathy is required. In order to cope effectively, the professional therefore needs to learn as wide a repertoire of responses as possible. The skilled practitioner must develop a large repertoire of behavioural elements which can be applied as the situation demands.

Sequences of behaviour

In most social situations there is a particular behavioural sequence which should be followed by those taking part. Argyle *et al.* (1981) argue that many encounters can be accounted for in terms of the following five-episode progression:

1. greeting
2. establishing the relationship and clarifying roles
3. the task

4. re-establishing the relationship
5. parting.

Investigating doctor-patient communication, Byrne and Long (1976) identified six phases which occurred in the majority of consultations. It is obviously important for professionals to be aware of the sequence of interaction episodes in different situations, to ensure a smooth communicative encounter.

Physical environment

The nature of the physical environment, in terms of the layout of furniture and fittings, lighting, heating, colour etc., can have a distinct influence upon the behaviour of individuals. For example, people feel more comfortable and tend to disclose more about themselves in 'warm' environments (soft seats, concealed lighting, carpets etc.). Furthermore, individuals feel more secure on 'home territory', than in unfamiliar environments. Doctors, health visitors and district nurses find patients more at ease in their own homes as opposed to the health clinic. Hospitals can be particularly disturbing for some patients, owing to the nature of the ward environment, with little personal space or privacy, bright lights, intrusive noise and few personal possessions. In such situations, the patient is likely to feel that he has no control over his situation, and this can cause further distress (Hargie and McCartan, 1986).

Concepts

In every social situation, there is a range of concepts which must be understood by the interactors if the encounter is to be successful. For example, a visit to the cinema may entail a knowledge of the concepts 'queue', 'ticket', 'usherette' and 'interval'. Similarly, a patient visiting a dentist may need to be aware of the concepts of 'filling', 'plaque', 'crown' or 'bridge'. However, a common error made by some professionals is to wrongly assume that patients have a knowledge of all of the concepts necessary for understanding an interaction (Brown, 1986). Furthermore, health professionals have developed a jargon of specific terminology for various concepts, and need to ensure that such jargon is avoided, or fully explained in appropriate language, when dealing with patients.

Skills and difficulties

As mentioned earlier, the practitioner must be capable of effectively handling a wide range of situations, some of which will be much more difficult than others. For particularly difficult situations, special skills are required, and this should be given concerted focus during training. Dealing with aggressive patients, depressed patients, counselling terminally ill patients or their relatives, and communicating with psychiatric patients, are all situations which require detailed preparation, in terms of the difficulties which these situations present and the skills and strategies appropriate for handling them.

Language and speech

The final dimension of social situations relates to the degree of linguistic variation concerned. Certain situations require a higher degree of formality of language than others. Giving a lecture or addressing a committee meeting involves a more formal, elaborate use of language than, for example, having a chat with a colleague over coffee. Equally, changes in tone, pitch and volume of voice occur across contexts. Professionals, therefore, need to be capable of varying their language and speech patterns to meet the needs of particular situations.

These nine components of social situations play an important role in interpreting the behaviour of individuals during interpersonal encounters, and they should therefore be taken into consideration during CST programmes.

3.8 PERSONAL FACTORS

The final element of the interpersonal interaction model outlined in Fig. 3.2 concerns the personal factors of the individuals involved. Before we actually interact with others, we make judgements about them based upon various features of their appearance. There are four main personal factors which are immediately available to us when we meet other people.

Age

Although some people go to great lengths to camouflage their true age, this is one dimension which can usually be estimated fairly accurately by others, certainly within the main life stages of infancy, childhood, adolescence, early adulthood, middle age and old age. Generally, we hold stereotypes about individuals based upon their age, which can quite often be very inaccurate. For example, Wolinsky (1983) illustrates how some elderly people categorized as irreversibly senile, may actually be suffering from short-term depression which can be alleviated by psychotherapy. Feldman (1985, p.163) further reports that 'even some physicians, who might otherwise be expected to be sympathetic to the elderly, use the terms 'crones' or 'trolls' when talking about their elderly patients'.

The age of the practitioner is also an important factor. In some contexts older professionals may be viewed as being more experienced and competent than younger colleagues. However, in other situations, younger professionals may be preferred by patients. For example, studies by Foxman *et al.* (1982) and Simms and Smith (1984) have shown that young mothers prefer younger health visitors, with whom they can identify more readily. Thus, the ages of both the professional and the client are important considerations which can affect expectations and behaviour during interpersonal communication.

Gender

During interpersonal encounters, we tend to respond differently to, and hold differing expectations of, others, depending upon their gender (Stewart and Ting-Toomey, 1987). Such differences are emphasized from an early age, since male and female infants are dressed, and responded to, differently. These early experiences undoubtedly contribute to later differences in behaviour patterns, attitudes and values between males and females. However, the extent to which such differences are learned, or are innate, is as yet unclear, although it seems likely that both nature and nurture play an important part in shaping later gender patterns of behaviour (Archer and Lloyd, 1986).

In terms of nonverbal communication, females tend to smile more, require less interpersonal space, are touched more, use more head nods and engage in more eye contact than males. In addition, women are more skilled at interpreting the nonverbal behaviour of others (Mayo and Henley, 1981). These sex differences were exemplified in a study by Whitcher and Fisher (1979) into the reactions of males and females to pre-operative therapeutic touch. It was found that one single touch by nursing staff produced a positive, significant effect upon females' response to surgery, whereas it had the reverse effect for males. Gahagan (1984) interprets such findings in terms of dominance signals, in that high-status individuals initiate and control their touch patterns with low-status individuals. She suggests that males may therefore interpret touch in terms of dominance, rather than affiliative, signals.

Stereotyped images of sex roles persist within the health field, in that the vast majority of nurses are female, and senior positions in most professions tend to be held by males. However, the numbers of females have markedly increased in medicine, dentistry and pharmacy, and this will undoubtedly bring changes in attitudes to female professionals. The gender of both the professional and the patient clearly needs to be taken into consideration when evaluating interpersonal communication episodes.

Dress

Although one of the prime functions of clothing is to protect the wearer from cold or injury, it is clear that dress also serves a number of important social functions. The clothes we wear can signify group membership, gender, status, occupation, personal identity and personality. We carefully select our apparel when preparing for social encounters in order to portray a certain type of image to others. In professional contexts, however, this choice is often removed, so that in hospitals different professions are required to wear different types of uniform in order to portray a more corporate, neutral, image. In other settings, however, the professional has more control over personal dress. For example, a community pharmacist needs to decide whether or not to wear a white coat, while a doctor has to dress in such a way as to appear competent and efficient without being unapproachable.

Physical appearance

The final personal factor to be considered is the physical appearance of the individual, in terms of body size, shape and attractiveness. Physique can influence how people are perceived and responded to. For example, endomorphs tend to be viewed as warm-hearted, agreeable, good-natured, sympathetic and dependent on others; ectomorphs as quiet, tidy and tense; and mesomorphs as adventurous, forceful, self-reliant and healthy (Argyle, 1975). Height is also a significant element in judgements of males. Taller men tend to achieve more in our society in terms of occupational status, and social opportunities such as dating. Furthermore, males of higher status tend to be perceived as taller.

Attractiveness would seem to be a crucial feature in interpersonal communication. People who are rated as physically attractive are also seen as more popular, friendly and interesting to talk to (Kleinke, 1986). Thus, individuals rated as highly attractive tend to receive more eye contact, smiles, closer bodily proximity and body accessibility (openness of arms and legs), than those rated as low in attractiveness (Altman, 1977). However, attractiveness involves more than mere physical make-up, since factors which are relevant here include dress, cleanliness, personality and competence (Rosenblatt, 1977). This would indicate that less physically attractive practitioners may be successful and popular with clients by ensuring they have good interactive style and a competent, professional, approach.

These four factors related to the appearance of individuals need to be borne in mind in any evaluation of interpersonal interaction.

3.9 OVERVIEW

This chapter has been concerned with an examination of a theoretical model (Fig. 3.2) which can be directly applied to the analysis of interpersonal communication. This model highlights the importance of a number of inter-related processes, each of which contributes to an understanding of the nature and function of social behviour. The central processes in this model are: the goals of the individuals involved and their motivation to pursue them; a range of mediating factors including cognitions, emotions, values and beliefs; the responses of both parties; the feedback available during interpersonal encounters; and the ability of the individuals to perceive important cues from others, while being aware of their own behaviour. In addition, the role of various situational and personal factors was also emphasized.

While, for the purposes of description, analysis and evaluation, each stage of this model has been studied separately, it will be apparent that in reality the processes involved do not occur in isolation, but rather overlap and are inter-related and inter-dependent. Communication is a complex process involving a myriad of impinging variables some, or all, of which may be operative at any particular time. In order to attempt to interpret, and make sense of this process it is necessary to systematically study the central components involved (Kasch, 1986).

The model presented in this chapter provides a conceptual framework for interpreting face-to-face interaction and offers a necessary theoretical underpinning for programmes of CST. It represents a broad-based foundation upon which can later be built specific communication skills such as those presented in the following chapters of this section. Furthermore, it provides a wider perspective within which each of these skills can be evaluated.

4

Responding skills

4.1 INTRODUCTION

In this chapter, and in Chapters 5 and 6, a range of interpersonal skills and strategies pertinent to the needs of health professionals will be examined. Given the vast literature in the field of communication skills it is clearly beyond the scope of this text to incorporate a comprehensive review. Rather, a summative overview of the core skills will be provided, and their application to health contexts exemplified. The trainer is therefore recommended to pursue some of the references employed throughout the chapter for further information on each of the areas covered.

The skills presented are essentially responsive in nature in that they are usually employed in reaction to the behaviour of others rather than as a means of initiating and directing interaction. The responding skills incorporated here are nonverbal communication, reinforcement, reflecting, listening and self-disclosure. Information on each, and their functional significance in interaction, will be outlined, together with associated exercises which the trainer can use during training.

The selection of the skills and strategies included in this chapter, and in Chapters 5 and 6, has been based upon an analysis of investigations into communication within different health professions (e.g. Byrne and Long, 1976; MacLeod Clark, 1982; Saunders and Caves, 1986), coupled with a review of the recommendations contained in various texts on interpersonal communication for health professionals. Methods which can be followed in identifying such skills will be dealt with in Part Three.

4.2 NONVERBAL COMMUNICATION

During the past two decades, increasing attention has been devoted to the field of nonverbal communication. This has resulted in a voluminous amount of publications in this area, in the form of books, book chapters and research papers. Books on this topic have also been applied directly to the health professions (e.g. Blondis and Jackson, 1982). Given this vast array of publications, it is only possible in this chapter to present a brief overview of the topic in terms of the main components involved.

In a sense, it can be argued that nonverbal communication is not strictly speaking a *skill* as defined in Chapter 1. Rather, it is a distinct, and extensive, mode of communication which can be employed (with or without verbal accompaniment) when utilizing a range of other skills. For example, a nod of the head can be used to convey reinforcement, or an upright posture can help to display assertiveness. However, it is essential for the professional both to display skilled use of nonverbal behaviours, and to be able to interpret the nonverbal signals from others (Klinzing and Klinzing, 1985). For this reason, practitioners need to be introduced to the concept of bodily communication as a separate, and crucial, field of study.

Nonverbal communication can be defined as all forms of human communication apart from the purely verbal message. Thus the term 'nonverbal' encompasses both what is referred to as *body language*, namely movements of the head, hands, feet etc. (Wainwright, 1985); as well as vocalizations associated with the verbal messages, such as the tone, pitch, volume, speed, accent etc. of the voice. This latter aspect is usually referred to as *paralanguage*. Both of these dimensions will be examined briefly later in the chapter.

Since *Homo sapiens* is the only species to have developed a systematic language, we tend to concentrate primarily on the verbal messages which we convey. For example, we are taught from childhood to 'watch what we say', but are not really taught to monitor our body language. The result is that we generally have much greater control over the verbal, than the nonverbal, channel. Thus, most people find it much easier to lie verbally than nonverbally, and indeed a range of nonverbal deception indicators have been identified (Rozelle *et al.*, 1986). Another example of this is the fact that when the verbal and nonverbal messages are contradictory, we tend to believe the nonverbal aspects. Thus, if someone yawns, looks at their watch and says in a bored tone 'That's very interesting', the listener will not believe the verbal message. In this sense, 'actions speak louder than words'.

There are also clear nonverbal patterns of behaviour associated with various clinical states. It has been found that depressed and anxious patients can be identified purely by analysing their body language. Waxer (1974) found that judges were clearly able to identify five depressed psychiatric patients from five non-depressed counterparts on the basis of viewing silent films of both. Their judgements were based primarily upon the association of depression with a lack of eye contact, eyes looking down and away from the other person, down-turned mouth, downward angle of the head and absence of hand movements. In a similar study anxious patients were distinguishable by more self-stroking, twitching and tremor in hand movements, less eye contact and fewer smiles (Waxer, 1977).

Bull (1983) reports that other patient groups are also characterized by specific nonverbal behaviour patterns. Autistics, for example, display extreme gaze aversion, which may be employed in order to avoid any communication with others. Schizophrenics have been found to look less when discussing personal matters, although displaying normal gaze patterns when discussing neutral material. They also tend to be poorer at displaying emotional information nonverbally. In relation to psychopathy, it has also been shown that violent male offenders prefer greater interpersonal distance from others, use more hand gestures, look more and smile less than normals. This behavioural pattern, in turn, probably increases the likelihood of violent encounters with other males.

These findings indicate the importance of an understanding of nonverbal behaviour in terms of evaluating the behaviour of patients in a clinical setting. However, this aspect of communication serves a number of important functions.

Functions of nonverbal communication

There are six main functions of nonverbal communication:

1. *To replace speech* This happens in various situations, the prime example being sign language amongst the deaf and dumb. However, in many contexts a meaningful glance, a caring touch or a deliberate silence can substitute adequately for any verbal message.
2. *To complement the verbal message* In most instances this is the main function of nonverbal behaviour. If we say we are happy, we are expected to *look* happy. Similarly, the practitioner may give a demonstration to accompany a verbal explanation, with the use of appropriate hand movements, etc.
3. *To regulate and control the flow of communication* Turn-taking during social encounters is controlled by nonverbal signals. We do not say verbally 'I am now finishing. You can take over'. Rather we indicate this nonverbally by stopping speaking, raising or lowering the final syllable, and looking directly at the listener. Similarly, dominant individuals maintain their dominance by speaking more loudly, choosing a position of control (e.g. the top end of a table as with the board chairperson) and interrupting others.
4. *To provide feedback* During social encounters it is necessary to monitor the nonverbal reactions of others in terms of whether they are still listening, are worried, have understood what has been said, and so on. Health professionals should be sensitive to nonverbal forms of feedback, and during CST should be encouraged to develop their ability to interpret this information from others, while being aware of the nonverbal feedback which they themselves are providing. This latter dimension has been shown to be of crucial importance in health contexts. Patients often know

little about their condition and fail to fully comprehend the technicalities of explanations they receive. As a result, they place great importance upon the nonverbal cues emitted by practitioners in order to deduce information (Friedman, 1982).

5. *To help define relationships between people* This can be clearly observed in the hospital setting where uniforms are used to indicate the role, function and status of various professionals. This is often a useful dimension, since it facilitates identification and circumvents role confusion between professionals, although at times it can also cause confusion as, for example, when a hospital pharmacist wearing a white coat is 'seen' by patients to be a doctor.

6. *To convey emotional states* Emotions are recognized primarily on the basis of nonverbal behaviour. It is generally agreed (Siegman and Feldstein, 1987) that what is referred to as *social meaning* (attitudes, emotions etc.) is conveyed nonverbally. This is an important function, since saying verbally to someone 'I dislike you' may lead to overt aggression, whereas this message can be conveyed by more subtle nonverbal methods (looking less, orienting the body away from them etc.) with less likelihood of a confrontation.

Components of nonverbal communication

The above six functions can be achieved by coordinating a range of nonverbal behaviours. The main elements of nonverbal behaviour are as follows:

1. *Touch* In health settings, two different types of touch can be distinguished. Firstly, functional touch, in which the professional has to make physical contact with the patient in order to carry out a particular task (e.g. giving an injection, taking blood pressure etc.). Secondly, therapeutic touch, where the professional uses body contact to comfort or console a patient. Research into the use of these two types has produced equivocal findings. For example, the use of therapeutic touch by nursing staff at the preoperative stage has been found to be effective in producing a positive response to surgery among female, but not male, patients (Whitcher and Fisher, 1979). In another study, it was found that the more often physicians touched their patients during consultations, the less satisfied the patients were with the doctor, and the less they understood what they had been told (Larsen and Smith, 1981). This later study focused upon initial doctor/patient contacts, and this may partly have accounted for the findings. Touch tends to increase as a relationship develops, and thus from a 'strange' doctor the use of this behaviour may well be offputting and distracting for patients.

These findings emphasize the importance of a consideration of the context in which the touch occurs, when evaluating its appropriateness. For example the accompanying verbal message should complement the type of touch given (Montagu, 1978). In addition, the gender of the recipient needs to be considered, since males may perceive touch as an indicator of status or dominance, whereas females are less likely to construe it in this way (Henley, 1977). The form of touch employed also is of importance, since it has been found that a light 'incidental' touch, where the recipient was unaware of being touched, produced more positive perceptions of the environment in which this behaviour occurred (Fisher *et al.*, 1976), and also increased the compliance of the recipient to a request (Willis and Hamm, 1980).

2. *Proximity* This refers to the interpersonal distance which people maintain when interacting with one another. Hall (1959) identified four proximity zones, namely the intimate zone (0–18 inches); the personal zone (18 inches–4 feet); the social/consultative zone (4–12 feet); and the public zone (12 feet +). These distances relate to direct face-to-face interaction, so that we might be sitting beside a stranger at a lecture and yet not feel threatened in any way due to the absence of eye contact.

Large variations from proximity norms can cause discomfort, as exemplified by descriptions of individuals at opposite ends of the interpersonal distance continuum as either 'pushy' or 'stand-offish'. During social encounters we do not like others to invade our personal space without permission. This space enables us to maintain our personal dignity, respect and independence. However, it has been found that there is a status difference with regard to interpersonal distance, in that high status individuals can approach low status individuals quite closely, but low status individuals will usually seek approval before closely approaching people of higher status (Lott and Sommer, 1967). (Another example of status differences and personal space can be seen in the fact that higher status people occupy larger offices!)

Interestingly, in hospitals, patients on general wards often do not have any real personal space, in that practitioners can, and do, come within their intimate zone without seeking permission. This, in turn, may increase patients' sense of vulnerability and lack of control over their destiny (Oland, 1978). Professionals need to be aware of this, and, where possible, seek permission from patients before actually entering their personal zone. As a rough guide, French (1983) suggests that 'An area of two feet around a patient's bed and bedside locker could be viewed as his personal space' (p.53). Furthermore, Porritt (1984) points out that patients can suffer distress through being moved from a bed with which they have become familiar, to one in another ward area. Humans, like all animals, become familiar with a particular territory and feel more secure there. Thus, where it is essential to move a patient, Porritt advises staff to prepare the patient well in advance.

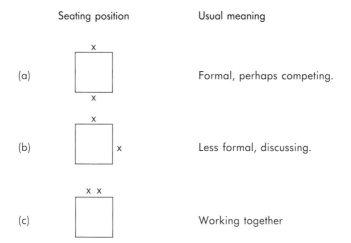

Fig. 4.1 Seating orientations.

3. *Orientation* This refers to the spatial positions which people take up in relation to one another. For example, in Fig. 4.1, position (b) would be the most appropriate for a doctor-patient consultation, since it is friendlier than (a) yet maintains a degree of formality which most patients will expect, as opposed to (c) which is more informal. However, if a doctor is explaining a detailed procedure she may well invite the patient to adopt the (c) position.

Height is another important aspect of orientation, in that it is usually associated with dominance. Hence, expressions such as 'He is above him at work', 'She is high up in the organization', 'He is someone to be looked up to', reflect the link between status and height. In hospitals, patients can feel particularly vulnerable when confined to bed, especially if staff with whom they interact remain standing. This can be overcome quite simply by sitting down on a chair beside the bed, especially if the interaction is more than just a fleeting visit. Similarly in paediatric contexts it is important for practitioners not to tower over children but rather to come down to their level when interacting.

4. *Posture* The posture which we adopt when sitting or standing can convey information about our attitudes, emotions and status. Interestingly, Goffman (1961) observed that at staff meetings in a hospital, the higher status individuals adopted the most relaxed postures, indicating that they were confident and in control of the situation. When seated, a forward leaning posture by doctors has been found to be associated with higher patient satisfaction (Larsen and Smith, 1981), as opposed to a backward lean, with the head tilted back.

Estimates of whether other people like us, or are interested in what we have to say, are influenced by their posture. A closed posture with arms and/or legs crossed often signals that the person is defensive or does not wish to become too involved in an interaction, whereas an open posture with hands and legs uncrossed tends to be interpreted as a signal of warmth, acceptance and willingness to participate (Egan, 1986). Furthermore, when two people are getting on well together they often adopt identical postures, a process known as posture-mirroring. This is a technique which can, in certain instances, be employed by the professional to convey to patients that they are 'with' them.

5. Body movements. This encompasses movements in three main regions of the body:

(a) *Hands and arms* Movements here, commonly referred to as gestures, can be either communicative or self-directed. Communicative gestures serve a useful function during social encounters, since they facilitate the transmission of messages from one person to another. Indeed, Graham and Heywood (1975) found that when subjects were not permitted to use gestures, when attempting to describe line drawings of two dimensional shapes, their speech patterns were affected in terms of an increase in speech hesitancies and pauses. Self-directed gestures, on the other hand, can be distracting for others and are often a sign of tension. Such gestures include ring twisting, hand wringing, nail biting or self-stroking. People who display extremes of self-directed gestures tend to be viewed as anxious or neurotic.

(b) *Head and shoulders* Slow head nods are usually taken as a sign of interest and willingness to listen, whereas fast head nods are interpreted as conveying impatience with the speaker. Likewise shaking the head slowly usually means ' I don't really agree' whereas shaking the head very quickly means 'I definitely disagree'! There are a range of other meanings which may be associated with various head positions in certain contexts, for example: head tilted slightly forward, eyes looking up through eye brows (submissiveness); head tossed in the air (defiance); head tilted to one side (listening). Movements of the shoulders are clearly more restricted in terms of communication, though we can shrug our shoulders to indicate that we do not know what is being asked, or stiffen our shoulders to convey tension.

(c) *Legs and feet* This region of the body is not typically used intentionally to communicate during interpersonal interaction (Patterson, 1983). But noticeable movements of the legs and feet are often interpreted by others as signs of unease, similar to self-directed gestures. Together, these have been referred to as 'social leakages', whereby the individual subconsciously displays evidence of tension or nervousness. These signals may be interpreted as a lack of confidence or as signs of deception, depending upon the context (Rozelle *et al.*, 1986).

6. *Facial expressions* One of the main functions of the face is to communicate emotional states, and facial expressions are therefore of vital importance during interaction between professionals and patients, in terms of the communication of affective information (Rand, 1981). Ekman and Friesen (1982) identified a total of forty-six 'single action units', or separate facial movements, such as 'wink' (orbicularis oculi), 'lip corner puller' (zygomatic major), 'inner brow raiser' (frontalis, pars medialis) and 'nostril compressor' (nasalis, pars transversa and depressor septi alae nasi). Clearly, the variety of combinations of two or more of these facial action units allows for an enormous number of overall facial expressions. However, perhaps the most important of these in many instances is a combination of interest in the patient, coupled with a smile to indicate receptivity and friendliness. Likewise, practitioners may need to control their facial expressions by, for example, not showing disgust when changing an infected wound or interacting with a patient with halitosis.

7. *Gaze* Eye contact is very important in our society, since it is usually a pre-requisite for any interaction, in that initial eye contact conveys a willingness to participate with another person. In western society, the listener usually looks at the speaker about twice as much as the speaker looks at the listener (Argyle, 1975). However, dominant or aggressive individuals tend to look more while speaking. Furthermore, the degree of eye contact engaged in depends upon the situation. Two young people in love may stare caringly at one another, whereas the same degree of gaze between two males may be the prelude to physical aggression. Conversely, the absence of eye contact may convey embarrassment, disinterest or deception.

   When dealing with patients, it is important to display appropriate levels of gaze, since too much or too little eye contact can be disconcerting. In the Larsen and Smith (1981) study mentioned earlier, it was found that greater use of eye contact by a doctor was associated with lower patient satisfaction during first-time visits. In this instance, the increased doctor gaze may have heightened the anxiety of patients when dealing with an unfamiliar physician. Interestingly, psychiatrists may put patients on a couch and sit in a chair behind them, to help reduce any possible embarrassment which patients may feel in discussing personal matters.

8. *Appearance* This includes both the physical make-up of the individual, and the clothes, jewellery, etc. which they wear. As discussed in Chapter 3 this is an important dimension of communication, since we make judgements about the nature, character and disposition of individuals based upon their appearance (Kleinke, 1986). However, some aspects of appearance can be manipulated more easily than others. For example, dress and hair colour can be controlled, whereas height can be adjusted only

slightly. It is important for health professionals to portray an appropriate image in terms of appearance so that they 'look the part' when interacting with patients.

9. *Paralanguage* This refers to *how* something is said as opposed to *what* is said. Indeed, the manner in which a verbal message is spoken will directly affect the meaning of that message, in that slight alterations in the tone, pitch, volume, speed, or emphasis on certain words, can change the overall meaning being conveyed. Davitz (1964), for example, found that a range of separate emotions could be accurately communicated by changing paralanguage when reading a neutral passage. Furthermore, Scherer (1972) found that a range of voice stereotypes could be identified, so that for example, flatness in the voice was associated with masculinity, sluggishness and coldness; males with tense voices were viewed as older, unyielding and cantankerous; whereas women with tense voices were seen as young, emotional, highly strung and less intelligent.

There are also speech styles associated with different settings. In this way, sports commentators on TV, clergymen saying prayers in church, and auctioneers selling goods, all have distinctive speech patterns. Health professionals, however, are required to display a range of speech styles. For example, the style associated with informing a patient of a terminal illness or death of a relative, will be markedly different from that associated with telling a young woman who has been trying to have a baby for several years that she is pregnant. Thus, sensitivity and flexibility are required in terms of appropriate use of paralanguage.

These nine features of nonverbal communication are important dimensions of most interactive episodes. Although these aspects have been separated for the purposes of analysis, it is obvious, however, that they are in fact interrelated. Not only should these nonverbal features complement one another when communicating with others, they should also be consistent with the verbal messge.

4.3 REINFORCEMENT

From a very early stage of development the importance of social rewards, in the form of verbal and nonverbal reinforcement, can be observed. The smile of the infant is an important reinforcer for the mother and, likewise, the smiles, caresses and soothing vocalizations of the mother are crucial to the mother-child bonding process. Furthermore, the social reinforcers of the mother are linked to the satisfaction of basic biological needs in the child, and they therefore attain a significant role very early in life. Thus, when the child is being fed, changed or kept warm, it is also receiving social reinforcement.

This association between social and material rewards is a common one.

The child who wins a race or passes an examination will usually receive some form of material reward, but will also receive praise and attention from peers and from significant others. This therefore strengthens the link between social and material reinforcers. As Skinner (1953, p.78) puts it 'The attention of people is reinforcing because it is a necessary condition for other reinforcements from them'. Over time, social reinforcement in itself acquires value for the individual even in the absence of more tangible rewards. As a result, the use of praise, encouragement etc. can be implemented to influence the behaviour of others.

Although the term reinforcement was introduced by Pavlov (1927), it is the more recent work of Skinner (1969, 1976) which has influenced interest in this concept as a social skill. As Skinner (1971, p.199) points out, reinforcement, in this sense, is based 'on the simple principle that whenever something reinforces a particular activity of an organism, it increases the chances that the organism will repeat that behaviour'.

It is obvious that this latter Skinnerian application of the concept of reinforcement has direct implications for human behaviour. Thus a young male who is interested in a young female will give her concerted attention in the form of eye contact, smiles, nods and verbal rewards, in order to encourage her to continue talking to him. Similarly, if we tell a joke at work and our colleagues reward us by laughing, we are more likely to tell another joke than if they frowned or declared that they were not amused! In this way, behaviour is shaped by the positive or negative consequences which ensue.

Functions of reinforcement

The use of social reinforcement serves a range of purposes, including:

1. *To encourage the involvement of the other person* In order to obtain maximum participation during interaction, it is necessary to reinforce other people when they are communicating with us. Without such reinforcement, their level of participation will decrease markedly. Indeed, one of the problems with many psychiatric patients is that they give little or no reinforcement to others. As a result, they receive fewer communications, which in turn increases their social isolation (Hargie and McCartan, 1986).

2. *To demonstrate interest* We pay greater attention to, and reinforce more, people who are of interest to us (Hargie *et al.*, 1987). For this reason, if people do not reinforce us, we in turn feel that they are not really interested in us. Thus, Kasteler *et al.* (1976) found that patients who felt their doctors were not interested in them were more likely to change to another doctor. Similarly, Nelson *et al.* (1975) found that schizophrenics were more likely to comply with treatment if they perceived their

physicians as being interested in them. Conveying interest is therefore an important function of reinforcement.

3. *To develop and maintain relationships* At the initial stage of relationship development people reciprocate high levels of reinforcement. Once a relationship has been established, reinforcement levels may subside. However, if reinforcement ceases, the relationship is likely to terminate. In health contexts the amount of reinforcement given will depend upon the setting. A patient who only occasionally sees her doctor, pharmacist or health visitor will expect more concerted attention than a patient in hospital will expect from a nurse on the ward.

4. *To provide reassurance* Although in certain instances reassurance can be employed to decrease behaviour, as when the professional reduces the anxiety of a patient who may be mistakenly concerned about his well-being by reassuring him that he is quite healthy, it also can have a re-inforcing potential. The very fact that the professional has taken the time to reassure the patient will probably encourage the patient to return to that person again. This will be especially true if the practitioner reassures the patient that he was very wise to seek professional advice. Patients are often worried about their condition, the prognosis and the ability of medical staff to help them overcome their difficulties. Often, such worries are based upon mistaken beliefs or mis-information and their fears can genuinely be allayed by the practitioner. Leigh and Reiser (1980, p. 294) define reassurance as consisting 'of a general optimistic and hopeful attitude and specific statements based on data and/or experience designed to allay exaggerated or unfounded fears of the patient'. Such reassurance should obviously be genuine, since false reassurance may well be counter-productive.

   Di Matteo and Di Nicola (1982) emphasize the importance of a re-assuring, reinforcing, 'bedside manner' for practitioners, especially during ward rounds after which there is evidence to indicate that patients often report feeling anxious, upset, depersonalized, and even dehumanized with resulting adverse changes in their physical condition.

5. *To convey warmth and friendliness* Individuals who are perceived as being warm, friendly and approachable, display much higher levels of verbal and nonverbal reinforcement than those who are perceived as cold or aloof. A number of studies have shown that patient satisfaction and compliance with treatment are positively related to perceptions of practitioners as being warm and friendly (e.g. Becker *et al.*, 1972; Kincey *et al.*, 1975). Thus, it is important for practitioners to employ appropriate re-inforcers to demonstrate a warm, friendly approach when dealing with patients.

6. *To help to control the topic of conversation* By selectively reinforcing particular aspects of the other person's communication it is possible to increase the incidence of these elements. This phenomenon is known as

the 'Greenspoon effect' following a study carried out by Greenspoon (1955) in which he demonstrated that by using the reinforcer 'mm-hmm' on each occasion during interviews when the interviewee used a plural noun, the total number of plural nouns used by interviewees gradually increased. Following this study, a range of similar investigations were conducted, confirming that the responses of interviewees could be subtly manipulated, through the selective use of reinforcement, to encourage them to discuss at greater length areas which were targeted by the interviewer. Quite often health professionals subconsciously use this technique to encourage patients to discuss certain matters, but not others. Indeed, a review of recordings of interviews by Carl Rogers, the well known advocate of non-directive counselling, found that in fact he differentially (and presumably unintentionally) rewarded certain categories of client utterance (Truax, 1966). It is therefore clear that reinforcement can be applied in such a manner as to control the topic of conversation.

Behavioural components of reinforcement

There are a wide range of verbal and nonverbal behaviours which can be employed in order to reinforce others. Nonverbally, most of the behaviours described in the previous section can be used in this way. For example:

1. *Touch* can be reassuring and comforting, as when the practitioner holds the hand of a worried patient or puts an arm around a bereaved person. With young children, touch can be very reassuring and rewarding;
2. *Proximity* is also a form of reinforcement, in that we tend to stand or sit closer to people whom we like and want to be involved with;
3. *Orientation* can also be manipulated to reward others. For instance, sitting down beside a patient rather than standing, or arranging chairs to encourage participation;
4. *Posture* can be utilized to convey interest and acceptance. Thus, when seated, a forward lean is usually taken as a sign of attentiveness;
5. *Head nods* have been reported to be the most common form of non-verbal reinforcement used to indicate listening (Rosenfeld and Hancks, 1980);
6. *Gaze* is also crucial, in that if someone is not looking at us, we take it as a strong sign of disinterest. Likewise, we usually look more at those whom we like;
7. *Appearance* can also be regarded as a reinforcer, since we take great care to dress and groom ourselves for important occasions with important people (e.g. on a first date or for a selection interview). The appearance of practitioners should therefore show respect for the patient;
8. *Paralinguistic cues* can strengthen the reinforcing potential of statements, so that verbal reinforcement should *sound* genuine. Furthermore, the use

of 'mm hmm' would seem to be the most frequently used reinforcing vocalization (Rosenfeld and Hancks, 1980).

These nonverbal reinforcers are usually combined with overt verbal reinforcement. There are five main types of verbal reinforcers:

1. *Acknowledgements* These are words or phrases which are employed in order to acknowledge the response of another person. Examples include: 'Thank you'; 'OK'; 'I see'; 'You are correct'. These acknowledgements are not very strong reinforcers but they are often expected as part of basic courtesy, and if not given can leave the person feeling aggrieved. Thus, if we open a door for someone who walks through without saying 'Thank you', we tend to feel somewhat annoyed!

2. *Compliments* It is rewarding to be told that some aspect of our personal appearance is worthy of positive comment. This can be particularly true in the health field where statements such as: 'You are looking well'; 'You haven't changed a bit'; 'I like your hair style'; 'That's a lovely dress', can be very rewarding especially where a patient may feel dejected or lacking in self-esteem.

3. *Supportive comments* Phrases such as 'That must have been very difficult'; 'You have every right to feel like that'; 'I agree entirely', can be employed to convey to another that they are speaking to someone who will offer encouragement, support and concern. This is very important when discussing personal and emotional matters. This form of reinforcement can also be gainfully employed where a patient is exerting effort worthy of reward. For instance, a physiotherapist may say to a patient who has nearly completed a set task 'Keep it going. Come on, you're nearly there!'

4. *Evaluative comments* Here, rewards are given for some effort another person has made. Thus a nurse may say to a young boy who has valiantly withstood crying when receiving an injection, 'Well done! You're a very brave little man!' Similarly, a physiotherapist may say to a patient making her first tentative steps following a stroke, 'Great effort! You're really coming on remarkably well'. Such forms of encouragement are invaluable in many health contexts.

5. *Response development* This involves paying careful attention to what someone is saying, and ensuring that their responses are built upon where appropriate. In this sense, developing and extending the topic of conversation raised by a patient is a potent form of reinforcement. As Crow (1983) points out, where a topic shift is to be made this should be preceded by a disjunct marker ('Can I ask you a different qeustion?' 'Before I forget . . .'). However, such disjunct markers should not be over-used.

These are the main verbal and nonverbal components of the skill of reinforcement. The importance of this skill has been highlighted in a review by Cairns (1986) who iterates that 'the way one person responds and reinforces another is a significant aspect of the communication between the people that leads to attraction, friendships or even more intimate relationships' (p.136). Health professionals should therefore be aware of the potency and beneficial effects of the appropriate use of reinforcement. There is evidence to suggest that this skill should be incorporated into CST programmes, since studies of doctor-patient (Verby *et al.*, 1979) and nurse-patient (MacLeod Clark, 1982) interactions have indicated a dearth of practitioner reinforcement. Furthermore, studies of speech therapist-patient interactions have found 'positive reinforcement' to be one of the most important skills as evaluated by the therapists themselves (Saunders and Caves, 1986).

Exercise 4.1 can be employed by the trainer to encourage trainees to focus upon the skill of reinforcement, and generate a wide range of behaviours which can be employed as rewards during social interaction.

Exercise 4.1 Reinforcement

Aim

To sensitize trainees to the range of verbal and nonverbal reinforcers which can be utilized during interpersonal encounters.

Instructions

This exercise is not suitable for very large groups of trainees. It involves subdividing the class into dyads or triads, and asking each subgroup simply to list, on a sheet of paper, as many examples of verbal and nonverbal reinforcers as they can within each of the reinforcement categories described in this chapter. Thus, trainees should note as many examples as possible of where touch, proximity, orientation etc. could be employed, and should then itemize as many examples of acknowledgements, compliments etc. as they can generate. Each subgroup should be given a specific order for listing examples (e.g. Group 1 could begin by examining 'Touch'; Group 2 'Proximity' and so on) so that a wide variety of examples will be generated. The subgroups should then be given a set time limit for completing the task.

Discussion

Using the blackboard, or the OHP, the trainer should take each reinforcement category in turn and obtain from the groups as many examples as possible. This procedure is followed until all of the categories have been covered. During this feedback session the trainer should raise, for various examples, issues such as:

1. The differential use of reinforcement with different age groups
2. Gender differences in the use of reinforcers
3. Cultural factors
4. The application of examples to health contexts.

4.4 REFLECTING

Reference has already been made to the multi-dimensional nature of communication (Chapter 1). People can communicate at either a factual or a feeling level. When responding to others, we can decide to focus specifically on either one of these levels, or can take both into account. As Fig. 4.2 illustrates, one technique which can be used to respond to patients is that of reflecting, whereby the practitioner, using his own words, feeds back to the patient the main elements of the latter's previous communication.

Where the emphasis is solely upon reflecting back the factual component, this is termed 'paraphrasing' (or 'reflection of content'); where it is solely upon feelings it is known as 'reflection of feeling'; and where both facts and feelings are involved this is referred to as 'reflection'. Crute (1986), neatly exemplifies the above distinctions in relation to a health visitor–client interaction:

> Client: 'I just don't understand my mother-in-law. One minute she's very kind and good to me, and the next she's treating me terribly'.
> Health Visitor: 'So, she's very inconsistent with you (Paraphrase). You feel confused (Reflection of feeling).'

Here, taken as a whole, the health visitor's response is an overall reflection, although either the paraphrase or the reflection of feeling could have been employed in isolation, had she decided to focus primarily on facts or emotions respectively.

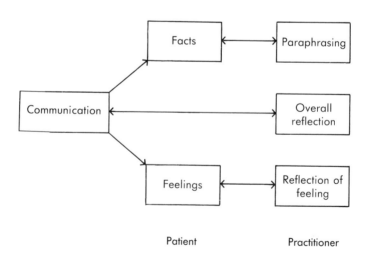

Fig. 4.2 Reflecting.

As Dickson (1986), in reviewing this skill, noted, there is some conceptual confusion concerning the actual term 'reflection'. For example, Hein (1973) in her discussion of nurse-patient communication defines reflection as simply echoing the actual words used by the patient, and uses the term 'restatement' to refer to the process of reformulating the patient's verbalizations in the nurse's own words. French (1983), on the other hand, conceives paraphrasing as involving the activity of putting the patient's statements, thoughts and feelings into one's own words. However, in this chapter the distinctions mentioned earlier will be utilized, and reflection will be regarded as involving the following steps:

1. Recalling and restating the speaker's message correctly;
2. Identifying the main factual and/or feeling aspects being expressed;
3. Translating these factual and/or feeling components into one's own words;
4. Verbally reflecting the essence of these facts and/or feelings;
5. Monitoring the reaction of the other person, to judge the accuracy of the reflection.

The use of reflection as an interviewing skill originated with the development by Rogers (1951) of client-centred, non-directive counselling. Here the emphasis is upon allowing the client to lead the interaction, and dictate the topics to be discussed. The counsellor is viewed as a facilitator, encouraging the client to talk through and sort out his own problems, and as a result, the use of more directive techniques such as questioning is eschewed.

Although reflection as a skill was identified within the field of client-centred therapy, this skill is also frequently employed in a wide range of interview settings (Hargie *et al.*, 1987). Indeed, it is commonly regarded as a skill which can be most gainfully employed when accompanied by other interviewing skills (Hargie, 1986), including certain types of questions (Chapter 5). As Hein (1973) puts it, in the health context, reflection 'in particular needs to be used in conjunction with other skills ... Used exclusively, it can generate antagonism and frustration from our patients' (p.46).

Functions of reflecting

The main functions of the skill of reflecting can be summarized as follows:

1. *To demonstrate interest in, and involvement with, the patient* Reflection is in fact a form of response development which, as discussed in the previous section, is in turn a potent form of reinforcement. It is quite difficult to listen to someone, assimilate what they are saying, and then immediately reflect this back to them using different terminology. The ability to do so is clear evidence of careful listening and this is therefore

appreciated by clients. However, as Ivey and Authier (1978) observe, this ability often takes time to develop, and trainers may need to devote concerted time and effort to ensure that trainees acquire an effective grasp of this skill.

2. *To use a patient-centred approach* In their analysis of doctor-patient consultations, Byrne and Long (1976) identified a continuum of interactive styles ranging from doctor-centred at one end to patient-centred at the other. At the latter end, one of the techniques employed was that of reflecting. However, Byrne and Long, while recognizing the value of a patient-centred approach, found it was seldom used by doctors. Livesey (1986) attributes this finding to the probable fear by doctors of losing control of the consultation, and of being involved in protracted interactions with patients. However, as Livesey iterates, these fears are groundless since control can be subtly maintained within a patient-centred approach; and very few consultations will involve complex problems requiring lengthy interviews. Furthermore, in discussing doctor-patient interactions Shorter (1985) identified two main conditions which were necessary for successful consultations, namely where:
   (a) The doctor showed an active interest in the patient;
   (b) The patient had an opportunity to tell his story in a leisurely, unhurried manner.

3. *To check for accuracy of understanding* Reflection is a useful skill for ensuring that both the practitioner and patient fully understand the patient's communications. In this sense, it allows the practitioner to periodically seek feedback from the patient, since following a reflection the patient will indicate verbally and/or nonverbally whether it has been accurate. This can also be valuable from the patient's point of view. Where the patient is talking through a complex problem that he has not fully sorted out in his own mind, the use of practitioner reflections may enable him to identify central thoughts, ideas and feelings in a new and meaningful fashion, thereby providing new insights and a deeper more accurate understanding of his own situation.

4. *To highlight certain facets of the patient's communciation* By reflecting back particular parts of the message received, the practitioner is, in effect, encouraging the patient to discuss these more fully and is thereby using a form of selective reinforcement. As already mentioned, such selection may involve an exclusive focus upon either facts or feelings. Within these two domains, of course, there may be further selectivity. One of the most commonly cited advantages of reflection is that it allows, and indeed encourages, the exploration of feelings (e.g. Cormier and Cormier, 1979; Porritt, 1984). The use of reflection of feeling conveys to the patient that it is acceptable for him to have such feelings and that the practitioner is willing to discuss them (Fritz *et al.*, 1984).

5. *To show respect for patients and their concerns* The willingness to allow

patients to freely express themselves, coupled with the use of practitioner reflections to demonstrate concerted listening, is an indicator that patients are valued and worthy of attention. This, in turn, facilitates the process of relationship development.

6. *To demonstrate empathy* In his analysis of the dimension of empathy in doctor-patient interactions, Authier (1986) highlights the central role of reflections in communicating an awareness and understanding of the patient's perspective. Since empathy is defined by Rogers (1975, p.3) as '... pointing sensitively to the "felt meaning" which the client is experiencing in this particular moment, in order to help him focus on that meaning and to carry it further', it is clear that the skill of reflection will be a core technique in conveying an empathic approach.

Guidelines for the use of reflections

There are a number of points which need to be borne in mind when utilizing this skill:

1. *Avoid interpretations* Reflections involve rephrasing what the patient has said, not going beyond this to analyse or interpret the message received. As Hein (1973) asserts, when using reflections 'No new information is being sought at these times. Validity, clarity and understanding of the old (i.e. previous) information are the major aims of this skill' (p.46).

2. *Be accurate* While the occasional inaccurate reflection will not adversely affect a relationship, consistent inaccuracy will indicate a total lack of understanding. In particular, it is important to gauge the correct level of emotion to reflect back. Trainees can be sensitized to this problem by having them distinguish three levels of emotion, namely low, medium and high. This can be achieved by giving them a few examples as follows:

Low	*Medium*	*High*
Annoyed	Angry	Furious
Pleased	Delighted	Ecstatic

Trainees can then be asked, either individually or in groups to identify as many of these emotional continua as possible, and their responses written on the blackboard.

3. *Nonverbal considerations* As well as verbally reflecting, the practitioner should nonverbally reflect the patient's communication. This may involve adopting a similar facial expression, posture, body movements or paralanguage. At times it may be necessary to reflect feelings based purely upon nonverbal signals, and in such cases it is wise to allow an opportunity for the patient to correct possible misinterpretations by using

prefaces such as: 'It seems to me that . . .'; 'You appear to be . . .'; 'I get the impression that . . .'.

4. *Do not use stereotyped responses* One of the common errors made by inexperienced interviewers is to begin every reflection with 'You feel . . .' (Stuart and Sundeen, 1983). Other errors include either under- or over-using this skill, and using questions in the mistaken belief that they are reflections. This latter misconception can partly be overcome by developing the ability of trainees to clearly identify appropriate reflections. One method whereby this can be achieved is for the trainer to display on an OHP a number of patient statements, and for each statement ask trainees to write down a relevant paraphrase and reflection of feeling. The trainer can then ask individual trainees to call out their responses.

5. *Be concise and specific* A reflection should be a brief reformulation of the essence of what the patient has said. Where feelings are involved, there should be a feeling 'label' in the reflection. Thus, general statements such as 'Boy, have you got a problem!' are not reflections.

These are the main points which should be considered when using the skill of reflection. This is a very useful skill for practitioners to acquire since, as Dickson (1986, p.171) concludes, 'From the research reviewed it would seem that reflections, whether of fact, feeling or both, are perceived positively by both interviewees and external observers'.

4.5 LISTENING

In terms of responding skills, the ability to demonstrate effective listening is of prime importance. In fact, many of the behaviours associated with all of the skills in this chapter, and in Chapter 5, can be employed as indicators of listening. Given this widespread range of listening behaviours it is hardly surprising that Pietrofesa *et al.* (1978, p.243) in their discussion of counselling conclude that 'If we had to pinpoint a crucial helping skill, it would be the ability to listen'. Furthermore, Porritt (1984, p.80), in her analysis of nurse-patient communication, asserts that, 'Most life events, including admission to hospital, do not require highly skilled counselling but do require skilled listening'. It is therefore vital that health professionals have a sound knowledge of, and capacity for, effective listening skills.

Although several books have been written specifically on this topic (Wolvin and Coakley, 1982; Adler, 1983; Floyd, 1985), and indeed most texts on communication for health professionals include at least a chapter on it, there is no agreed definition of the term itself. Smith (1986) in reviewing definitions of listening highlights the fact that some theorists regard this as involving solely the reception of auditory information, while others view listening as encompassing the assimilation of both verbal and nonverbal messages. It is this latter perspective which will be adopted here, and in this sense listening can be defined as the process whereby one person demonstrates that he or she is paying careful attention to, and attempting to understand, the verbal and nonverbal signals being emitted by another.

This definition emphasizes the active nature of listening. It is possible to listen to someone (especially to their verbal messages) without showing that you are paying attention, in other words to listen *passively* (Steil *et al.*, 1983). However, in professional contexts it is necessary both to listen carefully and to indicate this verbally and nonverbally. Thus, the use of reinforcement, reflections, self-disclosure, probing questions and so on, are potent indicators of *active listening*. Active listening is also required to ensure that maximum verbal and nonverbal information is received from patients. As discussed in Chapter 3, concerted effort is essential during interpersonal interaction to ensure that the selective nature of the perceptual process does not result in vital social information being lost (See Fig. 3.4).

The listening process

When we listen to others, there are a range of mental processes operative. As we listen we attempt to evaluate what the speaker is saying, we plan what we are going to say in response, and we covertly rehearse (often subconsciously) our response. While these processes are an inherent part of interpersonal interaction, they should not interfere with the act of listening *per se*. Thus, we should not be concentrating so much on what we intend to say that we stop paying attention to what the speaker is saying.

In relation to the actual reception of verbal messages, there are three factors which should be borne in mind:

1. *Reductionism* We can only cope with a limited amount of information, and so if we are presented with too much detail it is necessary to reduce this in order to retain it. Again, care must be taken to ensure only less important elements are lost.
2. *Rationalization* This refers to the process whereby we attempt to make incoming data fit more easily with our own experience. To facilitate such assimilation we may rationalize it in three ways. Firstly, we may attribute different causes to those presented (e.g. the practitioner may regard the pain expressed by a 'hypochondriacal' patient as imaginary). Secondly, transformation of language may occur. There is an apocryphal story about the message 'Send reinforcements we're going to advance' being sent by troops at the battlefront along the line, and eventually arriving at headquarters as 'Send three and fourpence we're going to a dance'! Such acoustic confusions (Gregg, 1986) are not uncommon in reality, but can be potentially dangerous in the health sphere where products with similar sounding names can easily be confused. Thirdly,

there can be the addition of material, a classic example being gossip enlargement! As mentioned under the skill of reflection, care needs to be taken not to 'read too much into' what a patient is saying.

3. *Change in the order of events* Where the information received contains a chronological order or a set sequence, this can be mixed up. Thus, 'Take 2 tablets 4 times daily' may become 'Take 4 tablets 2 times daily'.

Obstacles to effective listening

In order to employ effective listening skills, it is necessary to be aware of a number of obstacles which can interfere with the listening process. These include:

1. *Speech/thought rates* The average rate of speech is between 125–175 words per minute whereas the average 'thought rate', at which we assimilate information, is between 400–800 words per minute. This differential means that we usually have spare thought time when listening to others. It is essential to ensure that this spare cognitive capacity is taken up with activities which facilitate listening, such as asking covert questions. For example, the Royal College of General Practitioners Working Party (1972) recommended the following covert questions for doctors to ask themselves:

> 'What must I tell this patient? How much of what I learned about him should he know? What words shall I use to convey this information? How much of what I propose to tell him will he understand? How will he react? How much of my advice will he take? What degree of pressure am I entitled to apply' (p.17).

Without concerted concentration it is probable that spare thought time will be filled with other mental processes unrelated to listening (such as day-dreaming).

2. *Distractions* Listening ability is impaired if the environment contains too many intrusive distractions which divert attention away from the speaker. This would include other people talking in the room, telephone ringing, radio or television in operation, and so on. Likewise, it is difficult to attempt to listen attentively to two separate sources simultaneously, and indeed this type of *dichotomous listening* should be avoided.

3. *Inattentiveness* Listening is hard work, and requires constant concentration. As a result, if the listener is tired, or has something preying on his mind, he is less likely to listen in an efficient manner.

4. *Mental set* The initial frame of mind of the listener and his preconceptions of the speaker, can influence how the latter's message is received and interpreted. Judgements about the speaker are often made on the basis of age, sex, dress, appearance, status etc. Similarly, patients are

often evaluated on the basis of ascribed stereotypes (hypochondriac, troublesome patient). In this way, more attention is paid to who is speaking rather than on what is being said. Good listeners need to ensure objectivity during social encounters.

5. *Individual bias* Listening can be impaired when an individual distorts the message being received, owing to his own personal situation. Thus the practitioner who is in a hurry may choose not to 'hear' a message because she knows it will entail an extended interaction with a patient. On the other hand, seriously ill patients, or their relatives, may choose to ignore unpleasant facts being detailed by the professional because they are too threatening or disturbing. Another example of individual bias occurs where someone does not listen simply because he wishes to speak, and get his own message across, regardless of what others have said.

6. *The speaker* Quite often the cause of ineffective listening lies with the speaker. If the speaker has a severe speech dysfluency, speaks at an extremely fast or slow rate, has a marked foreign or regional accent, or is being deliberately vague and evasive, it will be very difficult for the listener to cope.

7. *Blocking* Hargie *et al.* (1987) have identified a range of blocking tactics which a listener may employ when she does not wish to pursue a certain line of communication. These blocking techniques, which include referring the person elsewhere, responding selectively to only part of the message, or changing the topic completely, are utilized to divert, or terminate the conversation. It should however be realized that in certain instances blocking tactics may be used positively so that, for example, a pharmacist would be expected to refer a patient to see the doctor if he suspected a serious illness.

Active listening

During interpersonal encounters, the practitioner must make the effort not only to listen to others, but also to clearly demonstrate, both verbally and nonverbally, that he is indeed doing so (Klinzing and Klinzing, 1985). This is not so simple as it may sound, since as Burley-Allen (1982) points out, listening requires a great deal of effort and concentration to sort out the relevance of various points and to consider their possible relationships. In addition, listening can be a time-consuming activity which, in some health professions, may be regarded as a form of inactivity. For example, Hein (1973, p.171) noted that in nursing practice, listening 'often is supplanted by more immediate and visually apparent tasks or priorities. Listening skilfully during a nursing task is often a good utilization of time, but as a solitary activity (except perhaps with psychiatric patients) it is often considered unessential'. While this approach to patient care is changing, there still remains a residual attitude that listening is somehow synonymous with 'doing nothing'.

Yet, the skilled use of listening when interacting with patients is useful in order to achieve a number of functions including the following:

1. To focus specifically upon the verbal and nonverbal messages being communicated by patients;
2. To gain a full, accurate, understanding of the patient's situation;
3. To communicate interest, concern and sympathetic attention;
4. To encourage full, open and honest patient communication;
5. To develop a more non-directive, patient-centred style of interaction.

Fritz *et al.* (1984) argue that this skill is so important that the health practitioner who does not learn to listen effectively sets the course for a professional life filled with inefficiency, inaccuracy and shallow satisfaction. Trainers therefore have a particular responsibility to ensure that they inculcate in trainees a desire to listen carefully to patients. Conine (1976, p.160), for example, notes that, 'In the course of their education many physical therapy students have had little experience of being listened to, a factor contributing to a lack of appreciation for listening to others'. Thus, trainers should act as appropriate listening models for trainees to imitate during professional practice.

Listening, therefore, is a core skill for health professionals. In reviewing studies which have examined doctor-patient interactions, Di Matteo and Di Nicola (1982) found that in almost every instance the doctor talked significantly more than the patient, yet most physicians believed that they spent much more time listening to their patients than talking to them. These findings underline the need for more concerted training in listening skills. Wolff *et al.* (1983) suggest ten main points that should be borne in mind to facilitate effective listening:

1. don't stereotype the speaker
2. avoid distractions
3. arrange a conducive environment (adequate ventilation, lighting, seating etc.)
4. be psychologically prepared to listen
5. keep an open, analytical mind, searching for the central thrust of the speaker's message
6. identify supporting arguments and facts
7. do not dwell on one or two aspects at the expense of others
8. delay judgement, or refutation, until you have heard the entire message
9. don't formulate your next question while the speaker is relating information
10. be objective.

Exercise 4.2 can be employed to demonstrate to trainees the difficulty in listening to and recalling even quite a short message, and the necessity, therefore, for careful, concerted listening during professional encounters.

Exercise 4.2 Listening

Aim

To highlight to trainees some of the difficulties involved in effective listening, and facilitate discussion as to how listening ability can be improved.

Materials

Duplicate copies of the 'Passing the message' exercise for all class members.

Instructions

Ask for (or select!) six volunteers from the class to leave the room, before instructing the remaining class members that they are to act as observers and will be required to record how the message changes upon each re-telling, by using the Observation Sheet as instructed. Then ask the first volunteer to come into the room and give him/her the following instructions: 'I am going to read you a message only once. You must not ask any questions and are not allowed to take notes, but just listen carefully and attempt to remember it. You will then have to pass this message on to the next person who comes in. You must also give that person the same instructions which I have just given you. Is that clear?' Then proceed to read the message slowly. The second volunteer is now taken back into the room and listens to the message from the first volunteer. This procedure continues until the sixth volunteer receives the message, and is asked to relate it to the entire class.

Discussion

Obtain feedback from the observers as to when the message became distorted. Usually, a lot of information is lost initially since there is simply too much to remember. As well as being *reduced*, the message is also usually *rationalized* (see under section 4.5 'The listening process'). The volunteers should then be asked what problems they faced in this exercise, and a general class discussion can then ensue as to how the listening process could have been improved. This would include the volunteers being allowed to ask questions, asking for information to be repeated, taking notes, not having the distractions from an audience etc. If time permits, the exercise can be repeated with a new message, new volunteers, and a change in the rules to allow interaction between speaker and listener (i.e. asking questions, or seeking clarification). This demonstrates the importance of active listening since the second exercise will normally illustrate improved listening effectiveness.

PASSING THE MESSAGE

OBSERVATION SHEET

MESSAGE: Please tell Natasha Simpson that Justin Hollins called. The computer she ordered, DX 9175, cannot be delivered before Christmas, but the one she left in for repair, TY 3268, has a disc malfunction and could be ready before then. If she could ring me before Thursday, on extension 4027, we can discuss this, and also negotiate financial details concerning our continued electronic maintenance service.

Please note:

Under the appropriate number for each volunteer place a tick (√) when the words are repeated correctly. Otherwise leave blank or make a brief note of what was actually said.

	1	2	3	4	5	6
Please tell						
Natasha Simpson						
Justin Hollins called						
The computer						
She ordered						
DX 9175						
Cannot be delivered before Christmas						
The one she left in for repair						
TY 3268						
Disc malfunction						
Could be ready before then						
If she could ring me						
Before Thursday						
Extension 4027						
Negotiate financial details						
Continued electronic maintenance service						

4.6 SELF-DISCLOSURE

In order to make accurate diagnoses about patient's illnesses, it is necessary to encourage them to openly and honestly disclose personal details about their condition and their situation. As Smith and Bass (1982, p. 157) put it:

'Patients and new employees in a health-care setting must often be encouraged and helped to recognize some of the situations in which extra self-disclosure is necessary. Physicians and other health professionals often need to know personal or intimate details about a patient to make a diagnosis and either to prescribe or to carry out treatment. The patient's willingness to disclose himself may be crucial'.

Self-disclosure, in this sense, can be defined as the act of verbally and/or nonverbally communicating to others some dimension of personal information. Thus, self-disclosure can be nonverbal, in that it is possible, for example, either to hide feelings such as happiness, sadness, anger etc., or to express them through the use of facial expressions, gestures, and so on. Most texts on self-disclosure, however, tend to emphasize the verbal component of this skill since this aspect is less prone to misinterpretation, whereas we can be mistaken in our judgements about the nonverbal behaviour of others.

A knowledge, and skilled use of self-disclosure is important for health professionals for two main reasons. Firstly, they should be aware of the factors which will encourage patients to fully present, and openly express, their needs. Secondly, practitioners need to be sensitive to situations in which it is apt for them to self-disclose to patients, thereby presenting a 'human face'. The use of self-disclosure by professionals can be divided into two main categories. As Hargie and Morrow (1988) point out, practitioner self-disclosure can be about one's own personal experiences, or about one's personal reaction to the patient's experiences (although Danish *et al.* (1976) argue that technically the former is a *self-disclosing* statement whereas the latter is a *self-involving* statement).

Both of these types of self-disclosure can be appropriate, depending upon the circumstances. The first type can be used to reassure patients that they are not alone in their situation, and can demonstrate shared experiences. However, it should not be taken to extremes, or to what Yager and Beck (1985) term the 'We could have been twins' response! The second type keeps the focus of attention firmly upon the patient, and indicates a willingness to become involved in his experiences.

Elements of self-disclosure

Three main elements of self-disclosure have been identified (Derlega and Grzelak, 1979) and these need to be considered when evaluating the effectiveness of this skill in professional contexts.

1. *Informativeness* This relates to the amount (total number) of disclosures made by the individual and to their depth (or intimacy). There is a relationship between psychological adjustment and self-disclosure, in that people who are not well adjusted tend to be either extremely high or low disclosers. For example, clinically depressed patients will be very reticent about imparting personal information, whereas neurotic patients generally are quite verbose in providing details of their personal affairs. The depth of self-disclosure increases as a relationship develops. During initial social encounters with strangers, disclosures tend to be fairly superficial but gradually become more intimate as a relationship grows. This underlines the importance for practitioners of developing a good relationship with patients.

2. *Appropriateness* Self-disclosures are most frequently used between people of equal status, followed by disclosures from low-status to high-status individuals. The least frequent usage is from high- to low-status, so that too much self-disclosure from professionals to patients would not be deemed appropriate (Hargie *et al.*, 1987).

3. *Accessibility* Certain individuals will be more inhibited than others at presenting personal information. This may be due to personality differences (e.g. extroverts will disclose more than introverts), upbringing (i.e. the child may be taught not to reveal too much of their business to others) or culture (some cultures encourage more disclosure than others). With embarrassing, intimate problems, practitioners may find more difficulty in accessing complete disclosure. Often patients will present a problem which is not in fact the primary problem, and health professionals need to ensure therefore that they encourage patients to disclose fully, thereby getting to the heart of their true concerns.

Influencing factors

Self-disclosure will be influenced by a range of factors pertaining to the speaker, the listener, the overall relationship, and the situation itself (for a fuller review see Hargie *et al.*, 1987).

1. *The speaker* Research findings indicate that, generally, self-disclosure increases with age although the most problematic stage seems to be that of mid-adolescence when disclosure is at a minimum. Overall, females disclose more easily and at a greater depth than males. Interestingly, first born children seem to disclose less than their siblings, a finding attributed to the possibility that with later born children parents will have developed more experience of child rearing, coupled with the fact that younger children are usually able to seek support from their older and therefore higher status brothers and sisters. As mentioned earlier, personality differences affect disclosure, as does ethnicity (so that for

example Americans tend to disclose more than comparable groups from Europe or the Middle East).

2. *The listener* As a general rule, people tend to disclose more to members of the opposite sex. However with intimate problems, patients may prefer to deal with a practitioner of the same sex. Disclosure also increases if we perceive the listener as attractive, either in respect of physical appearance, or in terms of holding similar values, beliefs, attitudes etc. We also will disclose more to people who are friendly, accepting and empathic.

3. *The relationship* Trust is a crucial factor in encouraging self-disclosure from patients, who will confide more in practitioners in whom they have developed confidence. Reciprocation of self-disclosures at a similar level is the norm in most relationships although, as already pointed out, in the professional context the patient will do most of the disclosing. However, Gallagher (1987), in reviewing the use of self-disclosure in counselling, concludes that there is a considerable body of research evidence to support the finding that counsellor self-disclosures encourage client self-disclosures. In the health context, Weiner (1980) has emphasized that appropriate practitioner self-disclosure is beneficial in fostering a positive relationship with patients. Yet, on some occasions, patients may seek advice from a professional with whom they are not acquainted. This has been likened to what is known as the 'stranger-on-the-train' phenomenon, wherein two people who meet on a long train, or plane, journey, and realize they are unlikely ever to meet again, will disclose quite intimate personal information (Thibaut and Kelley, 1959). One advantage of so doing is that there is not the likely embarrassment of interacting with that individual again, having initially disclosed a great deal of very personal information.

4. *The situation* Patients will disclose more where there is greater privacy. Thus, a doctor's surgery will be more conducive to self-disclosure than a public hospital ward or pharmacy shop floor. Moreover, 'warm' environments with potted plants, carpets, curtains and effective use of colour and lighting, promote greater self-disclosure. Furthermore, where people find themselves in a crisis situation, such as prior to surgery or following bereavement, they are also more liable to divulge their personal feelings. Finally, people who feel isolated or 'cut off' from the rest of society, for example patients in a hospital ward, tend to engage in more self-disclosure.

Functions of self-disclosure

Given the above aspects, it will be clear that self-disclosure serves a number of important functions in the health setting. These include:

1. To open conversations. (e.g. 'Hello. My name is Mary Hilton. I'm a pharmacist here at the hospital and I would like to talk to you about the medicines you are currently taking . . .');
2. To encourage reciprocation. As Archer (1979, p.47) points out, 'the most frequently demonstrated determinant of disclosure is disclosure itself';
3. To provide reassurance. Sometimes a patient may feel foolish having to discuss a particular problem. Here, a reassuring disclosure from the professional can be of great benefit;
4. To share common experiences. This is useful to demonstrate to patients that you are 'on the same wavelength', and can empathize with them;
5. To express concern for others;
6. To facilitate self-expression. It can frequently be therapeutic for patients just to be allowed to talk things through with a caring professional;
7. To develop relationships. Self-disclosure is crucial to the development of relationships since as Taylor (1979, p.122) iterates, 'self-disclosure leads to liking and liking leads to self-disclosure'.

An awareness of the skill of self-disclosure is therefore crucial for health professionals. Di Matteo and Di Nicola (1982, p.107), in reviewing the importance of practitioner self-disclosure, conclude that:

> If it is appropriate in timing, dosage and content, self-disclosure can enhance the therapeutic retationship and hence patient co-operation . . . a limited amount of practitioner self-disclosure has been found to promote clients' perceptions that the therapist is genuine . . . to increase clients' self-disclosure . . . strengthen interpersonal attraction and social influence . . . (and during first visits) increases the chances of clients returning for a second session.

Practitioners can also increase the level of self-disclosure from patients by establishing a relationship of trust, confidence, acceptance and empathy; by ensuring an attractive, professional, appearance; by providing a warm private environment in which intimate matters can be discussed freely; and by dealing with patients in a relaxed, unhurried style.

Exercise 4.3 can be utilized to introduce trainees to the concept of self-disclosure within the context of a practitioner-patient interaction. An inventory which can be used to measure the self-disclosure level of trainees is provided by Derlega and Chaikin (1975).

Exercise 4.3 Disclosure

Aim

To sensitize trainees to some of the important elements of self-disclosure.

Materials

Blank acetates and felt-tip pens.

Instructions

Divide the total class into small groups each comprising three or four trainees. Each subgroup should then generate a number of low-, medium- and high-level self-disclosure statements, some of which in each category should be health-related. Examples can be given as follows:

LOW LEVEL DISCLOSURES   – 'I have a headache'; 'My name is Phillip'.
MEDIUM LEVEL DISCLOSURES – 'I have trouble passing water'; 'I'm separated
                                                     from my husband';
HIGH LEVEL DISCLOSURES   – 'I have AIDS'; 'I've tried to commit suicide
                                                     twice'.

Having generated a range of such disclosing statements and listed these on the acetate the groups should then evaluate some of the difficulties which would be faced by patients when disclosing each health statement, of either a medium or high level, to the practitioner. Some examples can be given to stimulate trainees (e.g. The patient may find it embarrassing having to disclose 'I have trouble passing water' to a practitioner of the opposite sex). However, the onus should be put upon trainees to generate specific difficulties for each statement, and to then suggest methods whereby these difficulties might be dealt with.

Discussion

Each subgroup in turn (or a spokesperson) comes to the front of the class and presents the acetate detailing the disclosing statements. They then relate the difficulties which they have identified, and their suggested methods for coping with these difficulties. At this stage, other groups should be asked for their comments, and a general open class discussion should ensue concerning the problems presented by each self-disclosure.

4.7 OVERVIEW

This chapter has examined five skills central to effective practitioner–patient interactions. These skills, namely nonverbal communication, reinforcement, reflecting, listening and self-disclosure, are essentially responsive in nature. They are particularly useful in encouraging patients to participate fully in consultations. Together with the skills provided in the following chapter, these are the core communication skills used by health professionals. As such, they should form the basis of CST programmes. The intention of this chapter has been to provide a brief overview of the central facets of each skill, and the trainer is recommended to pursue further some of the references employed throughout the chapter.

5

Initiating skills

5.1 INTRODUCTION

This chapter extends the analysis of communication skills covered in Chapter 4, by focusing upon those areas where the practitioner generally initiates the interaction or plays a leading role in it. The initiating skills included here are questioning, explaining, opening interactions, closing interactions and assertiveness. Again, it is the purpose of this chapter to provide a summative overview of each skill, which should act as a useful *aide memoire* for the trainer to consult. While the skills are discussed in relation to health situations, the reader is strongly advised to pursue some, or all, of the references used. When taken in conjunction with the responding skills reviewed in Chapter 4, these two chapters provide a synopsis of the core interpersonal skills which have been identified to date (Hargie *et al.*, 1987).

5.2 QUESTIONING

The ability to use questions effectively would seem to be a core skill for most health professionals. Almost every text on communication in this sphere devotes a significant portion of space to this skill. It has also been the focus of a number of research investigations. One fairly obvious reason for this degree of interest is the rationale that before appropriate advice on medication can be given, the practitioner must obtain all relevant information from the patient. The most direct method of obtaining information is to ask questions, and therefore a knowledge of the nature, functions and types of question is of particular importance in facilitating accurate diagnosis.

However, given that the skill of questioning has a high face-validity, there is a danger that practitioners will rely too heavily upon, and indeed even mis-use it at the expense of effective communication with patients. In discussing this issue, for example, Dillon (1986, p.114) states that often, 'In doctor–patient interviews, the doctor is observed to speak almost nothing but questions, to ask numerous, response-constraining questions (yes/no, multiple choice), at a staccato pace with incursions into patient turns, and with an even briefer pause between the patient's answer and the doctor's next question – as little as one-tenth of a second'. A similar use of questions by nurses was reported by MacLeod Clark (1982) in her studies of nurse-patient communication.

Hargie *et al.* (1987) argue that health professionals frequently use questions to manipulate patients and maintain control of the interaction. In most social situations it is the person with high status and power who asks the questions. Thus, questions are asked by lawyers in the courtroom, by teachers in the classroom, by detectives in interrogation rooms and so on. In all of these settings clients do not ask many questions, and in fact are often discouraged from so doing. West (1983) reports similar outcomes in a study of 21 doctor-patient interactions where it was found that doctors posed over 90% of the total number of questions asked. It was further discovered that, when patients did ask questions, many of these were marked by speech disturbances indicating that they felt uncomfortable requesting information from the doctor. West (1983, p.99) therefore concludes that, 'patient-initiated questions are dispreferred in medical exchanges'. Likewise, in their analysis of doctor-patient interactions, Stimson and Webb (1975) found that patient requests were posed in the impersonal form such as, 'What can be done?' or 'Is there anything that can be done?' rather than in the personal form of 'What can you do?' or 'Is there anything you can do?' again indicating a reluctance to ask direct questions of the doctor.

These results are somewhat disconcerting, given that there would seem to be distinct positive advantages which can accrue from encouraging patient questions. Roter (1977), for example, found that an experimental group of patients who were encouraged by a health counsellor to formulate questions they would like to ask prior to consultation with their doctor, asked more questions and subsequently demonstrated higher appointment-keeping ratios, than a control group who were given no such counselling. Later results also demonstrated that the earlier in the consultation the first question was asked by the patient, the more questions they asked overall, the shorter was the time the consultation lasted and the higher was the appointment-keeping ratio (Di Matteo and Di Nicola, 1982).

Clearly, health professionals need to ask questions of their patients. Equally, however, they should also expect and encourage patients to ask questions of them. By so doing, they can develop a style of interacting which allows patients to negotiate their own needs, and become active participants in the health care process.

Definition and functions

A question can be defined simply as a request for information whether factual or otherwise. Such requests can be nonverbal and may take the form of raised eyebrows, a quizzical facial expression or the use of a high pitched vocalization ('hmmm?'). However, most requests for information are verbal, and it is this aspect which will be focused upon. Questions serve a number of important purposes for the practitioner, including the following:

1. to obtain precise information from patients
2. to open interactions (e.g. 'How are you today?')
3. to diagnose particular difficulties which patients may be experiencing
4. to focus attention upon a specific area
5. to assess patient condition and their knowledge and understanding of it
6. to maintain control of the interaction
7. to encourage maximum participation from patients
8. to demonstrate an interest in the patient
9. to help create enlightenment (e.g. 'Did you know that . . . ?')
10. to facilitate the discussion of attitudes and feelings.

Types of questions

There are a number of different types of question which have been identified. Rudyard Kipling recognized the main categorizations in the lines:

I keep six honest serving men,
(They taught me all I know);
Their names are what and why and when,
And how and where and who.

The main categories of questions are closed, open, leading and probing.

Closed questions

These are questions which restrict the respondent to a one– or two–word answer. In this way, they limit the options available to patients; in other words they *close* down the available scope for the response. There are three types of closed question:

1. *The identification question* Here the patient is expected to identify a piece of information and present this as the response, e.g. 'Where exactly is the pain now?' 'When did you first notice the swelling?' 'What type of contraceptive do you use?'
2. *The selection question* This form of closed question requires the patient to select one from two or more alternatives, and as a result is sometimes referred to as 'forced-choice'. Examples include 'Would you prefer aspirin or paracetamol?' 'Is it worse at night or in the morning?' 'Is the pain at the front or the back of your knee?'
3. *The yes/no question* In this instance the patient is simply expected to respond either 'yes' or 'no'. For example: 'Does it keep you awake at night?' 'Have you been physically sick?' 'Do you have any difficulty passing water?'

Closed questions are particularly useful in obtaining limited pieces of factual information. They are also easy for patients to answer, and can therefore assist patients who are unused to talking at length. As Hein (1973, p.34) puts it: 'Often patients with a limited vocabulary, minimal education, or lack of culturally enriching experiences are more comfortable in responding to closed questions.' However, when overused, closed questions can be counter-productive, in that they have been shown to be a powerful influence for controlling, and blocking the development of conversation (Bradley and Edinberg, 1982; MacLeod Clark, 1982). They can also be frustrating for the more articulate patient who is capable of elaboration without constant questioning.

Open questions

This type of question allows the patient much more scope in determining the response. In this sense, the answer is left *open* to patients who can therefore more easily negotiate their own needs. Open questions are broad in nature and require more than a one, or two, word answer. However, there are degrees of openness in that some open questions allow more scope than others. Morrow and Hargie (1985b) give the following examples to illustrate how a questioning sequence can gradually become more restricted:

How has your new medication affected you?
What types of problems has it caused?
What sort of pain have you had?
What is the pain like now?

Open questions tend to produce longer responses than closed questions (Hargie *et al.*, 1987), and indeed it may be a fear of patients answering at length, or giving irrelevant information, which results in practitioners relying heavily on the closed type of question. Both types of question can, of course, be useful. Where time is limited, and an urgent diagnosis required, closed questions are often appropriate, whereas if patients are being encouraged to express feelings or attitudes open questions would be more apt.

Leading questions

These are questions which, by the way they are worded, lead the patient to give a response which the professional expects to receive. There are four types of leading question:

1. *Conversational* Here the question anticipates the response which the patient would probably have given. The conversational lead is used to stimulate the flow of conversation e.g. 'Isn't this lovely weather we're having?' When they are used appropriately they have been shown to facilitate the development of rapport (Dohrenwend and Richardson, 1964).

2. *Simple* These are straightforward leads which clearly exert pressure upon the patient to acquiesce to the practitioner's viewpoint. MacLeod Clark (1984) in her study of nurse-patient interactions gives some examples of simple leads employed by nurses including: 'There, that didn't hurt, did it?' 'You're all right, aren't you?'
3. *Subtle* In this instance the question may not be immediately recognized as leading, since subtle leads use a particular wording style in order to influence patients. For example, Loftus (1975) found that when people were asked 'Do you get headaches frequently, and if so how often?', the average response was 2.2 headaches per week. However, when the word 'occasionally' was substituted for 'frequently' the average figure given was 0.7 headaches per week. A range of similar studies have confirmed how subtle changes in question wording can influence the responses obtained (Dillon, 1986).
4. *Implication* This form of leading question either requires the patient to respond as expected or accept a negative implication. Examples would include: 'I'm sure you weren't stupid enough to drink alcohol when you were taking these tablets, were you?' 'As an intelligent person I would assume you didn't have any trouble following the instructions, did you?'

The latter three types of leading question need to be used with caution since they may 'put an individual in a defensive position . . . there is a rather clear suggestion of manipulation . . . (and) . . . an increased probability that inaccurate information will be given'. (Fritz *et al.*, 1984, p.97).

Probing questions

These are follow-up questions which can be employed to encourage the patient to develop a particular theme. Probes can be open, closed or leading. The main types of probing questions are as follows:

1. Clarification. 'What exactly do you mean?' 'Could you describe it?'
2. Justification. 'What makes you think that?' 'Why do you say that?'
3. Exemplification. 'What type of pain is it?' 'When has this happened in the past?'
4. Extension. 'Go on' 'Then what happened?'
5. Accuracy. 'You definitely took one tablet every day?' 'It is only sore at night?'
6. Echo. This involves simply repeating in an inquisitive fashion the last few words uttered by the patient e.g. Patient: 'It has been very painful for the past three days.' Practitioner: 'Three days?'
7. Nonverbal. The practitioner can indicate a desire for further information by raising or lowering his eyebrows, or uttering vocalizations such as 'Oh?' These, and other forms of nonverbal behaviour, can be used as probes.

Related factors

There are other facets of questions which need to be considered. These include:

Prompting

When the patient either does not answer or gives an answer which is clearly unsatisfactory the practitioner can prompt, to encourage a more meaningful response, in one of three ways:

1. By either restating the question or rephrasing it in parallel language;
2. By rephrasing the question using simpler language;
3. By reviewing material previously covered to remind the patient of the context in which the question is being asked.

Pace

The use of pauses is important. The professional can pause after asking a question, and after receiving a response. There is evidence to suggest that by pausing in this way it is possible to increase the amount of talk-time of the respondent (Rasmuson, 1987). It also ensures that the interaction does not become like an interrogation with continual rapid-fire questioning.

Multiple questions

This involves asking two or more questions simultaneously. Walton and MacLeod Clark (1986) found that patients reported being unable to formulate a reply when asked more than a single question. Despite this, they note that nurses frequently ask multiple questions and give the following example: 'Come on, take your trousers off. How do you like your pillows? Do you want the back rest out or not?'. Such questions only serve to confuse the patient and decrease the probability of receiving accurate information (Fritz *et al.*, 1984). They should, therefore, generally be avoided.

Structuring

Where a number of questions are to be asked of a patient it is important to prepare him in advance by informing him why these questions are being asked. This allows the patient to get mentally prepared for what is to follow, as well as making him more amenable to responding (providing he accepts the reason given as valid). Another facet of structuring involves combining together all questions relating to one specific topic before progressing to a different area.

Affective questions

Numerous studies of interaction in health contexts have indicated that it tends to be essentially task-centred focusing upon physical symptoms. MacLeod Clark (1982) found that only 1.3% of all nurse-patient communication is concerned with emotional or psychosocial matters. Similar findings have been reported in studies of doctor–patient interaction (Helfer, 1970; Verby *et al.*, 1979). Indeed, Maguire (1981) suggests that a dearth of questions which are related to the affective domain is the main reason for the poor rate of detection of psychosocial problems in patients. Thus, the use of affective questions, which specifically relate to the emotions, attitudes and feelings of the respondent, should be an important aspect of focus during CST.

The skill of questioning is of vital importance for all health professionals who need to learn to identify the range of types of questions available and their likely effects upon patients. There is evidence to suggest that practitioners may become fixed in their style of interacting soon after qualifying (Maguire *et al.*, 1986). It is therefore crucial for trainees to develop an effective style of questioning prior to qualifying, and this should be an important task for trainers during CST. Exercise 5.1 can be employed by trainers to illustrate the disadvantages of closed, as opposed to open questions.

Exercise 5.1 Questioning

Aim

To highlight some of the differential effects of open, as opposed to closed, questions.

Instructions

This is a short, easily executed exercise. Inform the class that you are about to play the role of a patient presenting an illness. What they are required to do, is to ask only *closed* questions in an attempt to ascertain exactly what the illness is. Ask someone in the class to count the total number of questions employed. As 'patient' you should only answer the questions as they are asked, and should not volunteer any information beyond this. The illness can be of various types, although we have found that even a simple one such as pruritis can produce a large number of closed diagnostic questions. Repeat the exercise a second time using a different illness, but on this occasion allow class members to ask open questions.

Discussion

Evaluate the differences between the two types of questioning strategies in terms of (i) total time taken (ii) effort on the part of the practitioner and (iii) patient satisfaction. This exercise neatly illustrates some of the advantages of using open questions during patient consultations.

5.3 EXPLAINING

All health professionals have to give explanations to patients, and it is therefore important to address this aspect of practice during CST. There is firm evidence that patients value the effective communication of information by practitioners (Faulkner, 1984). At the same time, however, patients have been found to express more dissatisfaction with the explanations given by doctors than with other dimensions of medical service (Cartwright and Anderson, 1981). Yet the benefits for the patient of receiving, and comprehending, a full account of their condition are well documented (Ley, 1983). In an early review of studies examining patient compliance, Davis (1968) reached the conclusion that, although there was not complete agreement on exactly how the doctor–patient relationship affected compliance, most investigators recognized the importance of appropriate communication and explanation. In a more recent review Di Matteo and Di Nicola (1982) also demonstrated how patients who were well informed by their practitioners were more satisfied with the medical care they received; less likely to discontinue treatment; experienced less stress prior to difficult medical examinations and procedures; and seemed to actually benefit more from treatment.

Given these findings, it is somewhat disconcerting to note that information-giving to patients is not one of the strengths of many health professionals. Indeed Wallen *et al.* (1979) found that less than 1% of the total time spent on information exchange between doctors and patients was devoted to doctor explanations. In noting the consistently reported failure of doctors to provide adequate explanations to patients, Livesey (1986, p.89) takes the somewhat depressing view that, 'so frequent is this failure, that it is difficult to avoid making the conclusion that it is more by intention than by chance.' Maguire *et al.* (1986), however, attribute this failure to lack of training and assert that, 'Some young doctors do discover for themselves how best to give patients information and advice, but most remain extremely incompetent. This is presumably because they get no training as students in this important aspect of clinical practice. This deficiency should be corrected, and competence tested before qualification to practise' (p.1576).

The importance of effective information-giving to patients has also been noted in studies of speech therapists (Saunders and Caves, 1986), pharmacists (Morrow and Hargie, 1987b), physiotherapists (Dickson and Maxwell, 1985), health visitors (Crute, 1986) and nurses (MacLeod Clark, 1982). The trainer, during CST, should therefore attempt to ensure that trainees develop an awareness of, and expertise in, a range of techniques central to the effective use of the skill of explaining.

Definition

In everyday usage the verb 'to explain' has two meanings. One of these emphasizes the *intention* of the explainer ('I explained it to him but he was too stupid to understand') while the other highlights the *success* ('I explained it to him and he was able to do it'). In professional contexts it is the latter usage which is employed, and in this sense, to explain is to give understanding to another person. Thus, if the recipient does not comprehend what he has been told, we would argue that the problem has not been fully explained.

However, there are two levels of explanation:

1. Level 1. At this simple level, explaining involves giving information of a descriptive or prescriptive nature, and involves telling, describing or instructing. For example: 'I am giving you a prescription for Paracodol which you should take instead of the soluble aspirin you are taking at the minute. I'm also giving you Fybogel to keep your bowels active.'
2. Level 2. At this more complex level an explanation provides understanding in the mind of the listener, by going beyond simple description to reveal causes, make links, give reasons, demonstrate relationships etc. For example: 'You should stop taking soluble aspirin since these will upset your ulcer and cause you pain. I will give you soluble Paracodol which you can take for your headaches. These will do the same job as the aspirin but will not affect your ulcer. However, they can cause constipation, so to keep your bowels active I am also giving you Fybogel, a natural fibre medication.'

Types of explanation

Explanations can be divided into three main categories:

1. *Verbal* This type of explanation usually occurs where no aids are available and so the practitioner has to rely solely upon her verbal skills.
2. *Illustration* Here audiovisual aids are employed to facilitate explanation. This is useful where the information being conveyed is difficult to relate in purely verbal terms. Illustrations can also help to underline the most important elements in an explanation. Many products (suppositories, inhalers etc) are accompanied by illustrative diagrams and these can be employed by the professional to 'talk through' an explanation with a patient (Sause *et al.*, 1976). Alternatively, where such commercially produced aids are not available, Livesey (1986) suggests that to help explain certain types of problem for patients it is often useful for the practitioner to draw a simple diagram which can be executed very quickly. The advantage of illustrations is evidenced by the maxim: 'One picture is worth one thousand words.'
3. *Demonstration* Where the information being imparted relates to a practical activity, the use of a demonstration by the practitioner can be of particular benefit, since it has been said that 'One demonstration is worth one thousand pictures.' As Hargie *et al.* (1987) emphasize, an important

part of any demonstration should be allowing the recipient to attempt the procedure as soon as possible. This is underlined by the old Chinese proverb: 'I hear and I forget. I see and I remember. I do and I understand.'

Functions of explanations

Depending upon the context, the skill of explanation serves a number of purposes, namely, to:

1. provide information
2. simplify complexities
3. correct mistaken beliefs
4. give advice
5. aid patient compliance
6. highlight the important elements of any procedure
7. offer reassurance and reduce uncertainty
8. justify one's actions and recommendations
9. increase patient satisfaction
10. ensure patient understanding.

Features of explanation

A number of reviews of the central features of the skill of explanation have been carried out (e.g. Ley, 1982b; Brown, 1986; Hargie *et al.*, 1987), and there is general agreement about the nature of the component elements.

Planning

In some instances, the practitioner will have more opportunity to plan an explanation than in others. When planning, consideration should be given to three aspects:

1. The identification of the key elements in the problem to be explained;
2. The relationship between these elements and how they can best be linked during explanation;
3. The ability level, background knowledge, and possible reactions, of the recipient of the explanation.

Presentation

This is the crux of any explanation. How the explanation is presented will determine how successful it is. Good explanations have been likened to good bikinis in that they should both be brief, appealing, cover the essentials and the best parts should stick out! More specifically, success in explanation can be achieved through a number of techniques:

1. *Speech fluency* Messages are more easily understood when delivered in a clear, fluent style, with the use of short sentences and an avoidance of 'ums', 'ers', etc.
2. *Reducing vagueness* As Kitching (1986), in his discussion of pharmacist-patient interaction, illustrates, the ambiguity of terms such as 'plenty', 'a lot', and other similar expressions can cause confusion for patients and should therefore be avoided. In other words, the practitioner should use specific, rather than vague, expressions.
3. *Pausing* By using pauses appropriately, the professional can move at a moderate pace and thereby ensure that he does not cover too much material too quickly. Research evidence also illustrates the importance of speaker pauses in facilitating the understanding and recall of information by listeners (Rasmuson, 1987).
4. *Using appropriate language* Health professionals, like all groups of professionals, have a specialized terminology which can facilitate communication within the profession. However, the use of such 'jargon' should be avoided when dealing with patients, or if technical terms are used they should be concisely explained. Another pitfall to avoid is the use of middle class (elaborated code) language with working class (restricted code) patients. Indeed Pendleton and Bochner (1980) report that doctors offer fewer explanations to lower social class patients in the belief that they do not require, and could not comprehend, too much detailed information.

   Another danger is that of 'talking down' to patients. In their study of nurse-patient communication, Walton and MacLeod Clark (1986) found that one of the main criticisms voiced by patients was that nurses' and doctors' approach was condescending in that they were often treated like children. It should be realized, for example, that at the age of 2 years the average child has a vocabulary of over 400 words, at six years 2500 words, and by the age of 14 years this reaches 50,000 words (Kopp and Krakow, 1982). Thus, even young children, and in particular adolescents, are quite capable of understanding appropriate explanations from practitioners.
5. *Providing emphasis* Important parts of a message can be emphasized verbally and/or nonverbally. Verbal emphasis can be achieved by repetition of the important points, by using verbal cues ('This is very important . . .'; 'What you must never forget is . . .'); and by verbal foci ('First . . . Second . . .'; 'major'; 'crucial' etc). Emphasis can also be achieved nonverbally by, for example, raising or lowering the volume of voice; and by hand gestures, facial expressions, sudden body movements etc.
6. *Using examples* These relate new and unfamiliar concepts to situations with which the listener is already familiar. Livesey (1986) illustrates how the use of simple analogies, which may technically be inexact, can facilit-

ate understanding. He offers the following suggestions: 'the heart is a simple pump with one-way valves, atheromatous arteries may be likened to furred up water pipes, and brown fat stores are radiators which burn up calories and radiate heat' (p.92).

7. *Summary* It is often useful to briefly recap the main points covered, especially if an explanation has been quite lengthy. This helps listeners to assimilate and retain the information presented.

8. *Expressiveness* Hargie and Morrow (1987) report that the manner in which an explanation is delivered can influence its effectiveness. In particular, the demonstration of enthusiasm, concern, friendliness and humour by verbal and nonverbal means can make an explanation more appealing and interesting for the listener.

9. *Structuring* Explanations should follow a logical sequence, moving from the known to the unknown and from the simple to the more complex. In order to do so it is necessary to ascertain at the outset what the patient already knows or believes. Yet there is evidence that doctors rarely explore patient knowledge and beliefs (Tuckett *et al.*, 1985). Structuring also involves informing patients in advance of what is to be said, so that they can 'tune in' to the explanation.

Feedback

The definition of explaining given earlier emphasized the importance of its success, and in order to evaluate whether an explanation has been successful it is necessary to obtain feedback from the listeners. This can be achieved by the following methods:

1. Attending to the nonverbal expressions of listeners to identify signs of confusion, puzzlement or bewilderment;
2. Asking listeners if they understand. The danger here, of course, is that many patients are likely to respond in the affirmative regardless of whether they understand or not;
3. Asking specific questions designed to test comprehension. To overcome the likelihood of any embarrassment, the practitioner can take the blame for any possible failure by using expressions like: 'I don't know whether I explained that very well, can I just check ...'; 'This is quite difficult and I may have gone too quickly ...';
4. Asking patients if they have any questions;
5. Asking listeners to summarize the explanation, or complete a procedure if a practical task is involved.

It is clear that the skill of explaining is central to effective communication in health contexts. Practitioners will have to explain to patients the nature of an illness and its aetiology, the treatment being prescribed and its effects, the prognosis, and, often, what other professionals have said to them! Research has indicated that patients frequently misunderstand, or forget, information which they receive from practitioners, with potentially serious consequences for their own well-being. To overcome this problem, concerted training in explaining skills is required during CST.

In order to demonstrate to trainees some of the difficulties involved in giving explanations, a simple exercise which can be utilized is to divide the class into small groups. Give each group an index card bearing the name of a concept which they will have to explain to the rest of the class (with the proviso that they do not mention the name of the concept, or use the 'blank' technique, e.g. 'The Beatles sang "All You Need is *Blank*"' for the concept 'Love'). Concepts which can be employed here include 'Blasé'; 'Dogma'; 'Pragmatic' 'Hostile', etc. Allow each group three minutes to prepare their explanation and then take each group in turn and ask them to present their concept, while the rest of the class members try to guess what it is. When all the groups have presented their concepts, hold an open discussion on the difficulties presented by the task, and the techniques employed to facilitate explanation in the light of these difficulties. The implications of this exercise for giving explanations to patients should also be discussed.

5.4 OPENING AND CLOSING

Two important parts of any interaction are the opening and the closing stages. Research on human memory indicates that we tend to remember best what we experience first and last in any sequence (Murdock, 1962). Perhaps it is for this reason that we have developed elaborate greeting and parting rituals during social encounters. If people are more likely to remember what we do when we meet them or just before we leave them, then it follows that we should devote time and effort to these interactive phases. Indeed, it is interesting to note that even very young children are taught by their parents to be aware of the importance of 'hellos' and 'goodbyes'! In health contexts, the practitioner should therefore take cognisance of the impact which can be made at the beginning and end of encounters with patients.

Opening skills

During the first few minutes of an interaction people make judgements about one another, which can then influence how they perceive one another and how they interpret each other's behaviour (Arvey and Campion, 1984). Such judgements when made by patients can be based upon factors such as the physical appearance, dress and grooming of the practitioner, their verbal and nonverbal behaviour and the lay-out of their office. This is especially true when the professional is meeting the patient for the first time: there is truth in the maxim, 'You don't get a second chance to make a first impression'. Once a good relationship has been developed with a patient, the practitioner may be excused the occasional hurried introduction, but during initial encounters this will not be acceptable and a more relaxed, attentive and receptive style will be appreciated.

The significance of the opening segment of patient interviews has been emphasized in most texts on communication in the health professions. Heath (1986, p.25) has identified the following sequence at the beginning of doctor-patient consultations: 'Greetings are exchanged, identities checked, the patient establishes an appropriate spatial and physical orientation, and the doctor sorts out equipment and documentation, not infrequently reading the medical card'. However, Livesey (1986) argues that with many doctors little effort is devoted to this process of 'meeting, greeting and seating'. He speculates that this is because for the physician the next patient is just one of many to be interviewed, but argues that the doctor should always remember that for the patient the consultation is 'one-off', special and perhaps even anxiety-provoking. In recognizing this point, Shuy (1983) states that: 'The medical interview can be cold and frightening to a patient. If the goal of the physician is to make the patient comfortable, a bit of personal but interested and relevant chitchat, whatever the cost in precious time, is advisable. The patients are familiar with normal conversational openings that stress such chitchat. The medical interview would do well to try to move closer to a conversational framework' (p.200).

There is evidence, however, that practitioners could improve their greeting skills considerably. Studies of health visiting have shown that patients often did not know the name of their health visitor (Robinson, 1982), and complained about the lack of welcome given to them by the health visitor during visits to clinics (Field *et al.*, 1982). Similarly, Maguire and Rutter (1976) found that doctors frequently failed to introduce themselves at the beginning of interviews with patients. Furthermore, Maguire *et al.* (1986, p.1575) in a study of the consultation skills of young doctors, report that, 'Few doctors explained the purpose of the interview or the time available. They had questioned the value of this mode of beginning as students and still rejected it'. As a result, Maguire *et al.* recommend that more attention be devoted to the importance of opening skills during medical training.

In discussing the vital role of such skills during nurse-patient interactions, French (1983) proposes that the nurse should complete some or all of the following tasks at the beginning of an encounter with a patient:

1. Tell the patient what she is going to do, and what is going to happen;
2. Give reasons why any information being sought is necessary;
3. Ask if the patient has any misgivings, and answer any questions by providing a full explanation;
4. Advise the patient what he has to do and what is expected of him;
5. Check the accuracy of any information already collected, where appropriate;
6. Gain the attention and co-operation of the patient.

Hargie *et al.* (1987) provide a review of a range of techniques which can be employed to good effect at the beginning of interactions. These include:

1. *Arranging an appropriate environment* This encompasses the reception area and waiting room. If these are bleak, cold and uninviting this can have an initial off-putting effect upon patients. Likewise, the practitioner's office should be arranged in a co-operative fashion (Chapter 4, 4.2). Where possible, 'creature comforts' should also be provided, including a soft chair, a cup of tea or coffee and reasonable heating and lighting.

2. *Appropriate greeting behaviour* This may involve meeting the patient at the door, shaking hands, smiling, engaging in eye contact, the use of non-task comments (e.g. about the weather), and offering a seat.

3. *Motivating the patient* By appearing interested, concerned and attentive at the outset, the practitioner helps to motivate the patient to participate fully in the consultation. As Livesey (1986) points out, if a doctor is still making notes about a previous patient, does not look up from the notes and merely grunts a welcome, this can certainly be de-motivating for patients!

4. *Checking details* This can involve introducing oneself, checking the patient's name, stating one's function (this is especially important in the hospital where the patient may be meeting a host of different health professionals), reviewing any previous information which may have been gathered, ascertaining the expectations of the patient, outlining the objectives of the interaction and informing the patient as to what exactly is about to happen. Exercise 5.2 can be employed to demonstrate to trainees the importance of giving accurate instructions in advance of a task, and how such instructions can influence the performance of individuals.

Exercise 5.2 Giving instructions

Aim

To highlight for students the importance of advance instructions in the effective completion of a task.

Materials

Duplicate one copy of the attached 'INSTRUCTIONS TEST' sheet for each trainee.

Instructions

This exercise should be completed prior to any lecture on the skill of opening. Inform the trainees that you want to 'Wake them up' before giving your lecture.

Accordingly, you are going to administer a test which measures how quickly they can follow instructions. Give the following guidelines 'I am going to distribute this test *face down* to everyone. Do not turn it over until I tell you to do so. You will have a total of *three minutes only* to complete the test. This will be carried out under strict examination conditions, so if you finish the test quickly please remain silent. There is to be no talking for the next three minutes. (Distribute the test). Turn the sheet over. Please start ... NOW'.

Discussion

Some trainees will complete the test exactly as instructed. However, most will be fooled by the above emphasis upon time, coupled with the first instruction which emphasizes the importance of working rapidly. Discuss with the class what effect the prior instructions had upon their performance, and the implications for giving instructions to patients.

INSTRUCTIONS TEST

1. Read everything before doing anything *but work as rapidly as you can.*
2. Put your name in the upper-left-hand corner of this paper, last name first.
3. Circle the word 'paper' in sentence two.
4. Underline the words 'sentence two' in sentence three.
5. Draw a circle round the title of this test.
6. Write the name of your country *backwards* _____
7. In sentence four draw a circle round the word 'underline'.
8. Draw an 'X' in the lower right-hand corner of this paper.
9. Draw a circle round the 'X' you have just drawn.
10. Count out loud backwards from ten to one.
11. Write your date of birth in the top right-hand corner of this paper.
12. Speak out loud your first name.
13. Write down the tenth letter of the alphabet _____
14. Now that you have read the instructions carefully, do only what sentences one and two ask you to do. Ignore all other instructions.

Closing skills

As well as paying attention to how interactions are opened, professionals need to arrange a smooth, effective closure. However, this can often be more difficult, since the nature and content of a closing sequence is dependent to a large degree upon what has taken place during the inter-action. Furthermore, the practitioner cannot simply decide to terminate the interaction without the agreement of the patient, since to do so would be likely to cause resentment, pique or anger. Rather, as Heath (1986, p.150) observes in relation to doctor-patient communication, 'Bringing the consultation to an end is a progressive, step-by-step process in and through which doctor and patient co-operate and co-ordinate their actions'. On occasions this process can be difficult, particularly where what Byrne and Long (1976) refer to as the 'By the way ...' syndrome occurs, whereby a patient introduces a new, often important, problem just as the interaction is about to end. The professional is then faced with the difficult decision about whether to discuss this problem or arrange another consultation with the patient in the immediate future.

Livesey (1986), however, argues that in doctor-patient consultations physicians often terminate their interviews before the patient expects it, and that the usual manner in which this is achieved is by handing over a prescription. Livesey believes that this state of affairs is due to both the pressure under which a doctor may be working, and to the mistaken belief that what patients really want are prescriptions. He suggests that by encouraging patients to participate early on in the consultation, the 'By the way ...' phenomenon can be circumvented, and a smooth closure effected. In discussing the techniques associated with closing interactions in a skilled fashion, Hargie *et al.* (1987) identify the following central methods:

1. *The use of closure indicators and markers* In order to convey to the patient that the time is approaching when the interaction will terminate a variety of verbal and nonverbal behaviours can be employed as closure indicators. These include breaking eye contact, looking at a watch, writing a prescription, organizing papers together, orienting towards an exit, and utterances like: 'Well we've covered just about everything ...'; 'Oh dear, is that the time ...'. As Owen (1983) in discussing health visitor-patient communication, notes, these behaviours are useful since the patient needs some warning that the practitioner is about to draw the proceedings to a close. When the interaction is finally terminating, this is underlined by the use of final closure markers such as standing up, shaking hands, tearing a prescription from the pad and handing it to the patient; and making utterances such as 'Good-bye'; 'I'll call in again tomorrow'; 'Come back and see me if the pain persists', etc.

2. *Summarizing* At the end of an interaction it is often useful for the practitioner to provide a summary, reminding the patient of the main points covered. As Hein (1973, p.49) in discussing the use of summaries, remarks, they are, 'a capsule review of the content and feelings discussed during an interview ... (they) ... allow time not only for review, but also for patients to begin adjusting to the end of the interview. Just as summaries give evidence of progress, they also give evidence of the areas needing development'. In their detailed analysis of social closure, Albert and Kessler (1976) describe the summary as an 'historicing act', in that it refers to the interaction as something that has already happened, and in this way signals that the encounter is at an end.

3. *Obtaining feedback* In the Maguire *et al.* (1986) study of the consultation skills of young doctors mentioned previously, one of the identified weaknesses of this group of physicians was their failure to check that the

information they had obtained from patients was accurate and reflected key problems. One of the important closure skills is, therefore, ensuring that both parties are in agreement about what has been discussed and what decisions have been taken. This is sometimes referred to as a procedure of 'checking out'. It can be accomplished by the use of appropriate questions by the practitioner, and by inviting the patient to make comments or ask questions about anything that has been discussed.

4. *Making future links* This refers to the 'what happens next' element. It may involve a simple statement such as 'OK Mrs Rodgers, I'll call back tomorrow to see you at the same time'; or 'Take these tablets for a week and it should clear up. If not, come back and see me'. However, a patient at the pre-operative stage of surgery, for example, may require much more detailed discussion and analysis about the procedures involved and their likely effects.

5. *Motivating the patient* On occasions, it is useful for the practitioner to motivate and encourage the patient at the end of a consultation. For example, a physiotherapist may end a session by underlining for a patient the importance of following a set exercise routine, or a doctor may stress the continued benefits of not smoking to a patient who has recently given up cigarette smoking.

6. *Reinforcing the patient* The process of relationship development and maintenance can be enhanced by providing the patient with appropriate rewards at the end of an interaction. These may be task-related, as when a dentist says to a young child 'You were very brave', or a health visitor says to a mother coping with her first baby 'You are doing really well'. On the other hand they may be non-task-related reinforcers such as 'I really enjoyed talking to you'; 'Thanks for the tea. Your home-made cake was delicious'. By employing such reinforcers the practitioner can give patients a sense of achievement, as well as facilitating the development of rapport with future encounters in mind.

7. *Using non-task statements* Once the substantive business has been conducted, it is often appropriate for the professional to make some comment unrelated to the actual task itself. As Crute (1986) points out, such comments are usually about the weather, although they may relate to holidays, traffic problems etc. By taking the time to engage in such dialogue the practitioner is thereby highlighting the social, as opposed to the purely task, dimension of her relationship with the patient.

Opening and closing skills are clearly crucial to the effective delivery of health care by all practitioners. In her review of these skills, Saunders (1986, p.175) states that, 'While most people can recall the difficult openings and closings they have experienced, few can clearly and systematically analyse how the difficulties have been overcome, if indeed they have'. For this reason it is vital, during CST, for trainees to be sensitized to the importance of these two phases of any interaction, and to recognize the variety of strategies which can be implemented to ensure that opening and closing skills are effectively executed.

5.5 ASSERTIVENESS

The ability to assert oneself skilfully is crucial to effective interpersonal functioning in many situations. However, within the health professions it would seem that certain groups find this skill quite difficult to implement. Morrow and Hargie (1987a), for example, found that pharmacists rated assertion skills as the most important, yet most difficult to put into practice, especially when dealing with other professionals and with ancillary health-care workers. Likewise, McIntyre *et al.* (1984) found that nurses were quite unassertive when compared to other professional groups, but that, following an assertion training programme, they demonstrated a significant improvement. Findings such as this underline the fact that 'assertion is a *skill*, not a 'trait' that someone 'has' or 'lacks''. (Rakos, 1986, p.408).

A number of definitions of assertiveness have been proposed, and all of these emphasize the core components as comprising standing up for personal rights, respecting the rights of others, and expressing thoughts and feelings openly and honestly. However, to fully understand the meaning of this skill, it is necessary to distinguish between four main styles of responding, namely nonassertive, assertive, aggressive and indirectly-aggressive:

1. *Nonassertive style* Here the individual hesitates, speaks softly, avoids eye contact, denies his true feelings, does not express opinions, avoids contentious issues, is subservient, appeases others, accepts blame needlessly, is self-effacing and apologetic, fidgets frequently and generally lacks confidence.
2. *Assertive style* In this approach the person responds immediately, speaks in a firm yet conversational tone, expresses true feelings, maintains eye contact, gives opinions, addresses contentious issues, is self-respecting, protects the rights of both parties, seeks equality with others and generally conveys confidence.
3. *Aggressive style* This style involves interrupting others, speaking loudly and abusively, glaring at others, vehemently expressing opinions, fuelling contentious issues, seeking superiority over others, not being concerned with the rights of others, being self-opinionated and generally overbearing and intimidating.
4. *Indirectly-aggressive style* This style involves a range of behaviours such as sulking, huffing and pouting, using emotional blackmail (for example, crying in order to make someone feel guilty) and employing Machiavellian tactics to subtly manipulate others. It may also involve deflected aggression, such as banging doors, or drawers, shut.

In discussing these four styles, Hargie *et al.* (1987) give the following example of each style being used in response to someone smoking in a designated 'No Smoking' zone.

1. Not mentioning your discomfort, and hoping that someone else will confront the smoker. (Nonassertive)
2. 'Excuse me, but do you realize that this is a "no smoking" area? Cigarette smoke affects me quite badly, so I'd be grateful if you would not smoke here.' (Assertive)
3. 'Hey, you, there's no smoking allowed in this area. Either put out or get out!' (Aggressive)
4. Coughing loudly and vigorously waving a hand towards the smoker, as if to fan the smoke away. (Indirectly-aggressive)

Of these four styles, assertion is generally agreed to be the most effective in most instances. People who are either directly, or indirectly, aggressive may initially get their own way, but they will be disliked, whereas nonassertive individuals are often viewed as weak, incompetent and easily manipulated. Assertive people, on the other hand, are respected and are seen as competent, strong, fair and confident. The use of assertiveness can therefore serve a number of functions, namely to:

1. maintain and protect personal rights
2. recognize the rights of others
3. make reasonable requests
4. withstand unreasonable requests from others
5. handle unreasonable refusals
6. avoid unnecessary conflict
7. confidently, and openly, communicate one's own position.

Types of assertion

A distinction can be made between three main types of assertion.

1. *Direct assertion* This involves a short, straightforward statement in support of one's personal rights.
2. *Indirect assertion* Here the person does not actually confront the issue, but rather indirectly states his or her point of view.
3. *Complex-direct assertion* In this situation, the individual uses an embellishment to 'soften' the assertion. The main types of embellishment are: an *explanation* for being assertive; showing *empathy* towards the other person; the use of *praise*; giving an *apology* for any negative consequences; or suggesting a *compromise*.

Recently, one of the authors received a telephone call from a colleague at another institution inviting him to present a paper at a Conference, but for various reasons he did not wish to accept this invitation. Using this scenario, the three types of assertion can be exemplified in the following responses:

1. *Direct*: 'No, I can't undertake such a commitment at this time';
2. *Indirect*: 'Phew ... I've got so much on my plate at the minute; I have a deadline to meet on two books and I know I have another commitment around that time ...';
3. *Complex-direct*: (a) 'I couldn't undertake this commitment, since I am behind with the deadline for a forthcoming book, and I already have another speaking engagement in June'. (Explanation);
   (b) 'I know you have a lot on your plate organizing the Conference, but ...' (Empathy);
   (c) 'It's really nice of you to ask me and you know if I could do it for you I would ...' (Praise);
   (d) 'I'm sorry to give you more problems in organizing speakers, but ...' (Apology);
   (e) 'I can't undertake this, but I have a colleague whom I think could ...' (Compromise).

Generally, the use of complex-direct assertion is recommended, since direct assertion can seem like aggression, whereas indirect assertion can lead to further pressure to relent (Linehan and Egan, 1979). Furthermore, a number of the above embellishments can, of course, be used in combination to protect the relationship with the other person.

Assertion techniques

There are a number of techniques associated with the use of assertion.

1. *Escalating assertion* Rimm and Masters (1979) recommend that the initial assertion should be at the level of the *minimal effective response*. In other words, the person should use only the minimum amount of assertiveness which could be successful at the outset, but gradually escalate the degree of assertion as required to ensure a successful outcome. For example, a health professional dealing with a 'pushy' salesman may respond as follows:
   (a) 'No, thank you, I don't want to place an order for these'.
   (b) 'As I have already said, I *do not* wish to order any of these'.
   (c) 'Look, I am not going to discuss this any further. Please leave now'.
2. *Confrontive assertion* This is required when someone's actions do not concur with their words, and the individual is forced to confront them with this discrepancy. For example, a ward sister may say to a nurse 'You said you would bed bath Mrs Johnson before 3.30. It is now 3.45 and you still have not done so. Would you please do so immediately!'
3. *Progressive assertion* Rose and Tryon (1979) have identified three stages of assertion. These can be exemplified in relation to a situation where someone is being continually interrupted:
   (a) Description of the behaviour – 'Excuse me, that is the third time you have interrupted me'.

(b) Description, plus indication of non-compliance – 'Excuse me, that is the third time you have interrupted me. I find it very disconcerting'.

(c) Description, non-compliance, plus request for behaviour change – 'Excuse me, that is the third time you have interrupted me. I find it very disconcerting. Would you please let me finish what I was going to say'.

Rose and Tryon found that ratings of assertiveness increased as individuals progressed from simply using the first stage through to employing all three stages.

4. *I-Language assertion* Kolotkin *et al.* (1983) report findings which indicate that the use of self-reference pronouns ('I', 'me' etc.) underline the fact that a response is intended to be assertive, whereas the use of 'You' statements is associated with aggression. Compare, for example, the following statements: 'I am upset by what has happened'; 'You have upset me by what you have done'.

5. *Process factors* The way in which assertive behaviour is executed is also important. For example, this may involve arranging, or altering, the environment to make the situation more conducive to assertiveness. Thus, a community pharmacist may invite a dissatisfied patient to discuss his grievance in a private area away from the main shop floor. Likewise, a doctor may select a central seating position at a case conference, thereby increasing his ability to influence the proceedings.

Other process skills include seeking the opinion of a third person who is known to hold a similar view on any particular issue; asking for more time to consider a request; and using rewards (praise, encouragement etc.) to reduce any negative feelings engendered by assertiveness and also to help maintain, and protect the relationship. Finally, the nonverbal behaviour of the asserter is very important, and should include medium levels of eye contact, direct body orientation, upright posture, smooth use of gestures when speaking yet inconspicuous when listening and the use of smiles which serve to emphasize that a response is intended to be assertive and not aggressive.

Covert aspects of assertiveness

There are three main covert elements involved in assertiveness.

1. *Knowledge* In order to be assertive it is necessary to know *what* one's rights actually are as well as knowing *how* to protect them. Indeed, we often consult the opinions of others to ascertain whether our rights have been infringed upon (e.g. 'Has he the right to ask me to do that?'). As Porritt (1984, p.105) states 'If you have not thought about your rights as a health professional and the rights of others now is the time. Once you hold beliefs about your rights and their accompanying responsibilities you will find it easier to act in a way which expects those rights to

be upheld and also accepts the responsibility attached to any action you take'.

2. *Perceptions* People may be unassertive owing to mistaken perceptions, such as perceiving unreasonable requests as being reasonable, or perceiving a tyrant as being a 'strong boss'. Such individuals need to learn to be more accurate in judging the behaviour of others or they may be viewed as 'easy touches' who can easily be manipulated.

3. *Beliefs* Some people are submissive as a result of mistaken beliefs, such as believing that they must always do what their superiors tell them. Again, a learning process is necessary here in order to educate the individual to develop a more realistic set of beliefs.

Influencing factors

A range of factors influence the degree, nature and effectiveness of assertion. The gender of both parties is important, since it is often easier to be assertive with someone of the same sex. In the health context, it is difficult to be assertive with seriously or terminally ill patients and their relatives, with physically or mentally handicapped people and with the elderly. It is also more difficult to be assertive with close friends and with people of higher power and status. Similarly, practitioners will often find it more difficult to be assertive in the patient's home as opposed to the health clinic. There are also cultural differences, in that some cultures value this skill whereas others may emphasize values of humility, tolerance and subservience (Furnham, 1979), and this will have obvious ramifications for the professional who works in a multi-racial society.

All of the above factors are important in that they contribute to the fact that some professionals will find it relatively easy to be assertive in many situations, whereas others will find it difficult to be assertive in any. However, the skill of assertiveness is important for every health professional. As Briggs (1986), in describing a two-day course on assertion skills for nurses, points out, 'Assertion training is about improving personal, and thereby professional, effectiveness. It is concerned with the building of self-confidence and esteem, and the ability to translate this into improving communications and relationships' (p.24).

Exercise 5.3 provides details of an exercise which can be employed by the trainer to encourage trainees to develop their awareness of assertiveness, and distinguish this approach from other response styles. Gambrill and Richey (1975) provide details of an assertion inventory, which has been subsequently adapted by Kagan *et al.* (1986) for use in the training of health professionals.

5.6 OVERVIEW

The focus of this chapter has been upon the skills of questioning, explaining, opening interactions, closing interactions and assertiveness. We have termed these 'initiating skills', since they are used primarily in contexts in which the practitioner takes the lead during interaction with patients and other professionals. When taken in conjunction with the skills covered in Chapter 4, this provides a coverage of the central skills of interpersonal communication in health situations. The purpose of this chapter has been to provide a summative overview of each skill, and the trainer is advised to pursue some of the references given throughout the chapter for further information on the skills. In the following chapter we examine higher-order interactional strategies which build upon the skills covered in this chapter and in Chapter 4.

Exercise 5.3 Assertiveness

Aim

To encourage trainees to identify, and discriminate between, assertive, non-assertive, and aggressive styles of responding.

Materials

Blank acetate sheets and felt-tip pens. Two (or more) prepared acetates or hand-outs depicting a situation where assertive skills are required. One of these situations should relate to the professional situation, whereas the other can be of a more generic 'life' situation. For example (1) 'You are a nurse on ward duty. A consultant is dealing with a female patient whom you know to be sensitive and shy. He is being markedly abrupt and rude with her and you can see she is visibly upset and close to tears'. (2) You have loaned £30 to a close friend who promised to pay it back the following week. Four weeks have now passed and there has been no mention of the money at all. You do not need the money urgently, but are worried about never receiving it if you do not raise the issue'.

Instructions

Having presented the scenarios divide the class into small groups. Provide each group with blank acetates and felt-tip pens. Each group is ten requested to generate and list on the acetate, an assertive, a non-assertive and an aggressive response to each of the given statements, and to discuss the possible outcomes of each type of response.

Discussion

Each subgroup in turn, or a spokesperson, comes to the front of the class and presents the acetate detailing the three types of response. They also discuss the anticipated outcomes of each response. At this stage, a general class discussion should be encouraged, concerning the identification of response styles, and the implications of employing each style in different contexts.

6

Interactional strategies

6.1 INTRODUCTION

This chapter builds upon the preceding two chapters, in that it examines three interactional strategies, each of which is dependent upon the effective implementation of a number of the interpersonal skills covered in Chapters 4 and 5. A strategy in this sense can be regarded as a planned course of action featuring elements of various social skills which are combined and implemented in order to achieve a particular goal. Strategies are therefore situation specific. For example, in a context where a patient is worried or distressed and needs to talk through a problem, the practitioner might usefully employ a counselling strategy. Counselling is, in fact, the first strategy analysed in this chapter, the other two being interviewing and influencing. These three strategies will be reviewed in terms of their applications to the work of health professionals.

6.2 COUNSELLING

The importance of counselling as a legitimate strategy for health professionals' is increasingly being recognized (Hargie and Morrow, 1987b). Unfortunately, the term 'patient counselling' is often used to mean simply all forms of practitioner-patient interchange, or more specifically situations in which the practitioner gives advice. Indeed, the term counselling frequently has this latter meaning in everyday usage (e.g. investment counsellors). However, in relation to professional interaction, counselling should be regarded as a therapeutic process which involves:

> helping someone to explore a problem, clarify conflicting issues and discover alternative ways of dealing with it, so that they can decide what to do about it; that is, helping people to help themselves (Hopson, 1981, p.267).

As this definition illustrates, counselling is definitely not simply about giving advice. Rather, it involves developing a relationship with the patient which will eventually allow him or her to fully discuss feelings, emotions and thoughts in order to make personal decisions. In other words, patients are encouraged to mobilize their own expertise and employ their own resources in searching for a solution to their own particular problems. The counsellor does not take the role of an expert who already has the answers, but instead devotes time and effort to actually finding out exactly how the patient feels, and to attempting to understand fully the patient's situation. In this sense, the counselling strategy is altruistic in that the emphasis is upon patient 'self-empowerment' through exploring and negotiating their own needs with no overtly directive guidance from the practitioner.

As Gallagher (1987) illustrates, the development of counselling as a widely researched and well established therapeutic activity has resulted in the establishment of a range of full-time and part-time counsellors in various settings (for example, full-time student counsellors in colleges, or part-time counsellors in organizations such as Samaritans, Marriage Guidance Council etc.). Within the health domain, however, most professionals utilize counselling as a sub-role, so that the practitioner may employ this strategy as an alternative form of intervention when dealing with patients (Nurse, 1980).

There are a number of different forms of 'helping' which the practitioner can use including:

1. counselling
2. giving advice (e.g. advising a patient to stop smoking)
3. giving information (e.g. informing a patient that smoking increases the risk of coronary heart disease)
4. taking direct action (e.g. dressing a wound)
5. teaching (e.g. showing a recently diagnosed diabetic how to use a hypodermic syringe)
6. offering sympathy (e.g. following a bereavement)
7. giving reassurance (e.g. where a patient is mistakenly worried about his well-being)
8. systems change (e.g. a GP may change her appointment system to ensure she is more readily available to attend to patients in distress).

All of these are valid and valuable helping strategies and one or more of them may be effective depending upon the context. However, they all serve different purposes. Hopson (1981) has identified the main functions of counselling as being to help patients to:

1. enter into a relationship where they feel accepted and understood and are therefore prepared to talk openly about their problems

2. achieve an increased understanding of their situation
3. discuss alternative courses of action
4. make a decision about what to do
5. develop specific action plans
6. do, with support, what has to be done
7. where necessary, adjust to a situation that is unlikely to change.

It should be realized, however, that there are a range of theoretical perspectives on counselling, each with its own conceptual underpinning linked to practical implications for dealing with the counsellee (for a useful review of these see Ivey *et al.*, 1987). In this chapter it is not possible to review these differing perspectives, but rather we will present some general information central to the overall process of counselling *per se*, together with a sequential analysis of the stages involved in this strategy.

In addition to being aware of the nature of counselling, an important factor for the practitioner is knowing *when* to implement it. Inskipp *et al.* (1978) argue that counselling may be required when someone wants to make a choice, make a change or sort out confusion. Typical situations in which patients or their relatives might be in need of this form of help would include following a loss of some kind (such as bereavement or amputation of a limb) or when receiving bad news (such as terminal illness or the need for major surgery). As Stewart (1983) iterates, counselling is generally indicated when emotional factors are causing problems for the individual. It has already been pointed out in this book that practitioners are often reluctant to deal with emotional and psychosocial dimensions of patients' problems. One possible reason for this may be the lack of training given in how to handle such problems (Bernstein and Bernstein, 1980). Indeed it may be for this reason that, in one survey of family practice residents carried out in the USA, counselling was ranked as the most important subject matter available from the behavioural sciences (Shienwold *et al.*, 1979).

Counselling stages

There are four main phases involved in the counselling process, namely attending, exploring, understanding and action. In order to gain a fuller understanding of the overall process, it is useful to examine each of these stages separately.

Attending

At this stage the practitioner needs to pay careful attention to the patient by demonstrating an active listening style (see Chapter 4). In particular, the manner in which the interaction is opened will have an important bearing upon how the patient responds (Chapter 5, 5.4) If the professional conveys the impression of having the time, disposition and energy to devote to the consultation, then the patient is more likely to enter into a counselling relationship. Patients frequently open the discussion with a 'presenting' problem, and will often only reveal their real problems when encouraged to do so (Chapter 4, 4.6). It is therefore important to be aware of verbal and nonverbal signals which patients may emit to indicate a desire for a deeper level of discussion (Nelson-Jones, 1983). Furthermore, the portrayal of warmth, which involves communicating a liking for the other person and an indication of being willing to spend time with them, is crucial to the establishment of a good rapport conducive to a helping encounter. The use of verbal and nonverbal reinforcers would seem to be central to the communication of warmth (Chapter 4).

Exploring

Following the initial relationship-development phase, the next step is to attempt to gain a full and accurate understanding of the patient's situation. This necessitates allowing the patient to present his own position with as little direction as possible from the practitioner. One way this can be achieved is through the use of reflections which to a large extent permit the patient to control the flow of the discussion (Chapter 4). Where questions are used, it is generally agreed that these should be open rather than closed, thereby again placing minimum restrictions upon the respondent (Long *et al.*, 1981). A third skill which is important at the exploration stage is the use of spaced reviews. By employing this type of intermittent summary, the practitioner can ensure that both parties are in agreement about the information presented, before moving on to explore further issues.

Understanding

Before progressing to the final stage, it is imperative to ensure optimal awareness by both parties of issues, thoughts and feelings raised during the exploratory phase. The practitioner will need to demonstrate empathy, by showing that he can see the world through the eyes of the patient. Authier (1986) concludes from a review of research that the behavioural components of empathy include good eye contact, close seating distance, a forward lean, the use of touch when appropriate, concerned facial expressions, the use of reflections of feeling, self-disclosure and confrontation. The latter technique necessitates tactfully, yet firmly, drawing attention to conflicting or contradictory aspects of the patient's communications. Self-disclosure is also important. This can either be about experiences which the practitioner has had which are similar to those being described by the patient, or it can involve commenting upon how the practitioner feels about the patient's situation. The patient also needs to feel accepted and the practitioner therefore must demonstrate positive regard, which involves being non-judgemental and treating the patient with respect. In addition, there must be genuineness in that the counsellor should be without façades, and should not be simply playing a role. Rather, congruence should exist between how the counsellor feels about, and how he responds to, the counsellee (Rogers, 1951). In other words, honesty, sincerity and altruism are essential attributes for the counsellor.

Action

By this stage, the patient should have fully explored, and achieved a full understanding of, his problem and be ready to take action to alleviate his situation. The patient needs to be the decision-maker, with the practitioner acting in a supportive role. Thus, the patient should know what he wants to achieve, and the steps which have to be taken to achieve his goal. He should also be aware of those factors which will either facilitate (benefits) or hinder (barriers) goal achievement. Success in goal achievement usually occurs where the benefits clearly outweigh the barriers (Egan, 1986). Action may also include educating the patient to enable him to achieve his goal, and teaching can therefore be a final part of the counselling process. For example, a female who has had a mastectomy will need to be taught how to use appropriate cosmetic aids. However, such teaching should never preclude, or be a substitute for, counselling. A final aspect of the action stage may necessitate referring the patient elsewhere for specialist advice and guidance.

Effective counselling

While a considerable volume of research has been conducted in this field, there is no easy answer as to what exactly constitutes effective counselling. This is because success in this sphere is dependent upon a range of factors, such as the type of patient, the nature of the problem and the time available. In relation to the latter dimension, counselling may be a long process involving a series of interactions between practitioner and client, or might be satisfactorily concluded in a single encounter. One difficulty faced by many practitioners, of course, is the lack of time available to enter into a therapeutic helping relationship on a long-term basis.

However, there is evidence to indicate that many patients only require one interview in order to relieve emotional distress, and that the result of encouraging patients to ventilate their feelings and emotions is a decreased dependence upon medical services (Follette and Cummings, 1967). In the past there would seem to have been an over-emphasis upon drug treatments for emotional problems, in the form of tranquillizers, with often disastrous results. However, the need for other 'non-medical' approaches, such as counselling, is increasingly being recognized. These alternative approaches need not always be time-consuming. As Bernstein and Bernstein (1980, p.188) point out: 'The time required for counseling is unlikely to be more than that taken up by repeated medical visits. The few patients who require long-term counseling could be referred to more appropriate sources'.

Indeed, it is also recognized that some health professionals will have more time available for counselling than others. For example, health visitors may be able to devote more time to patients than would doctors. Likewise, those working in a hospice setting will regard counselling as being central to their communication repertoire with patients and their relatives. In hospitals, resident social workers can also undertake intensive counselling with patients. Another approach is for the practitioner to arrange for a specialized professional to be available if required. Hodges (1977), for instance, has described how such collaboration has worked between a psychologist and a physician sharing the same practice.

Counselling would therefore appear to be a crucial strategy for health professionals. It has been found that by recognizing, and showing a willingness to discuss, the emotional and psychosocial issues pertaining to a patient's illness, the practitioner not only improves the overall relationship but often also actually contributes to the physical well-being of the patient (Faulkner, 1984). It is hardly surprising, therefore, that Marson (1985, p.41) asserts that: 'all nurses require first level counselling skills. Those working with the dying, the chronically sick, the elderly and in psychiatry, probably need to develop more advanced skills'. We would support this viewpoint. Basic programmes of CST should aim to develop the general ability of practitioners to communicate effectively. At a more advanced level, the special problems posed by specific groups of patients can be given concerted attention.

In concluding this section it is useful to highlight the main factors which would seem to contribute to successful counselling. As Authier (1986) notes, this occurs where: the practitioner is able to participate completely in the patient's communication; fully understands how the patient feels and successfully communicates this understanding; follows the patient's line of thought; and treats the patient as an equal co-worker on a common problem.

6.3 INFLUENCING

An important dimension of the role of every health practitioner is to, at one time or another, influence patients to pursue a recommended course of action. This may occur when initially explaining, following diagnosis, what action the patient will be expected to take, or if resistance is shown and objections raised to the proposed treatment it may be necessary to employ persuasion techniques to overcome such objections (Hargie and Morrow, 1987c). In this section, we will be concerned with this type of direct inter-personal influence as a social strategy, rather than with, for example, wider mass media campaigns aimed at securing changes in health behaviour.

Raven and Haley (1982, p.427) define social influence as 'a change in the cognitions, attitudes, or behaviour of a person (target) which is attributable to the actions of another person (influencing agent)'. In attempting to influence others we can utilize a range of what Miller *et al.* (1987) refer to as 'compliance-gaining message strategies'. A knowledge of the range of influencing tactics which can be used to increase patient compliance is clearly of importance for health professionals, given the wealth of research evidence currently available to indicate that patients frequently do not follow advice about medication or changes in life-style (Brigham, 1986).

This type of social influence and persuasion is an emergent area of study within the field of psychology. A number of books have been devoted to this topic (e.g. Tedeschi, 1972; Roloff and Miller, 1980; Clark, 1984; Cialdini, 1985; Zanna *et al.*, 1987) and there has been a proliferation of research articles published in this sphere during the past decade. This interest is hardly surprising given the pervasive nature of the process of influencing, which occurs at all levels, from a child attempting to persuade his parents to buy him an expensive toy, to a doctor trying to convince a patient with a serious alcohol problem of the necessity to stop drinking. Depending upon the context of the interaction one or more tactics may be employed to obtain compliance.

Influencing tactics

A number of tactics have been identified, and the remainder of this section is devoted to an overview of those methods which have been shown to be effective in influencing others.

Power

Six types of social power which can be exerted by practitioners have been identified (Raven and Rubin, 1983). Power, in this sense, can be regarded as the potential ability of the influencing agent to gain the compliance of the target. The six bases of power available are:

1. *Expert power* Most health professionals are regarded as 'experts' by the lay population, in that they possess expertise or knowledge which others do not have. However, in terms of inter-professional communication, there is also a hierarchy of expert power so that, for example, nurses

have been shown to follow the commands of a doctor regarding medication for a patient even when these instructions violated hospital policy and were clearly and dangerously excessive (Hofling *et al.*, 1966). Expert power is underlined by three main factors. Firstly, the use of *titles* such as doctor, nurse etc. sets the professional apart from others. Secondly, the *clothing* worn by many practitioners clearly indicates that they have a specialized function. Thirdly, *trappings* can convey expertise, in the form of diplomas on the wall, large tomes on a bookshelf, stethoscope round the neck, and so on. Raven and Rubin (1983) illustrate how, in many instances, in order to maintain respect as an expert one not only has to display an impressive front, but must also carefully withold information and keep the source of one's knowledge a mystery. The use of this latter technique has obvious dangers for health professionals in terms of patient understanding of instructions (see Chapter 5).

2. *Information power* Here, the content of the message is the basis of the power. Thus, a dentist might persuade a mother to give her children fluoride drops by showing her the positive results of research studies comparing this course of action with a control group who received no fluoride drops. Another form of this type of power occurs when someone has access to information which another person either wishes to discover or does not want to be revealed. Bribery and blackmail respectively may be the result of such power!

3. *Legitimate power* In this instance, power emanates from the position occupied by the individual. In this way, a ward sister will have power over nurses, but if she retires she obviously relinquishes this power. The authority is vested in the role or position, not in the person. Interestingly, patients have legitimate power over practitioners, so that a doctor will be expected to help a distressed patient.

4. *Referent power* We can be influenced by others because we want to be accepted by them and be part of their group. One good example of this is dress, hair-style etc. among teenagers where there is often enormous pressure to conform to the current fashions. Likewise, television advertisers use famous people to sell products. Recently, this has been termed the 'Wannabe' phenomenon based upon thousands of teenage girls who wanted to be like the pop star Madonna. Practitioners can use referent power to influence patients by, for example, stating that the medication they are recommending has been very effective when used by many other 'caring mothers' (or other appropriate reference group). The process of demonstrating the acceptability of a medication or recommended course of action by referring to others has been termed 'social proof' and shown to be a highly successful technique (Cialdini, 1985).

5. *Reward power* This stems from the ability of the person to reward others if they comply with requests. A parent will have reward power over her children ('If you're good I will give you some chocolate'). A nurse

may comply with the sister's commands in order to receive a positive evaluation, and increase the chances of promotion.

6. *Coercive power* This is the converse of reward power, since it refers to the person's capacity to administer punishments. Policemen clearly have this form of power, and we are therefore likely to obey their requests to, for example, move our car from a restricted parking zone! Practitioners may wield reward and coercive power to the extent that patients are concerned about receiving positive social reinforcement from them, or are dependent on them for other rewards.

Fear

Boster and Mongeau (1984) itemize the stages involved in using fear as an influencing technique as being:

1. You are vulnerable to this particular threat;
2. If you are vulnerable, then you should take action to reduce this vulnerability;
3. To reduce this vulnerability, you must accept certain recommendations;
4. These are the recommendations you must accept.

In the health context, an example would be:

1. Having had one heart attack, your chances of having another are increased;
2. You should, therefore, take steps to avoid having a second attack;
3. There are a number of things you can do to reduce the risk;
4. You must stop smoking, take some exercise and change your diet . . .

In reviewing research into the effectiveness of fear-arousing messages, Sutton (1982, p. 323) concludes that 'increases in fear are consistently associated with increases in acceptance (intentions and behavior)'. Thus, the use of fear would seem to be a potent influencing technique. However, the success of this tactic is dependent upon three critical elements, namely (a) the magnitude and severity of the negative outcome, (b) its probability of occurring if no action is taken to avoid it, and (c) the likely availability and effectiveness of the recommended course of action (Rogers, 1984). The greater the extent to which these three factors are present, the more effective the fear message is likely to be. Equally, if any one of them is missing, then the message loses its efficacy (Boster and Mongeau, 1984).

Beck and Frankel (1981) make another important distinction between *response efficacy*, which refers to the effectiveness of the proposed response in reducing the threat, and *personal efficacy*, which is the perceived ability to carry out the response successfully. Thus, a patient may recognize the importance of giving up smoking, but may believe that it is something he personally could not do. Leventhal (1970) argues that where such a situation arises, patients may either feel hopelessness ('I'm probably going to get cancer anyway, so I might as well smoke and enjoy myself') or defensiveness ('This couldn't possibly happen to me'). Leventhal makes an important distinction between *fear control* and *danger control*. The former is concerned with the reduction of internal states and feelings of fear, whereas the latter involves coping with the environment and overtly responding in such a way as to reduce the danger which is present. To continue with the smoking example, the most effective danger control technique would be to stop smoking. However, individuals who respond primarily in terms of fear control can simply avoid negative messages about smoking, rationalize their behaviour (e.g. 'I know a man who smoked 60 cigarettes a day who lived to a ripe old age'), or as Fishbein (1982) demonstrates, smokers may convince themselves that while others may suffer as a result of smoking (general beliefs), they personally will not be adversely affected (personal beliefs). It is therefore important to ensure that patients are clearly shown, and capable of carrying out, danger control responses to overcome fear-arousing messages.

Moral appeals

Many people are susceptible to exhortations that they have a duty to carry out a particular course of action, and that if they do not fulfil their moral obligations they will feel guilty. Marwell and Schmitt (1967a; 1967b) identified the potency of *self-feeling* in either a positive ('You will feel better if you comply') or negative ('You will feel very bad about yourself if you do not comply') mode. They also illustrated the importance of *altercasting* in influencing others, either used positively ('A person with good qualities would comply') or negatively ('Only a person with bad qualities would not comply'). Another technique recognized by Marwell and Schmitt was that of *altruism*, where an appeal is made to the 'better side' of an individual (e.g. 'We are all depending upon you, please don't let us down'). A practitioner may employ moral appeals by reminding a patient that he has a duty to his wife and family, and that therefore he should take steps to modify his behaviour (e.g. to stop drinking). Interestingly, this form of moral appeal is used by insurance companies to sell life policies, with a high degree of success!

The relationship

We are more likely to be influenced by people we like, are friendly with or have a high regard for (Gergen and Gergen, 1981). For this reason, it is important for health professionals to develop and foster a positive relationship with patients. Most of the skills covered in Chapters 4 and 5 can be employed to build a conducive relationship. In particular, the skill of reinforcement can be very potent. Drachman *et al.* (1978) found that praise and compliments were effective techniques to employ when persuading others (even when the praise was clearly untrue). It would seem that the receipt of praise leads to liking for the sender, which in turn can facilitate the process of influencing (Flattery, it appears, may indeed get you every-where!). Furthermore, where the practitioner has similar attitudes and values to the patient, or has a common interest or hobby, this can also facilitate the relationship (Cialdini, 1985). Many salesmen are, in fact, trained to use this latter 'we have something in common' approach. When interacting with customers they are taught to search for clues as to the interests of the customer (e.g. golf) and use this accordingly (e.g. 'I hope the weather stays fine for the weekend so I can get a few rounds of golf . . .'). Using the patient's name is another useful strategy since, when not over-used, this can lead to positive evaluations of the practitioner (Kleinke, 1986). The attractiveness of the practitioner is important in terms of physical appearance and dress, since we are more likely to be influenced by attractive individuals (Chaikin, 1979).

Reciprocation

One way to influence other people is to use the 'trade-off' method, whereby an exchange of favours is arranged. This may take the form of *pre-giving* where the target person is 'buttered-up' by being given rewards before any requests for compliance are made (Miller *et al.*, 1987). This tactic is used by many sales companies when they give away free samples of their goods in the knowledge that this will increase their overall sales (Cialdini, 1985). Such a procedure puts pressure on an individual to reciprocate, since they tend to feel in debt to the giver. An alternative approach is to make a promise ('You do this for me now, I will do that for you later'). Practitioners can employ the reciprocation tactic by pointing out to patients the efforts they have made on their behalf, before requesting compliance with a re-commended course of action.

Logical argument

Raven and Rubin (1983) identify a number of features of arguments and the way they are delivered which tend to increase their persuasive appeal. The message conveyed should be fully comprehensible with clear conclusions being drawn and the important aspects repeated to underline them. (Chapter 5, 5.3). The advantages of the recommended course of action and disadvantages of the alternatives should be firmly stated, both at the beginning (primacy effect) and at the end (recency effect) of consultations. In terms of delivery, a reasonably fast rate of delivery (around 200 words per minute), an open posture and a 'powerful' authoritative speech style (few hesitations or expressed doubts, coupled with the use of *intensifiers* such as 'definitely', 'absolutely' etc.) increase the influencing power of an argument.

Scale of the request

Two separate approaches have been identified in terms of the scale of the initial request. The first is the 'foot-in-the-door' tactic, where a small response is required at the outset, and, if agreed to, future requests gradually increase in size. This technique has been found to be fairly successful, although if the costs of later requests are very high it may not be effective (Feldman, 1985). A doctor might use this technique by asking a patient to stop smoking for a day and gradually increasing the time span. Similarly, a physiotherapist will often ask patients to try to progressively bend a joint a little further. The second method is the 'door-in-the-face' tactic wherein a very large request is made in the knowledge that it is very likely to be refused. Then a much smaller request is made, and is likely to be successful. Thus a doctor might ask a reluctant patient if he would be willing to go into hospital for a week to undergo some tests. This request could then be scaled-down to a request to attend for only a morning as an out-patient.

Aversive stimulation

Here the target person is subjected to unpleasant experiences until he relents and agrees to a request. An everyday example of this is nagging by a spouse or child, aimed at wearing down the resistance of the target! A practitioner could obviously employ this technique with patients, but in a tactful fashion.

Scarcity value

Highlighting that an object or experience is in limited supply can influence people to seek it. Hence the appeal of 'limited editions' or 'once in a lifetime' opportunities. A parallel tactic is to indicate a time-limit on an offer (e.g. 'This sale ends on 19th January'). Thus, a patient might be encouraged to undergo an operation by being told that if she does not do so immediately it would be some considerable time before it could be arranged again.

These are the main influencing strategies which are available to health professionals. In utilizing these, it is useful to be aware of the five components involved in persuasion as identified by McGuire (1968):

1. Attention – the message must attract the attention of the target person;
2. Comprehension – the person must fully comprehend the message;
3. Yielding – the message must be accepted;

4. Retention – the person must remember the message;
5. Action – the person must implement any recommendations.

When attempting to influence and persuade patients, the practitioner should ensure that all five of the above components are adequately catered for in order to ensure a successful outcome. It should of course also be realized that numerous factors may have an effect upon patient compliance, including the illness (e.g. life-threatening or a minor irritant), the nature of the treatment (e.g. injections, oral administration, side-effects etc.), patient motivation and mental state, age, sex, race and so on. As Sutton (1982) points out, much more research is needed in this field before any firm conclusions can be reached with regard to optimum techniques which can be used to influence particular types of patients in specific contexts of practice.

6.4 FACT-FINDING INTERVIEWING

The third strategy which we will examine in this chapter is that of the fact-finding interview. There are a number of different types of interview which are carried out within health situations, and the nature and objectives of each type will vary depending upon the specific context. However, Sheppe and Stevenson (1963) have argued that all medical interviews have three general goals, namely (1) to establish a good relationship with the patient, (2) to elicit specific information from him, and (3) to observe his behaviour.

An interview can be defined as 'a specialized pattern of verbal inter-action – initiated for a specific purpose, and focused on some specific content area, with consequent elimination of extraneous material ... the role relationship of interviewer and respondent is highly specialized, its specific characteristics depending somewhat on the purpose and character of the interview' (Kahn and Cannell, 1957, p.16). The main elements of this definition have been itemized by Bernstein and Bernstein (1980) who identify four main characteristics of the medical interview:

1. It is held more for the benefit of the patient than the practitioner;
2. It has a specific purpose;
3. It is a formal interaction;
4. The interaction centres around the problems, needs or feelings of the patient.

All health professionals are involved in interviewing. For example, nurses conduct medical history interviews, hospital pharmacists interview patients to obtain drug histories and doctors carry out diagnostic interviews. It is therefore important to provide trainees with instruction in the methods and techniques of interviewing as part of CST. This is particularly important, since it would appear that to date this has been a neglected aspect of training (French, 1983).

Interview structures

A number of different types of interviewing structures have been identified (for a review of these see Richardson *et al.*, 1965). In relation to doctor-patient interviews, Gill (1973) has distinguished three main types. Firstly, the traditional short diagnostic medical interview focusing purely upon physical symptoms. Secondly, the detective type of personal interview which is much longer and deals with feelings, relationships and psychosocial dimensions of the patients well-being. Thirdly, what Gill refers to as the 'flash' type of interview which involves having a free-flowing interaction, without the doctor having any pre-conceptions, during which there is the chance that a flash of insight will occur in terms of sudden mutual understanding by doctor and patient about what has caused some of the problems faced by the patient.

Carlson (1984) has identified four types of interview structure applicable to health contexts:

1. *Nonstructured* Here the practitioner merely has a general idea of the topics and subtopics that could possibly be discussed. No exact questions are prepared in advance and there is no pre-designed order in which the interview is expected to progress. This format is quite close to the counselling strategy discussed earlier in the chapter.
2. *Moderately structured* In this type of interview, the major questions to be asked are decided upon before the interview is conducted. However, there is a degree of flexibility inherent in the interaction, in that while the questions to be asked have been worked out, these do not have to be posed in a set, pre-ordained order. Rather, they can be raised in the context of a more natural conversational style of interaction.
3. *Highly structured* Using this approach, the precise wording of all questions is decided upon in advance of the interview, and usually these are posed in a pre-determined sequential fashion. In most instances, they are written out and the practitioner reads them to the patient.
4. *Highly structured standardized interviews* In this instance not only is the exact wording and sequence of questions decided in advance, but the interviewee response options are also pre-determined. Almost all of the questions are closed, to allow a tight control of the interview. The questioning schedule for the interview really takes the form of a questionnaire to be administered orally rather than simply completed individually by the patient. French (1983) notes that an interview rather than self-completed questionnaire, is often necessary for three reasons. Firstly, while most of the points to be covered can be standardized in a closed format, there is usually a need for some degree of probing at certain points to allow for expanded information. Secondly, the practitioner may have to code answers into particular boxed categories, especially where computer analysis is to be conducted. Thirdly, the interview can

allow the practitioner to reassure and motivate the patient while at the same time clarifying any uncertainties regarding particular questions.

The interviewing structure to be employed will depend upon the goals of the interaction. If there is certain specific factual information to be obtained then the interview can be highly structured allowing the practitioner to direct and control the interaction. On the other hand, if the objective is to find out emotional as well as factual information and to gain as complete a picture as possible of the patient's situation then a less structured approach can be employed, thereby giving the patient a much higher degree of control over the content and direction of the consultation. The less structured approach also facilitates the establishment of rapport and the development of a conducive relationship.

Interview stages

There are five main stages which are of importance in interviewing:

1. *The pre-interview stage* Before the interview takes place the practitioner should take steps to ensure it will be as successful as possible. Carlson (1984) suggests a number of questions which the practitioner should ask himself at this stage: 'What is the general purpose of this interview?' 'What are my specific goals?' 'What are the ways in which I can best achieve these goals?' and 'Out of all the ways I could achieve my goals, what is the best way for the patient as well as myself to achieve these goals?' By asking questions such as these it is possible to obtain maximum benefit from the interview itself, since the practitioner will then know exactly what he wants to achieve and how best to do so. The preparatory stage also involves organizing a suitable environment for the interaction by providing as much privacy as possible, minimizing any possible interruptions or distractions (e.g. by ensuring telephone calls are intercepted if the interview is taking place in an office setting), and arranging suitable seating, ventilation and so on.

2. *The opening stage* At this juncture all the skills of meeting, greeting and seating the patient are crucial (see 'Opening' in Chapter 5, 5.4). It is essential for the practitioner to develop a good initial rapport with the patient to facilitate the exchange of information in the interview. The actual objectives of the interview should also be carefully itemized, the probable duration given, some idea of the main areas to be covered should be outlined, and the role of the patient explained. If the patient expresses concern or shows resistance at this stage there are a number of steps which can be taken. Klinzing and Klinzing (1985) recommend the following:
   (a) The purpose of the interview can be reiterated;
   (b) The benefits of co-operation should be underlined;

(c) The need to obtain the information requested should be stressed;

(d) The patient's fears should be fully identified and allayed. Where none of these tactics work, the interview may have to be postponed and, where necessary, another practitioner asked to conduct it. As Edwards and Brilhart (1981) point out, it is essential for the health professional to gain the confidence of the patient at the outset if the interview is to be successful.

3. *The information collection stage* This is the main body of the interview, during which a number of skills need to be effectively employed. The appropriate use of questions is essential to ensure active patient participation, accuracy of information received and a logical flow of conversation (Chapter 5 contains further information on questioning). The maintenance of rapport can be achieved through the apposite use of reinforcement and active listening, while in patient-centred interviews the skill of reflecting may be employed to allow the patient to influence the direction of the interaction and play a central role throughout (Chapter 4). An awareness of nonverbal communication is also crucial in terms of, firstly interpreting the cues being emitted by the patient and, secondly sending appropriate messages to the patient; likewise, techniques for encouraging maximum patient self-disclosure should be implemented (Chapter 4).

In many interviews it will be necessary for the practitioner to make notes. Where this is the case, the reasons for note-taking should be explained and the patient should be aware of what exactly is being written down. It would also seem that note-taking interchanged, rather than concurrent, with conversation is more effective in terms of remembering what has been said (Watson and Barker, 1984), as well as allowing for a more natural interchange. Gorden (1980) emphasizes the importance of providing 'transitions' which are used 'to provide specific material to act as a bridge from one topic to another' (p.356). This can serve to show the patient the relationship between the old and new topics, help to relate the new topic to the objectives of the interview, and prepare the way for a smooth change in subject matter. Transitions are therefore lead-ins to questions, which give patients time to fully assimilate the question itself.

4. *The closing stage* Drawing the interview to a satisfactory conclusion is an important skill for practitioners to master (Chapter 5, 5.4 has information on Closure). The patient should be prepared for the termination of the interview through the use of closure indicators (e.g. 'This is the final question . . . .'), and closure markers of either a verbal (e.g. 'Well, that's it . . .') or nonverbal (standing up, gathering papers together etc.) nature by the professional. Other components of the closing stage may include giving a summary of what has been covered, inviting and answering patient questions, providing rewarding statements ('You have

been very helpful'; 'I've enjoyed talking to you'), and making future links in terms of informing the patient how the information gathered will be used.

5. *The post-interview stage* After the interview the practitioner should check that all the information received has been recorded and correctly coded. At this final stage it may also be necessary to make further notes regarding the patient. As French (1983) points out, this is particularly true in the case of subjective judgements based upon the reactions of the patient throughout the interview. These activities should occur as soon as possible following the interview since a prolonged time delay may result in inaccuracy or distortion in the recording of what actually took place. By carefully checking the details of the interview at this stage it is also possible to quickly identify any material which may have been inadvertently omitted, or not fully covered, and return to the patient to obtain it.

Reducing bias

Steps should be taken to ensure the accuracy of information provided by patients. This can be achieved by attempting to reduce those factors which may bias the responses given. There is clear evidence to indicate that interviewees will often try to please interviewers by offering responses they believe are expected or socially desirable (Sudman and Bradburn, 1982). It is therefore important for practitioners not to lead patients, either directly or indirectly, to give certain types of responses. Thus, the questions asked should not be leading (Chapter 5), and the verbal and nonverbal reactions of the practitioner should be non-judgemental. Bias can be very difficult to eliminate, however, since it would seem that factors such as the age, sex, social class and race of the interviewer in comparison to the interviewee can have marked effects upon how the latter responds (Brenner, 1981). Nevertheless, all possible steps should be taken to maximize the objectivity of the interview. The language employed by the professional for example, should be appropriate to the level of the patient. For instance, Bradburn and Sudman (1980) illustrate how respondents reported having masturbated three times as often when a familiar, rather than formally correct form of wording was used for this activity. Likewise, the use of reinforcement techniques to establish a good working rapport has been found to be effective in eliminating bias in health interviews (Marquis, 1970).

Interviewing is clearly an important strategy for health professionals. As Elliot (1980), in discussing the evolving role of nurses, notes 'Among the skills needed for such an expanded role in nursing is a highly developed competence in interviewing' (p.xxiii). At the same time, this dimension of practice is perhaps one of the most difficult to master, and, in fact, Maguire (1981) found that both hospital doctors and senior medical students were deficient in this respect. Indeed, it has been argued that 'the diagnostic interview as practised by the physician is certainly one of the most complex and demanding of skilled interviewing techniques'. (Kahn and Cannell, 1957, p.258). If practitioners are to become effective interviewers it would therefore seem that time and effort will need to be devoted to this strategy during training.

6.5 OVERVIEW

This chapter has been concerned with three strategies central to the work of health professionals, namely counselling, influencing and interviewing. As with the skills covered in Chapters 4 and 5, the purpose of this chapter has been to offer a summative analysis of each strategy, and the trainer is recommended to pursue some of the references used for further information on these areas. When taken together, these three chapters provide an overview of the central skills and strategies employed by practitioners in various contexts of practice. A knowledge of the material covered in these chapters will facilitate an understanding of the overall process of CST as detailed in the remaining chapters of this text.

PART THREE

The process of communication skills training

In Part Three we turn our attention from matters of content *per se* to systematically examine the CST process. In discussing the training of professional skills, Hargie and Saunders (1983a) highlight the fact that while CST 'has been attracting growing interest in recent years, it is not a unitary concept, in that more than one alternative paradigm is available for those who may wish to implement a programme of social skills instruction' (p.151). As mentioned in Chapter 1, there are often wide variations between such programmes with regard to dimensions including the time devoted to training, the skills studied, the number of trainees participating, the use of methods such as roleplay, model videotapes, CCTV feedback, and so on. However, Hargie and Saunders identify three main stages in the instructional sequence which are essential to the effective implementation of programmes of this type. These stages are Preparation, Training and Evaluation.

At the initial preparatory stage it is necessary to identify those communication skills deemed most suitable to meet the needs of the particular group of trainees. With groups undergoing basic-level training, these will probably be the core skills outlined in the previous section. When CST forms part of continuing education and is designed to provide instruction of a more specialized nature e.g. communicating with the elderly, then more refined skills may be required. In either case, it is important for the instructor to be familiar with the general approaches and specific techniques which can be utilized to uncover the essential skill content prior to commencing CST. These issues of skill identification are dealt with in Chapter 7.

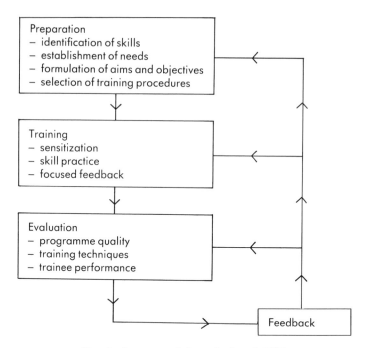

Fig. 1 A sequential analysis of CST.

The second major stage of CST is the implementation of the training programme. Here there are four main steps involved. It will be recalled from Chapter 1 that, in terms of communication competence, a distinction can be made between knowledge of communication ('knowing that'), ability to use it ('knowing how') and actually doing it (performance). This distinction is reflected in these four training steps. The first, skill analysis, involves introducing trainees to each of the skills, in turn, through the use of lectures, guided reading, etc., thereby providing background knowledge regarding components of skills, and their effects during various contexts of practice – in other words with ensuring that trainees 'know that'. The second step, skill discrimination, is concerned with illustrating the skills in operation through the use of model videotapes or other forms of demonstration, and is necessary to provide trainees with knowledge about 'how' to use the skill successfully. The overall process of skill analysis and discrimination is referred to as 'sensitization' and is fully described in Chapter 8.

The third and fourth steps of training are concerned with performance. Once trainees have learned to identify each skill, and understood its importance, the next step is to provide them with some form of practice opportunity to allow them to attempt to operationalize that knowledge. Various forms of practicals can be employed and these are reviewed in Chapter 9. Practice alone, however, is not sufficient for skill acquisition, since trainees also need to receive feedback as to the efficacy of their responses to enable them to monitor their performance and adjust it in an appropriate direction. A range of feedback methods and procedures are therefore detailed in Chapter 10.

In Chapter 1 various general approaches to training in interpersonal communication were outlined. In particular, such approaches can be divided into those which emphasize either 'thinking', 'doing' or 'feeling'. CST combines all three elements. The skill analysis step is broadly concerned with the cognitive component of skill learning, the skill discrimination and skill practice steps involve both observing and carrying out skilled performance, while at the feedback stage discussion encompasses the feelings of those involved in practicals.

The third stage of CST is that of evaluation. The instructor may wish to evaluate the outcome of training for a number of reasons. As part of student assessment, decisions may be arrived at as to competency to progress in the course, or ultimately to practice. Here there are two types of procedure which can be considered. Firstly, trainees can be assessed by direct, observational methods, perhaps dealing with patients in either real or simulated practice situations. Secondly, indirect methods can be implemented such as the use of questionnaires, written tests, essays or analyses of simulated consultations. The advantages and disadvantages of both alternatives are discussed in Chapter 11.

Evaluation exercises are sometimes conducted with the intention of reaching decisions not about those who have undergone training but about the programme itself. The overall quality of instruction can be assessed or the contribution of particular elements subjected to a more analytical scrutiny. Such feedback may take the form of formal or informal comments from trainees either immediately following CST or after a period of fieldwork at which juncture judgements about the relevance of the CST programme may more easily be made – especially in courses for pre-service trainees. Feedback can also be gauged from observation of trainees during interactions with patients, either by college tutors or fieldwork supervisors. By obtaining feedback from various sources, refinements to the CST programme are possible in order to strengthen its potential.

7

Identifying
communication skills

7.1 INTRODUCTION

The first phase of the CST process has to do with preparatory matters. This chapter addresses a key aspect of such preparation – that of identifying the most appropriate skill content to meet the needs of the particular group involved in training. Other wider issues of programme planning and design which must also be resolved as part of preparation will be taken up in Chapter 12.

The quality of practitioner-patient communication is fundamental to effective health care and the level of communicative ability of the practitioner can either help or hinder it. But what constitutes successful interpersonal communication? What distinguishes good performance from poor performance? How can skilled performance be recognized and analysed so that training programmes can be instituted to develop interpersonal competence? What are the elements of the interpersonal process which when integrated together form a co-ordinated whole, and result in the goals of each party being achieved? What are the interpersonal skills required by health-care personnel? What are the main skill deficits within these professional groups? Are there specific situations which require special skills?

This chapter is devoted to considering some of these issues and in particular to describing ways in which trainers can begin to identify key communication skills within their own professional domain and as a result design and implement appropriate training. The approach used will essentially be practical, thereby encouraging readers to reflect on, observe and undertake more extensive investigation of their own practice fields in order to establish a valid and clear picture of effective professional communication.

7.2 ESTABLISHING NEEDS

Producing a cogent learning experience can be thought of as representing a sequence of distinct stages. While there are variants on the basic theme, according to Cork (1987) most programme planning begins with what students need to learn; from this is derived the aims and objectives of training. Agreement on these matters enables the content and process of instruction to be selected. Relevant learning experiences are then contemplated and finally methods of evaluation affirmed. (The model of the CST sequence to be found in the introduction to this section is very much in accordance with this outline). Based upon a survey of literature on the topic emanating from the United States, Long (1983) also discovered that the most commonly cited first step in training provision was with determining learning needs.

It would, therefore, seem that the quest to identify the communicative content of training must begin with the recognition of a need for change. Present levels of knowledge may be regarded as inadequate, existing abilities deficient or current skills outmoded and incapable of meeting the demands now being placed upon the practitioner, or anticipated in the future. It is the realization of such states of affairs that produces the impetus for, and gives direction to, change through instruction.

But the concept of 'need', even from a curriculum design perspective, is by no means simple and unproblematic. On the contrary, it has produced considerable debate among educationalists. This has partly stemmed from imprecision in common usage thereby neglecting subtle semantic distinctions between it and similar concepts such as 'wants' and 'interests' (Jarvis, 1983).

According to Lawson (1975, p.37) we can think of 'need' in terms of 'a deficiency which can be remedied by the help of some educational process'. The recognition of this deficit often emerges from varying sources. Bradshaw (1977) termed 'felt needs' those that are experienced by the individuals concerned. Health-care workers may realize that they are poorly equipped to adequately provide the levels of care called for. This could be due to skills which have atrophied through lack of use, now being required, or the introduction of innovative techniques and therapeutic procedures necessitating new practices. Alternatively, the practitioner's role may have changed again making the acquisition of novel skills necessary.

If, however, total reliance were placed upon needs felt and expressed by learners as the sole criterion for instituting educational interventions, many who could benefit from such provision would be denied it. Some practitioners can be completely oblivious to their shortcomings. Learning needs are frequently defined by others including, for instance, administrators, professional bodies, educationalists, senior staff, etc. Indeed Armstrong (1982) draws attention to the fact that they are often 'imposed' from above in this way by postulating an ideological dimension. Nevertheless, and regardless of how they are arrived at, learning needs must be accounted for in the aims and objectives of the training intervention.

A further characteristic of 'needs' is that ultimately they reflect the uniqueness of the individual. It is highly unlikely that the requirements of any two learners will coincide entirely. The instructional implications are obvious. In this regard, Ellis and Whittington (1981) refer to clinical and curriculum approaches to skill identification and training. The former enables a tailor-made skills sequence to be derived from a focused assessment of the areas of strength and weakness of the individual trainee. 'In contrast, [the curriculum approach] produces an off-the-peg predetermined list thought appropriate for an entire group of trainees'. (Ellis and Whittington, 1981, p.49). The rationale here is, presumably, that if a general deficit has been identified amongst a particular professional group, and this sub-group belongs to that profession, then this sub-group is likely to share the deficiency and could consequently benefit from appropriate training.

CST programmes for health-care personnel are typically based on the curriculum approach although within the training process there is sufficient flexibility to cater, to some extent, for individual idiosyncracies. It is therefore unusual for an individual assessment of each prospective trainee to be conducted in accordance with some of the techniques discussed in Chapter 11; for entry into the programme to be determined on this basis; or for training to operate on a one-to-one basis. Rather CST is typically undertaken by a cohort of students in the same way as all other elements that are likely to constitute their course of study.

7.3 FORMULATING AIMS AND OBJECTIVES

Establishing learning needs is a prerequisite for deciding upon the broad aims and objectives of training. This in turn facilitates the subsequent task of arriving at the most appropriate skills to form the substantive content of the programme.

Aims are general statements of intention and purpose characteristically expressed in abstract terms (Jarvis and Gibson, 1985). With regard to CST, they should relate to the defining features of communication competence presented in Chapter 1, e.g. to promote relevant knowledge of, for instance, self, others, situations and/or interactive processes and techniques; to increase the ability to put such knowledge to use, and ultimately to improve communicative performance. Thus the aims of a programme intended for a group of occupational therapists could include:

1. To create an appreciation of the nature and process of skilled interpersonal communication;
2. To promote a knowledge and understanding of communication skills central to the practice of effective occupational therapy;

3. To develop an ability to utilize such skills in specific professional contexts;
4. To heighten a sense of critical awareness of self and others in particular situations in occupational therapy;
5. To stimulate participants to develop attitudes conducive to good communication practice in occupational therapy.

Objectives are more refined operational statements of the manner in which the preordained aims will be met. 'Educational objectives have a variety of functions. Perhaps the most important is that of guiding decisions about the selection of content together with learning experiences and of providing criteria on what to teach . . .' (Taba, 1962, p.197). A further discrimination between general and specific objectives can be made (Davies, 1976). General objectives represent an initial attempt to operationalize, in broad terms, the thinking underlying an aim. In the case of CST, they should accord with the features of skilled communication presented in Chapter 3, and include perceptual, cognitive, affective and behavioural dimensions. It is usually the latter performative component, nevertheless, which predominates in the identification of skill content and the operation of training.

By definition, general objectives are indeterminate and afford little insight into what precisely the trainee should be able to do, think, feel, etc., upon completing the programme. Specific objectives, in contrast, do permit such anticipations to be made (Davies, 1976). A list of competencies which the effective listener should be capable of demonstrating is presented by Smith (1986). From these a set of learning objectives relevant to the skill of listening, and at this level of specificity, can be deduced.

Table 7.1 Specific objectives of training in listening (based upon V. Smith, 1986)

At the end of the training programme, the group should be able to:

- attend with an open mind
- recognize main ideas
- perceive the speaker's purpose and organization of ideas and information
- recall basic ideas and details accurately
- discriminate between statements of fact and statements of opinion
- distinguish between emotional and logical arguments
- detect bias and prejudice
- recognize the speaker's attitude
- synthesize and evaluate by drawing logical inferences and conclusions
- recognize discrepancies between the speaker's verbal/nonverbal messages
- employ active listening techniques appropriately.

Such precision may be impossible however, under circumstances where it is by no means certain, at the onset, how best to achieve general objectives. In some specialized interactive contexts, for instance, little may be known initially as to how appropriate communication is effected at the practitioner-patient interface. Greater precision may have to await the identification of the skills content of training (Miles, 1987). It is to this that we now turn.

7.4 TOWARDS IDENTIFYING COMMUNICATION SKILLS

Clearly any attempt at determining social adequacy must be firmly grounded in the conceptual analysis of skilled communication outlined in Chapter 1 and extended in Chapter 3. A number of features were illuminated which have special significance for the task of identifying skills and which, therefore, merit further consideration at this juncture.

Content and consequences

Content refers to those observable aspects of behaviour which are believed to contribute to effective communication. They may be verbal or non-verbal but it is a somewhat arbitary decision whether they are significant components of skilled performance. Thus the content approach to analysing performance is limited. The consequences approach, in contrast, stresses the reactions to the behaviour by others. Here the emphasis is on eliciting positive reinforcement such that behaviour which produces such reactions is considered socially skilled. However, this perspective is also inadequate in that a nurse taking a principled, but unpopular, stand on a moral issue in contrast to her peers would be considered to be socially unskilled when in fact that would not necessarily be the case. It is therefore important to take both content and consequences into account in defining skill. As Arkowitz (1981) points out 'at a clinical level it is important to assess both what people do and the reactions which their behaviour elicits from others' (p.300).

Skills and situations

In any analysis of social skills it is important to consider the social context in which behaviour occurs, and its effect on behaviour; that is, the features of situations or social encounters which influence interpersonal communication. This is essential in that for CST to be most effective it needs to be both skill and situation specific (Argyle, 1983). Situations need to be measured, classified or analysed in some way in order to explain or predict the behaviour that occurs in them. Argyle *et al.* (1981) provide an analysis of social situations which identifies nine main components, namely goals, rules, roles, repertoire of elements, environmental setting, concepts, behavioural sequences, language and speech, and stressful or difficult situations requiring special skills (see Chapter 3). That social situations exist as regular events in society is due to the fact that they allow common needs to be met. The rules, roles, repertoire of elements and other features of situations are functional in that they make the process easier. For example, Argyle *et al.* (1981) suggested that the repertoire of elements in social situations is composed of four main units, namely verbal categories, verbal contents, nonverbal communication and bodily actions. Thus questioning as a behaviour would be considered as a verbal category or as a content free utterance whereas the question 'How has this medicine been affecting you?' could be described in content terms. Within the medical context Byrne and Long (1976), in an analysis of doctor/patient consultations produced a set of 55 categories of behaviour spanning verbal categories and content, nonverbal communication and bodily actions (Fig. 7.1).

Element	Example	
Verbal category	Questioning, encouraging, reassuring	
Verbal content	'How are you today.'	(questioning)
	'You've recovered remarkably well.'	(encouraging)
	'Everything is coming along nicely.'	(reassuring)
Nonverbal communication	Indicators of listening: eye contact, head nods, paralanguage etc.	
Bodily actions	Symbolic terminations: tearing off prescription form from pad; practitioner rising from seat and conducting patient to door.	

Fig. 7.1 Repertoire of elements in social situations.

Thus the characterization of the components of situations will be an important aspect of the identification of social skill in the health-care context. Moreover, it means that generalizations will tend to be avoided, recognizing that individuals may be skilled in some situations but not in others. Consequently, it demands that communication skill trainers be specific in their diagnosis of skill deficit, allied to the specification of which skill in which situation is most in need of training (Furnham, 1983b).

Single and sequenced behaviour

Discussion of the components of social situations prompts the question in the analysis of social performance should actions be assessed in terms of frequency of single elements of behaviour or as co-ordinated behavioural sequences? Similarly, how appropriate was the action within the actual context of the interaction? Measurement of the frequency of specific actions may lead to a misleading appreciation of a social encounter. Using a simple frequency criterion, an individual may be considered socially skilled because of his ability to initiate a large number of questions in rapid succession, yet the flow and expression of the questions within the context of the interaction may have produced a feeling of interrogation in the other person.

Arkowitz (1981) also pointed out that in measuring social skill, frequency counts of behaviour imply that it is better to have more of a 'good' behaviour (e.g. eye contact) and less of a 'bad' behaviour (e.g. speech disfluency). Yet an individual in any encounter who stared continually but spoke fluently may be considered less skilful than another person who gave less eye contact and an average amount of speech disruption. Thus, in identifying skilled behaviour there may well be a balance to be struck in assessing particular aspects of performance in that there may be optimal levels of certain behaviours in particular situations which simple analysis of frequency counts does not take into consideration.

With regard to the sequencing of behaviour it will be recalled Argyle *et al.* (1981) suggested that social encounters usually follow a five-episode behavioural sequence structure, (a) greeting, (b) establishing the relationship and clarifying goals, (c) the task, (d) re-establishing the relationship and, (e) parting. In their analysis of 2500 doctor/patient consultations Byrne and Long (1976) have presented a six-episode behavioural sequence to characterize the consultation as follows:

(a) relating to the patient
(b) discussing the reason for the patient's attendance
(c) conducting a verbal or physical examination or both
(d) considering the patient's condition
(e) detailing treatment or further investigation
(f) terminating.

Such a sequence may not, of course, always follow all of these steps in a fixed or set order. For example, the reason for the patient's attendance at surgery may be a follow-up to a previous visit such that part of the consultation is implicity known by both parties. However, the classification of behaviours into a progressive sequence is not only important but instructive in demonstrating how effective social interactions can be viewed as a series of appropriate, integrated and co-ordinated verbal and nonverbal actions intelligently carried out, with the purpose of achieving particular goals.

Overt and covert behaviours

In the examination of communication skill the focus of attention has tended to be on behaviours which are openly displayed. If the exclusive emphasis is placed on behavioural output, however, there may be a consequent neglect of the perceptual and cognitive processes involved. As described in the model of communication (Chapter 3) our cognitions and perceptions of social situations are crucially important in that behaviour will be influenced by our knowledge of social norms, our knowledge and understanding of response cues, our attention within any interaction, our ability to process information and predict and evaluate the consequences of particular types of behaviour.

Against this background it is therefore possible to classify unskilled behaviour as either due to a genuine behavioural deficit or rather to a misperception and misunderstanding of the situation. Indeed, if someone cannot 'read' a situation accurately then he or she will not be able to perform skilfully regardless of their behavioural repertoire. Thus in analysing practitioner/patient interactions it may well be valuable to try to identify why particular behaviours occur in order to ascertain the specific cognitive or perceptual processes which mediate them. Equally it may be important to examine with trainees particular mental frameworks that are likely to produce inappropriate behaviours (Exercise 7.1). As Kagan *et al.* (1986) have stated: 'It is important for us to bear in mind some of the sources of bias in person perception, and what our own tendencies to be consistent and/or to generalize are, if we are to begin to be able to make realistic observations, assessments and appraisals of our own interpersonal behaviour.' (p.81)

Exercise 7.1 Person perception

Instructions

Show a picture of an individual to a group of trainees. Then ask the following questions and compare the responses.

- How would you describe the person in terms of age, personality, occupation, marital status, interests, beliefs, values and attitudes?
- On what basis did you make these judgements?

For discussion

Did the conclusions reached concur? Why/why not?

- How does this exercise translate to the practice situation?
- Is it possible to identify any mental frameworks we have adopted?
- What actions do we need to take in order to achieve accurate and objective social perception?

Personal characteristics

A number of personal factors have a bearing on skilled performance. For example, the strategies that extroverts may use successfully in interpersonal interactions may not be effective for the introvert and vice versa. This has implications for communication skills training in that 'modelling the master' technique assumes that what will work for one individual will work for another.

Arkowitz (1981) highlighted physical appearance as an important element moderating social skill. Reference has already been made to this aspect of nonverbal communication and in particular to the ways in which appearance can be manipulated to enhance effectiveness in a given situation (Chapter 4).

Gender and age are two further personal elements which affect the interpersonal process. We tend to respond differently and have different expectations about the way others behave depending upon whether they are male or female and also depending on their age (Hargie and Marshall, 1986).

7.5 APPROACHES TO SOCIAL SKILL IDENTIFICATION

Over the last ten years there has been a more concentrated focus within the health professions on the communicative ability of practitioners. This has prompted a closer examination of what actually happens at the practitioner-patient interface, not only as it relates to the clinical elements of the interaction but also the communication behaviour of all those involved. The one is concerned with communication as a product, while the other emphasizes the process elements of interpersonal interaction.

In essence, the approaches to social skill identification fall into two main sections, namely, the trainer either identifies the skills by reflection or by observation. However, Ellis and Whittington (1981) have proposed three styles of approach namely the empirical, the analytical and the intuitive.

The empirical approach

This can be thought of as the traditional scientific method in that here skill identification involves systematic observation, recording, categorization and analysis of interpersonal interactions. It also involves experimentation to determine the relative importance of skill components and after training, measurement of outcomes. Obviously, one of the difficulties within such an approach is the establishment of a framework wherein objective analysis can be carried out. Indeed as has been previously iterated our perceptions of social interaction are coloured, at least in part, by our cognitive framework, such that in reality empirical analysis is more likely to be carried out within traditionally accepted skill categories which have been determined by reflection rather than observation! Thus, as Ellis and Whittington (1981) point out 'the pure application of the empirical paradigm has been tempered not only by pragmatism but by the logical necessity for pre-empirical analysis and theorising.' (p.29)

The analytical approach

This can be described as the theoretical approach to social skill identification. In essence it demands no observation or measurement but is the result of deductive processes based on the objectives of interpersonal communication. Thus, it may be considered that effective patient communication in the nursing context is to promote trust, confidence, and encourage patients to fully disclose their needs and problems. From this, rational discourse may produce a number of skill concepts, e.g. questioning, listening, empathy, which would be important elements to address within a skills training programme. Although this method is not considered ideal for social skill identification often the lack of empirical evidence has prompted its use.

The intuitive approach

This is very much the experiential approach, i.e. 'I've been in the situation and I found . . .'. It is therefore reflective in style and to some extent inductive in that as experiences are collated, possibly shared and discussed, it is possible to build up a picture of what are generic key skills and also what situations demand special skills. Moreover the results of the intuitive approach are often confirmed by empirical analysis. In the skill identification process there is therefore justification in using each of these methods depending on the facilities, time and personnel available. Indeed it is possible to produce useful lists of skills without necessarily undertaking empirical observation and analysis.

This is perhaps well illustrated with reference to the dental profession. Relatively little has been done by way of communication skill training for dentists particularly in the UK. However, some attempts have been made to identify the needs of dentists in relation to CST. The process of skill identification has been largely based on analytical and intuitive paradigms. Furnham (1983a) suggested that there are two different types of patient who have quite different attitudes to, and expectations of, their dentist and who by inference require different approaches in respect of interpersonal consultations. On the one hand there is the 'preventive' patient who is normally of high socio-economic status, is knowledgeable about dental health matters, has confidence in his dentist and is looking for professional dental skills and accompanying social skills. On the other hand there is the 'restorative' patient. These patients are usually of low socio-economic status, poorly informed about dental health, are poorly motivated as regards dental health and have negative attitudes to the dentist. During the consultation they seek primarily friendliness, reassurance and sympathy rather than professional dental skills.

Jackson and Katz (1983) presented a list of skills that need to be taught to, and mastered by, dental students prior to qualification. These fall into four main categories, namely giving patient attention, accepting and not judging the patient, reducing patient anxiety and presenting patient information. The authors suggest a number of behavioural patterns that need to be adopted to achieve the above objectives, e.g. reduction of anxiety may be effected by giving patients a source of control, i.e. hand raising, keeping the patient updated in what he/she will experience in the course of the treatment, talking at an even, relaxed pace and moving slowly and deliberately, keeping hands in sight.

7.6 METHODOLOGIES FOR COMMUNICATION SKILL IDENTIFICATION

Arising out of the three paradigms discussed above are a number of more specific investigative methodologies which can be employed to identify skills. These are outlined below together with a description of specific research initiatives that have been conducted within several health professional groups.

Task analysis

This is essentially a competence-based observational strategy designed to identify what the practitioner does. It involves a researcher literally following the practitioner around for a period of time and carefully noting what is being done. It therefore provides a detailed description of what actually constitutes, for example, nursing, medical or pharmaceutical practice. Obviously it would normally go beyond the interpersonal dimensions of practice but could be geared more specifically to the whole gamut of communicative behaviour. While this appears an attractive approach it suffers from the major disadvantage that it refers only to functional tasks and not to the level of skill with which people perform them. Thus task analysis items might specify 'interviews patients' 'advises on medicine administration', yet there is no indication of what is involved in these tasks or indeed what is required to perform these activities effectively. As Dunn and Hamilton (1984) state 'it tells what is done but gives no indication of how it is done' (p.138). Another disadvantage of this method is that it is likely to produce a long list of activities without any indication of their relative importance within the practice domain. On its own therefore its value in communicate skills determination is rather limited.

The Delphi technique

This technique utilizes a panel of experts or 'wise men' and is a useful and successful method of obtaining answers to questions which are issues of uncertainty, particularly professional behaviour/competence. It is regarded as a systematic procedure aimed at arriving at a reasoned concensus. This strategy involves the following main elements:

Selection of experts

This is critical to the technique since it is essential to attempt to bring together a panel of individuals who are most likely to have the relevant knowledge and experience concerning the objectives to be met. It should be recognized however that as far as social skill identification in a particular profession is concerned there may be no 'experts' in that field simply because the knowledge and experience of reputable individuals may be, and in many cases are, rooted in the cognitive and technical skills inherent in the profession and not in its social skills. Rapport (1983) has discussed the choice of experts and concluded that it is 'usually made on the basis of what may vaguely be called their reputations'. (p.164)

Formulation of competencies

Having selected a group of experts it is necessary to ask them firstly to define or formulate the general areas of knowledge, skills and attitudes necessary for effective interpersonal communication in the professional setting and secondly, to identify the specific competencies within this area. This is carried out individually and anonymously by postal survey of the panel of experts and therefore eliminates committee activity and also avoids the psychological influences of face-to-face debate.

Compilation of expert opinions

From the data generated by the group of experts the researcher is responsible for collating the information into a single composite document. All the information included in the returned lists should be included even if only one expert has entered a particular competency. Where specific competencies have not received unanimous support they should be marked with an asterisk.

Revision of opinions

Here the competencies compiled should be sent to all the experts with instructions to refer only to those asterisked and state briefly why in their opinion each of these competencies should be included or excluded in the final list. In addition, any new estimates of competency should be stated. Again the revised responses of the panel would be returned in confidence to the researcher for compilation. This process of listing, distributing, replying and collating competencies should be repeated until a consensus is reached and a final list of competencies drawn up based upon the additions and deletions.

Evaluation of competencies

The final list of competencies should be returned to the experts and again each of them individually asked to score on a five point scale how important each one is within the practice situation. The ratings should then be analysed and the results obtained indicate the principal competencies that a practitioner should possess in order to practise effectively. From this basis training strategies could be formulated to produce the competencies delineated.

These are the main elements of the Delphi technique which is characterized by its anonymity, independent participation with controlled feedback and statistical grouped response. For further information on this technique the reader is referred to the work of Linstone and Turoff (1975).

Critical incident survey

This technique is a more sophisticated method of collating behavioural data about the ingredients of skilled performance in the actual practice context. Here practitioners would be asked to reflect on incidents that they have been personally involved in or have observed, which reflected good or poor performance. Exercise 7.2 is a suggested schema for recording details of such incidents.

Exercise 7.2 Identification of critical incidents in practice

Instructions

Each practitioner should think of an incident or incidents in practice where poor/good interpersonal communication was apparent. The incident should be described below. The following questions serve to aid a full description of the event.

- Where did the event take place?
- Who were the individuals involved?
- What features of the individuals involved were important in the interaction e.g. deafness, emotionally upset etc?

- What actually occurred in the interaction?
- What was the outcome?
- Why was the interaction considered to be effective/ineffective?
- Finally, consider the implications of this incident to interpersonal communication performance.

Figure 7.2 illustrates a critical incident described by a pharmacist during a CST course. It should be remembered that such a technique is not designed to identify incompetent practitioners. Rather, the emphasis is on the incident as apposed to the individual. As the number of incidents reported increases it should be possible to perform some content analysis on them in order to cluster the information and thus predict essential areas of competence.

Pharmacist	A lady came into my pharmacy and complained that she had received the wrong tablets. As she was obviously quite concerned and upset I brought her into my dispensary to deal with the matter. In fact she hadn't received the wrong tablets but had, in accordance with her GP's prescription, been dispensed a generic form of her medicine which was coloured differently from the proprietary brand she normally received. I explained to her that although the tablets were coloured differently they still contained the same drug. However, she did not understand this. At the same time a local council worker was removing some empty cartons from my pharmacy and overheard the conversation. He politely interrupted and spoke to my patient – 'Mrs, if you go down the street to Coulter's garage you'll see five new Ford Escorts in the showroom. They are different colours but they are still Escorts. Your tablets are just the same.' My patient understood the analogy perfectly and left the pharmacy satisfied that she had received the correct medication. I thought 'Why couldn't I have used an illustration like that.'

Fig. 7.2 A critical incident report.

Within the pharmaceutical discipline Morrow and Hargie (1987b) have used a modified form of critical incident survey involving both empirical and intuitive paradigms to investigate the critical incidents in interpersonal communication in pharmacy practice. More specifically the study was undertaken firstly, to generate from pharmacists a comprehensive itemization of the interpersonal difficulties in the practice situation; secondly, to discriminate and conceptualize these difficulties into discrete categories; and thirdly, to investigate from the pharmacists' perspective the nature of the central interpersonal problems which they encountered. Exercise 7.3 is an adaption of the self-reported methodology used by these workers.

Exercise 7.3 Identification of factors influencing practitioner-patient interactions

Instructions

The trainer should prepare worksheets based on each of the three headings below. Each worksheet should be divided into two columns, one to chart the types of difficulties encountered and the other to list the actual communication problems that these difficulties pose. Each practitioner should complete an individual inventory and the pooled responses can then be collated, analysed and subjected to further peer review if required.

Types of 'problem' patients

Identify as many types of 'problem' patients as you can, e.g. the aggressive patient.

Identify the central communication difficulties that these people present, e.g. difficulty in reasoning with patient.

Types of patients' difficult problems

Identify as many types as you can and give two or three examples to illustrate types e.g. embarrassing problems: impotence, stammering, psoriasis.

Identify the central communication difficulties that these problems present, e.g. establishing a common language of understanding.

Miscellaneous factors

Identify as many factors as you can relating to the nature of the practitioner e.g. personality, attitude etc.

Identify any factors other than the above which may influence practitioner communication, e.g. environment.

Show how the factors identified opposite can influence the communication process, e.g. the shy practitioner finds difficulty in interacting with clients, or privacy may allow a patient to express his/her problem more freely.

From the data collected it was possible to undertake a qualitative analysis of pharmacist-patient interactions. A total of twenty-five different types of 'problem' patient who present communication difficulties for the pharmacist were reported. These included drug addicts, confused patients, handicapped people and illiterate individuals, among others. A closer examination of patient problems revealed that embarrassing, emotional/psychological and handicap situations together with terminal illness and financial problems appear to offer substantial challenge to the pharmacist in terms of satisfactory communication.

A content analysis of the actual communication difficulties suggested that these fell within four broad but overlapping categories, namely, nonverbal communication difficulties (e.g. interpreting nonverbal behaviour, establishing and maintaining eye contact, using sign language); difficulties in gathering and giving factual information (e.g. questioning, explaining, listening, providing reassurance); evaluative difficulties (e.g. recognition of patients' needs, assessment of patient understanding); and miscellaneous difficulties including ethical conflicts, diplomacy, alleviating embarrassment and imparting confidence.

Finally, a number of other factors which influence pharmacist interactions were identified including 23 features of the pharmacist (e.g. age, gender, integrity, friendliness, accessibility), 11 features of the practice environment (e.g. decor, layout, privacy, lighting) and 7 miscellaneous factors (e.g. time availability, lack of training in interpersonal communication, the prescription form).

Thus this investigation represented a first step in beginning to identify and analyse what actually happens at the pharmacist-patient interface allied to the highlighting of generic skills relevant to the pharmacy context, i.e. questioning, explaining, and also of the individual situations where special skills will be required for a successful outcome.

The main disadvantage of this approach is that the analysis of the data into distinct clusters tends to be somewhat subjective. However, this can be overcome by subjecting the analysis to a group of practitioners to test its appropriateness as a behavioural model of the work situation.

In our work with health visitors these practitioners have cited a wide range of difficult practice situations that pose substantial communication problems. Such situations have included, for example, marital disharmony, terminal illness, bereavement, the deaf patient, the stroke patient and the aggressive individual. The communication difficulties encountered in such situations were varied but the central difficulties focused firstly, on the problem of obtaining information from those patients who were unable to communicate effectively because of their illness/handicap; secondly, the difficulties of being able to persuade patients to change behaviours; and thirdly the difficulty of establishing and maintaining relationships with patients and helping them work through their problems. In terms of the actual skills required to communicate effectively in these situations explaining and counselling skills predominated.

Behavioural event interview

The behavioural event interview is an adaption of the critical incident survey. In this approach a number of practitioners in a given health profession are identified as being 'good' practitioners as judged by their peers. They are then interviewed in depth and asked to describe in detail some of the most critical interpersonal situations they have faced in practice. The interview should cover questions such as: 'What led up to the event?' 'Who were the individuals involved?' 'What was the purpose of the interaction?' 'What actions did you/the patient take?' 'What motivated your actions?' 'What were the outcomes for the parties involved?' 'How satisfied were the individuals concerned with the consultation?' Here the interest is focused on the goals of the individuals, the practitioner's perception of the event and the people involved, their thoughts, feelings and actions and the overall outcome, including any follow-up or future associated contact.

Following the interviews the practitioner should be asked what he/she thinks are the most important interpersonal skills required of a competent person engaged in that profession. One of the benefits of this approach is that it tends to highlight a wide variety of important and relevant situations which can be used for practical learning in the training situation by way of simulation exercises or case studies.

The second step involves repeating this exercise with a similar number of practitioners who are regarded as average performers. The final step involves an analytical treatment of the material generated through the behavioural event interviews in order to distinguish those competencies which are present, or absent in the interview records of good, as opposed to average practitioners. Because of the complexity of the task skilled analysts are needed (Spencer, 1979). However, the results should produce a detailed or specific 'behavioural code book' of interpersonal communication in the professional setting, thereby describing the competencies that predict performance.

Constitutive ethnography

This method, broadly defined, utilizes an empirical paradigm to identify and analyse the actual processes involved in interpersonal communication. It involves capturing a range of consultative events on video. Through subsequent rigorous analysis and description, salient patterns and regularities in the interactional behaviour of participants are revealed. In this way, tacit knowledge is illuminated which professionals possess but which they may not be able to articulate.

It is therefore possible to identify, for example, sequences in behaviour such as (a) asking a question; (b) clarifying the question if the response is inadequate; (c) prompting; (d) probing for further information, etc. It is also possible to begin to identify useful strategies for patient consultations which make the interaction more effective and more satisfying for the participants. Moreover, the importance of the nonverbal elements of behaviour can be determined and specific cues which moderate, control and facilitate interactions can be elicited, thereby giving direction to the elements of skilled performance which need to be developed or trained. Overall then the ethnographic technique, in relation to CST, is directed to analysing and identifying aspects of interpersonal behaviour which occur in social interactions in order to chart those skills and strategies which go to producing skilled performance.

Saunders and Caves (1986) have used some of the characteristics of the constitutive ethnographic approach to chart the communication processes within the speech therapy discipline. Here speech therapists were video-taped during actual patient consultations, with the recorded sequences sub-sequently subjected to peer analysis. Twelve therapists were involved in the study and the modal number of patients/children filmed was four per therapist. With adult patients the therapy sessions lasted from 45 minutes to one hour, with the children's sessions lasting from 20–40 minutes in length. (The reader is directed to this study for specific details of the analysis procedure).

The analysis yielded a detailed category system of behaviours exemplified by speech therapists during consultations together with the number of instances when these behaviours occurred. The categories delineated were presented either in terms of the function of the behaviour or as a more fine-grained analysis of the types of behaviour subsumed under a global category. (Fig. 7.3)

Furthermore, the analysis revealed firstly, the importance of using skills appropriate to the particular context of interaction. This was particularly

Global category	Sub-category	
Use of eye contact/ facial expression	To regulate the flow of interaction To maintain and demonstrate interest Modelling appropriate eye contact to monitor the patient's speech Maintaining eye contact to avoid underlining the patient's disability	Functional
Counselling – where patient shows stress of frustration	Methods of stress alleviation	Functional
	Pause in therapy task Humorous or light comment Instruction to relax Alerting to possible difficulties Explanation of reasons for difficulty	Methodological

Fig. 7.3 Examples of categories of behaviour in speech therapist-patient interactions.

true in the use of the generic skill of questioning in the process of encouraging patients to self-monitor their own speech patterns. Here the importance of asking specific kinds of open questions was highlighted allied to the actual timing of the questions. Secondly, the investigation indicated how one professional group can use a skill in a highly differentiated way. Speech therapists used some fifteen different types of cue in order to encourage patient participation in the therapy as well as using cueing techniques frequently during sessions. Similarly, positive reinforcement techniques were used widely to provide support, give praise and otherwise encourage patients during the treatment programme.

Variations of the ethnographic technique have also been applied to other health disciplines. For example, the work of Byrne and Long (1976) into doctor-patient communication still represents the most systematic, rigorous and extensive study of interpersonal verbal communication within the health field. The study represented 3½ years of recording and interaction analysis of almost 2500 audiotaped doctor-patient consultations from the United Kingdom, Holland and Ireland.

From the analysis of the recordings these workers identified 55 categories of behaviour which occurred consistently during phases of the consultation. These included, for example, giving recognition, apologising, reassuring, summarizing, and symbolic termination. Moreover, they identified consultation styles by clusters of scores in these 55 categories in specific phases of the consultation. They described doctors' styles along a doctor-centred to patient-centred range, and identified four diagnostic styles made up of a series of skills and seven prescriptive styles along the same continuum. (Fig. 7.4)

Byrne and Long also identified a number of negative behaviours exhibited by doctors, namely, rejecting patient offers, reinforcing self-position, denying patient, refusing patient ideas, evading patient questions, not listening, refusing to respond to feeling and simultaneous talking. Furthermore, Maguire (1984a) has drawn attention to the fact that within the medical discipline there is reluctance to cover more personal issues during the consultation, and to control the consultation by closed, rapid-fire questioning. This is reflected in the fact that doctors appear especially reluctant to cover the psychosocial aspects of illness as borne out by patient satisfaction studies, which show that such patients feel actively discouraged to disclose this type of difficulty (Maguire *et al.*, 1980b; Cartwright *et al.*, 1973). In addition Plat and McMath (1979) demonstrated key deficits in the communication performance of doctors during patient interviews, namely inadequate greetings and explanations, lack of understanding, support and reassurance, disinterest in patients' well-being and eagerness to close consultations thereby missing key leads. More recently, in a study of young doctors who had previously received CST, Maguire *et al.* (1986) demonstrated their lack of ability to give information and advice to patients.

Use of patient's knowledge and experience ... **Use of doctor's knowledge and skill**

	Clarifying and Interpretation	Analysing and Probing	Gathering information
Silence	Broad question	Direct question	Direct question
Listening Reflecting	Clarifying	Correlational question	Closed question
	Challenging	Placing events	Correlational question
Offering observation	Repeating for affirmation	Repeating for affirmation	Placing events
Encouraging	Seeking patient ideas	Suggesting	Summarizing to close off
Clarifying	Offering observation	Offering feeling	Suggesting
Reflecting	Concealed question	Exploring	Self-answering questions
Bringing patient ideas	Placing events	Broad question	Reassuring
Seeking patient ideas	Summarizing to open up		Repeating for affirmation
Indicating understanding			Justifying self-chastizing
Using silence			

Use of patient's knowledge and experience ... **Use of doctor's knowledge and skill**

Doctor permits patients to make decision	Doctor defines the limits and requests the patients to make decision	Doctor presents problem. Seeks suggestions and makes decisions	Doctor presents tentative decision subject to change	Doctor sells his decision to the patient	Doctor makes decision and announces it	Doctor makes decision and instructs patient

Fig. 7.4 Doctors' diagnostic styles (after Byrne and Long, 1976).

MacLeod Clark (1981, 1982) in analyses of audio- and videotaped nurse-patient interactions in surgical wards showed that trained nurses spent on average 1.43 minutes in these conversations. Furthermore, a content analysis of the conversation indicated that 75% of the verbal communication was concerned with some aspect of the treatment of care, 16.5% was related to 'intake and output' (ingestion and excretion), 5.5% to social chit-chat and 1.3% to emotional/psychosocial matters. Nursing behaviour was also observed to be positive or negative, i.e. nurses either employed techniques to encourage or reinforce conversations or techniques to block the development of conversations. Thus, asking closed or leading questions effectively controlled the interaction, while the avoidance or refusal to accept certain cues meant that professional 'distance' was maintained. In essence this research began to identify good communicative behaviour as opposed to poor communicative behaviour in so far as one encouraged trust, self-disclosure and contributed to allowing patients to negotiate their own needs, while the other actively discouraged 'in depth' communication.

From an analysis of recordings of nurse-patient interactions, Maguire (1985) suggested that the deficiencies in skilled interpersonal performance among nurses fall into four main categories namely, poor problem identification particularly as it relates to psychosocial morbidity, an overemphasis on physical illness and the practical aspects of care rather than patient feelings, needs or expectations, a perception that talking to patients is less important and less effective than the practical aspects of care, and finally specific skill deficiencies. These latter deficits include lack of structure during interactions, lack of technique, e.g. faulty questioning style, insufficient clarification of information, overcontrol in interactions and needless repetition. Furthermore, general skill deficiencies highlighted by Maguire concentrated upon the lack of precision in understanding patients' problems, inappropriate use and clarification of jargon, inappropriate questioning styles, inadequate recognition of and response to nonverbal cues, insufficient provision of information, inadequate support and reassurance and the lack of ability to handle difficult situations. The situations posing greatest communication difficulty for nurses predominately concerned the psychiatric and terminal care situations.

In summary, the research findings within the nursing discipline suggest that (a) nurses spend relatively little time engaged in verbal communication with patients; (b) this verbal communication tends to be superficial in nature and substantially task orientated; and (c) nurses employ strategies to avoid giving patients information.

The disadvantages of the constitutive ethnographic method are predictable. Firstly, there are the logistical problems of being able to videotape actual practitioner-patient consultations. Secondly, there are major ethical issues to be faced when 'invading' what are normally very private interactions. These will be discussed later. Thirdly, there is the lack of adequate safeguards against the investigator's subjective biases determining the aspects of interaction highlighted. Fourthly, there is the difficulty in obtaining consensus from peer review and analysis of the data. Fifthly, the problem of selecting individuals capable of interpersonal analysis of practice situations may be considerable and finally, the objectivity of analysis may be impaired because of the psychological influences existing in group debate and discussion. While these factors constitute risk to the whole skill identification phase, Saunders and Caves (1986) have argued that 'this risk may be worth taking as long as subsequent attention is given to the reliability and validity of the interaction sequences which emerge'. (p.32)

Other approaches

The methodologies described above utilize both qualitative and quantitative assessments of communication behaviour allied to the health care context. Obviously, adaptations of these general themes can be employed in order to identify communication skills. For example, it would be possible to draw from wider research in interpersonal communication by way of listing a number of communicative strategies. These could then be submitted to professional review in order to determine which strategies work most successfully in given practitioner-patient situations.

An alternative technique is the 'What would you do next?' approach. Here practitioners are presented with part of a written dialogue of a patient interaction, or shown a portion of a video sequence of a patient consultation, and asked how they would proceed with the interview, or alternatively how they would have conducted it from the outset. Exercise 7.4 is an example of this approach. From the responses it should be possible to chart an effective, situationally appropriate communication strategy, which could be used as a basis for communication skills training.

Exercise 7.4 What would you do next?

Instructions

The following is the initial part of a conversation between a nurse and a patient. The patient had originally been admitted to hospital for investigation following the discovery of a lump on her breast. It was found to be malignant and a mastectomy had been performed. Follow-up chemotherapy had also been instituted. Based on this trainees should be challenged to identify ways in which the overall interaction should be handled and the skills so required.

Nurse: Hello, Mrs —. How are you feeling today?
Patient: Not too good.

Nurse: Sister said you were feeling sick.
Patient: Oh, it's not the sickness. I wish that was all – (bursts into tears). What am I going to do? I never thought it would ever come to this . . .

7.7 ETHICAL AND CLINICAL CONSIDERATIONS OF INVESTIGATIVE METHODOLOGIES

Obviously in carrying out some of the above techniques there will be a number of practical considerations to be taken into account. These will include, for example, technological factors concerning the choice and actual use of audio- and video-recordings (Chapter 12), and also the time, personnel and financial commitment that would be required to undertake a major empirical research initiative. More importantly perhaps, are the ethical and clinical issues that confront the investigator using audiovisual methodologies to examine the dimensions of interpersonal communication at the practitioner-patient interface. It is therefore essential that the researcher be aware of these elements in order to afford 'protection' to all parties involved.

Any form of recording which makes the consultation between a patient and his practitioner a matter of permanent/semi-permanent and possibly public record, raises fundamental ethical questions. Moreover, any access to this relationship through the use of recordings for teaching or analysis purposes endangers its integrity. Thus firstly, do these methods, while providing potentially rich resources of material for research and instruction violate privacy and confidentiality? Secondly, while 'informed consent' is a process whereby patients accept a certain level of risk do they fully understand the implications of this commitment? Thirdly, does the act of recording a consultation affect the nature, content and outcome of the interaction itself, i.e. are there any 'clinical' ramifications to the use of these techniques? Obviously videotaping is a more comprehensive form of recording than audio-recording, and therefore by its very nature more revealing, such that ethical guidelines developed for this form of recording will undoubtedly cover the audio situation.

Figure 7.5 is an adaption of the proposals made by Block *et al.* (1985) to defining a method of ethical reasoning in respect of videotaping patient consultations in the medical context. The ethical principles underpinning the paradigm are those of autonomy, non-maleficence, beneficence and justice. Autonomy is concerned with respect for persons and recognizes the self-governing nature of the individual. Non-maleficence is a principle which serves to protect the individual and literally means 'do no harm'. Beneficence refers to a duty to confer benefits or further the wellbeing of another as well as helping them advance their important and legitimate

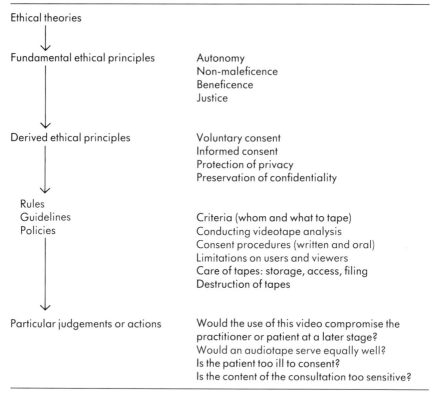

Ethical theories
↓

Fundamental ethical principles   Autonomy
│   Non-maleficence
│   Beneficence
│   Justice
↓

Derived ethical principles   Voluntary consent
│   Informed consent
│   Protection of privacy
↓   Preservation of confidentiality

Rules
Guidelines   Criteria (whom and what to tape)
Policies   Conducting videotape analysis
│   Consent procedures (written and oral)
│   Limitations on users and viewers
│   Care of tapes: storage, access, filing
↓   Destruction of tapes

Particular judgements or actions   Would the use of this video compromise the
                                        practitioner or patient at a later stage?
                                        Would an audiotape serve equally well?
                                        Is the patient too ill to consent?
                                        Is the content of the consultation too sensitive?

Fig. 7.5 A method of ethical reasoning applied to the videotaping of practitioner-patient consultations (adapted from Block *et al.*, 1985).

interests. Finally, justice is concerned with affording others their 'rights or dues'.

The whole area of privacy and confidentiality is substantially governed by the principle of autonomy where the individual has the right to control information about himself to the extent of who knows it. Thus patients share intimate information with their doctor, pharmacist, health visitor, etc., but would not want that information to go any further.

However, patients may authorize that information given in a consultation setting be used for research and educational purposes. This becomes informed consent and the practitioner must ensure that in giving such consent the patient is truly autonomous. It is therefore important that the patient is fully aware of what he is consenting to. For example, videotapes used purely for analysis in research are much more easy to control in terms of who will view them etc., whereas the consequences of using them for educational purposes are much more open and unpredictable and indeed potentially harmful, if individuals are recognized. Patients have therefore a right to know and be made aware of these situations.

Against this background it is crucial to ensure the voluntary and informed consent of the patient and prevent unauthorized access to the tapes and the information they contain. Within the patient care setting it is possible for patients to feel coerced into participting in such activities, and therefore, it is important to create a situation where the patient is free to say 'No'. Patients should not be allowed to feel under obligation to any of their health-care practitioners to do them a 'favour' by participating in any research or teaching project. Indeed Martin and Martin (1984) reported that patients were less likely to refuse video-recording of their consultation if they were asked by the doctor for their verbal permission on entering the consulting room rather than if they were asked to sign a consent form. Patients were also more willing to express their reservations about video-recording if asked to fill in a questionnaire at home rather than immediately at the surgery. Furthermore these workers found that even 11% of those who consented to recording actually disapproved of the technique.

Consequently it may be better if voluntary informed consent was obtained by someone other than the practitioner. As far as informed consent is concerned the patient needs to know exactly what is being recorded and to what use it will be put. This extends to knowing who will see the tape – other health workers, students, the public, and what the risks are of being recognized. Finally, tapes should be stored securely and access to them limited to those who are legitimately authorized to use them.

Following on from this, practical guidelines need to be formulated which can serve to establish a code of practice for the making and showing of practitioner-patient recordings. In addition a consent form will be required whereby all participants must give written consent to the use of the recording(s), in which they took part (see Hart, 1984).

One further associated feature of the ethical issues surrounding video- or audio-recordings is the effect that they have on the actual consultation itself. Pringle *et al.* (1984) in a comparison of video-recording alone, as opposed to a general practitioner trainer sitting in on a GP trainee consultation, showed that video-recorded consultations more closely related to the 'normal' situation than did the two-doctor consultation when stress levels of patients were measured. They also reported that patients who refused consent to be filmed were more highly stressed than those who agreed. Similarly, Martin and Martin (1984) reported that patients with anxiety, depression or problems relating to the breasts or reproductive tract were more likely to withhold consent.

Herzmark (1985) in a study of 295 videofilmed doctor-patient interviews compared to a control group of 185 patient interviews which were not filmed concluded that the actual videofilming process did not appear to affect to any great extent the consultation from the patients' point of view.

However, he did report, in some instances, lower rapport ratings between doctor and patient and also recognized the potential doctor anxieties of being seen to be 'doing the right thing'. The level of refusal to be recorded by patients was also reported, 10% in one practice and 2% in the other, one of the implications being that if large numbers of patients decline to be recorded in any investigation the resulting sample will be less representative of the population and thus the credibility of the results undermined. Furthermore, Servant and Matheson (1986) demonstrated that if the coercive elements of obtaining consent are reduced then the consent rates are substantially decreased, thus reinforcing the ethical dilemmas of this sort of investigation, confounding the representativeness of the study sample and strongly pointing in the direction that patients do mind being videotaped.

7.8 FURTHER CONSIDERATIONS

The results of research into skill identification within the health professions raises a number of issues. Firstly, are the findings from the samples reported typical, in general, of practitioners within individual professional domains? It might be argued that research which utilized an exclusive empirical paradigm is more likely to reflect the true situation. Yet only by resubmitting the data to further independent professional review and testing its reliability with new samples of patient-practitioner consultation data can the accuracy and precision of skill identification be guaranteed.

Secondly, there is the issue of validity in that the skills identified for effective performance have been those primarily generated by professionals themselves and therefore represent only one view of the situation. The question must be asked, 'Does the use of these skills actually promote patient gains in terms of satisfaction, compliance, improved clinical status etc?'. Thus there is a need to test practitioner behaviour related to patient 'health' achievement.

Thirdly, there must be the recognition that the training needs of one professional group may be markedly different from another, such that training initiatives need to be custom developed to retain face validity with practitioners, as well as optimizing the potential for patient gains during consultations.

7.9 OVERVIEW

This chapter has sought to explore the area of skill identification within the health professions. The content of training must reflect the aims and objectives of the programme which, in turn, emerge from the established needs of trainees. Attention was drawn to the nature of interpersonal skill and the various factors which influence identification procedures. Three major paradigms were described together with specific methodologies which can be utilized in skill identification studies, and consideration given to the ethical and clinical ramifications of such investigations. The practical applications of these techniques were illustrated from within the health disciplines together with a brief outline of the findings of this research. Finally, the implications of these results were presented particularly in relation to the reliability and validity of the data. Once skills have been identified, training proper can begin. The following three chapters are devoted to the training phase of CST.

8

The sensitization phase of training

8.1 INTRODUCTION

Training considerations constitute the second stage of the CST process. Here attention is devoted to the provision of a sequence of learning experiences, designed to promote the acquisition of those skills revealed by the sorts of identification techniques detailed in the preceding chapter. In keeping with the reductionist principles underlying CST, the complexities of interpersonal encounters are reduced by breaking the overall communicative performance down into a number of constituent skills. From a training point of view, students are typically introduced to these individual skills in a structured, systematic and progressive fashion until gradually, at the end of the programme, the repertoire of skills established can be synthesized into a complete and effective reconstitution of the targeted interaction.

The initial step in this training procedure is labelled 'sensitization' and is dealt with in the present chapter. At a broad level it is intended to sensitize trainees to the characteristics and rationale of this type of instruction, and to introduce them to the particular programme which they will follow. More specifically, by means of skill analysis and discrimination techniques including modelling, an understanding of the central features, functional properties and theoretical bases of each of the skills is engendered. Furthermore, the ability to successfully operationalize this knowledge in successful performance is promoted (Ellis and Whittington, 1981).

8.2 COMPONENTS OF SENSITIZATION

Essentially sensitization is the instructive phase of the CST paradigm, prior to practice, where trainees are provided with information which allows them to develop concepts of behaviour and set performance standards.

Instruction therefore involves, firstly, the transmission of substantive information or salient features about social behaviours, e.g. the labelling or description of behaviour and, secondly, the identification of performance goals or standards as a means of inducing or guiding trainees' subsequent performance.

Sensitization can be considered as comprising two main components, namely sensitization of the trainees to the actual programme of CST itself, and sensitization to the specific skill components that form the substance of training. This latter dimension of the process can be further characterized in terms of skill analysis and skill discrimination. In addition skill discrimination represents the behaviour modelling component of sensitization of which descriptive and demonstrative models are the instructive agents (Fig. 8.1). Each of these aspects will be discussed.

Sensitization to the training programme

At this stage trainees are alerted to the actual methodology of the training process in which they are about to participate including the theoretical antecedents which underpin the training techniques and strategies employed. Here it is important for the trainee to be introduced to the relationship between motor and social skills, which has provided a valuable analogy for the study and practice of interpersonal interaction. It is also at this point that the aims and objectives of the training need to be established in order to provide trainees with a clear view of what they should achieve, and also

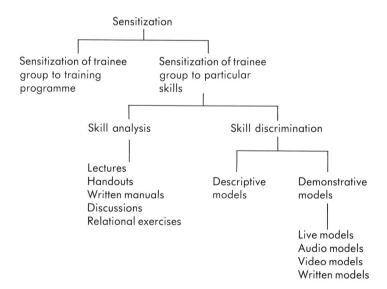

Fig. 8.1 Components of the sensitization phase of CST.

provide personal assessment markers during the CST course. Central to this aspect of sensitization is the fact that trainees need to be made aware that a participatory approach will be a key feature of the overall programme, the emphasis being mainly on experiential learning. Thus efforts should be made to encourage trainees to contribute to the process through, for example, group discussion, requesting and asking questions during lecture sessions and providing homework assignments. In addition, practical exercises which sensitize trainees to various dimensions of the communication process, within the context of health care, can be used to initially produce non-threatening participation. For example, exercises which explore the various dimensions of health and their implications for interpersonal communication can be used in this regard (Chapter 2). Another aspect of this phase, for example, is the use of video to film and then replay some group discussions, in order to allow trainees to get used to how they look and sound on film, prior to roleplay with CCTV. Further consideration of the use of video for such purposes is discussed in Chapter 9.

Skill analysis

At this stage of sensitization the skill is described to trainees in verbal form, involving the use of live or recorded lectures, handouts and background reading. Here the purpose is to provide the trainee with some theoretical understanding of the skill, outline its functions in designated contexts, present relevant research findings, and to analyse the skill in terms of behavioural components (e.g. the skill of nonverbal communication would include the behavioural components of positive facial expressions, touch, etc.). It should again be emphasized that this material needs to be presented within the framework of contemporary professional practice.

Lectures

Despite the fact that CST is often regarded as a 'high-tech' mode of instruction being commonly associated with the use of CCTV and video-recording facilities, the basic mechanism of skill analysis is undoubtedly the traditional lecture or lecturette. Although frequently maligned, Bligh (1971) concluded from available empirical evidence, that this teaching method was as effective as any other, with the possible exception of programmed learning, in the transmission of information. Several variants have been proposed by Jarvis and Gibson (1985) as being appropriate for teaching health professionals. The extremely teacher-centred nature of the 'straight lecture' may reduce its appeal for more mature groups of practising professionals. The 'lecture-discussion' tends to be a more attractive option. This may involve creating discussion groups to consider pre-selected questions arising from the preceding address. Alternatively more informal 'buzz' groups may be set up at different junctures in the course of the lecture to give trainees an opportunity to share their experiences, compare their understanding or air their opinions on some issue central to a targeted skill. Different audiovisual aids including 'trigger' audio or videotapes are a useful catalyst in promoting discussion among students and are used extensively as part of the sensitization procedure in CST.

Handouts and other readings

Often because of time constraints placed on CST it may be necessary to provide trainees with preparative reading prior to attending the course. Even if this is done it is necessary to review the material at the outset of training to consolidate its understanding. In addition it is helpful to prepare a checklist of the main features of the handout as an *aide memoire* and also as a reference guide for subsequent analysis of exemplars and roleplay situations. Care is also required in producing reading material in that psychological and sociological terms need to be adequately defined, especially for those trainees who have not had any previous background in the social or behavioural sciences. Further, it is important to introduce students gradually to, what for many will be a new area of training, otherwise they may feel overwhelmed by an unfamiliar topic. Useful sources of reading material are presented in Table 8.1.

Relational exercises

Relational exercises may be regarded as participatory activities that sensitize trainees to the actual components and use of skills without any recourse to professional knowledge or interactions. Essentially they may be described as games, puzzles, brain teasers, skill tests or creative exercises, which by their intrinsic nature vividly portray elements of the communication process. They are not designed for skill practice but rather to create awareness of the actual components of an individual skill. In this respect they are relational since the trainer can utilize these generic exercises to draw parallels with the actual practice situation. Thus, for example, in Exercise 4.2 the trainer can clearly illustrate the problems of listening within the context of an experiential, non-professional situation. The value of this approach is fourfold. Firstly, it is highly motivating for trainees in that they are keen to be seen to be successful in what appears to be quite straightforward exercises. Secondly, because the exercises do not directly draw on or test professional knowledge they are non-threatening and trainees can involve themselves fully in the experience. Thirdly, they are a potent method of ensuring that trainees actually remember core elements of the topic under discussion. Finally, this form of experiential learning allows trainees to pinpoint its relationship to their own professional practice, by drawing the links between simulated and real interpersonal communications. Simulation exercises are considered more fully in Chapter 9.

Table 8.1 Useful texts on interpersonal communication in the health professions

Carlson, R. (1984) *The Nurse's Guide to Better Communication*, Scott, Foresman & Co, Glenview, Illinois.

Faulkner, A. (ed.) (1984) *Recent Advances in Nursing*, Vol 7, Churchill Livingstone, Edinburgh.

French, P. (1983) *Social Skills for Nursing Practice*, Croom Helm, London.

Froelich, R. and Bishop, F. (1977) *Clinical Interviewing Skills*, C.V. Mosby, St Louis.

Hargie, O. (ed) (1986) *A Handbook of Communication Skills*, Croom Helm, London.

Hargie, O., Saunders, C. and Dickson, D. (1987) *Social Skills in Interpersonal Communication* (2nd edn), Croom Helm, London.

Kagan, C., Evans, J. and Kay, B. (1986) *A Manual of Interpersonal Skills for Nurses: An Experimental Approach*, Harper & Row, London.

Klinzing, D. and Klinzing, D. (1985) *Communication for Allied Health Professionals*, W.C. Brown, Dubuque, Iowa.

Ley, P. (1988) *Communicating with Patients*, Chapman and Hall, London.

Northouse, P. and Northouse, L. (1985) *Health Communication: A Handbook for Health Professionals*, Prentice-Hall, Englewood Cliffs, New Jersey.

Pendleton, D., Schofield., T. Tate, P. and Havelock, P. (1984) *The Consultation: An Approach to Learning and Teaching*, Oxford University Press, Oxford.

Porritt, L. (1984) *Communication: Choices for Nurses*, Churchill Livingstone, Edinburgh.

Purtilo, R. (1984) *Health Professional/Patient Interaction*, W.B. Saunders and Co., Philadelphia.

Smith, V. and Bass, T. (1982) *Communication for the Health Care Team*, Harper & Row, London.

Tähkä, V. (1984) *The Patient-Doctor Relationship*, ADIS Health Science Press, Sydney.

Thompson, T.L. (1986) *Communication for Health Professionals*, Harper & Row, New York.

Tindall, W., Beardsley, R. and Curtis, F. (eds) (1984) *Communication in Pharmacy Practice*, Lea and Febiger, Philadlphia.

Skill discrimination

This involves providing trainees with practical examples of the skill in action, thereby enabling them to critically analyse its behavioural components, evaluate its effectiveness and be prepared, in a particular practice context, to operationalize that information. This can either involve 'live' modelling where the lecturer enacts the skill in class or, more usually, videotape models of the skill being used. Alternatively audiotaped models could be used or written transcripts of patient-practitioner dialogues introduced to exemplify each skill, but it should be remembered in these latter cases that the nonverbal aspects of communication are substantially lost. Such models form the focus for group discussions during this phase and their use will be described in greater detail later in this chapter. That the acquisition of social behaviour is facilitated by imitating or modelling the behaviour of others has been well established (Bandura, 1977a). However, there is considerable work involved in preparing suitable exemplar models for a CST programme, the practicalities of which will be discussed in a subsequent section of the chapter.

Modelling stages

Modelling serves essentially three basic purposes. Firstly, it stimulates the learning of new skills or behaviours and secondly, encourages the strengthening or weakening of previously learned behaviour through disinhibition or inhibition of performance. Thus at one level it is creative in that it exposes the learner to a range of skills not previously known or practised. At another level it is actually therapeutic or developmental in that 'good' behaviour can be enhanced or refined while negative behaviours can be attenuated. A third purpose is that of response facilitation. The effect of this latter objective 'is to increase behaviours that the observer has already learned and for which there are no existing constraints or inhibitions. The effect of the model is simply to provide an information cue that triggers similar behaviour on the part of the observer' (Perry and Furukawa, 1986, pp.69–70).

Modelling theory and practice is based on the principle that people are influenced by observing the behaviour of others. Thus in viewing others, learning or reading about them, we gain information about their behaviour which may mean that our own behaviour is modified as a result. Bandura (1977a) has suggested that modelling requires an individual to attend to the behaviour of another, to remember what he has observed, to have the capacity to imitate that behaviour and to be motivated to subsequently enact it. Thus, attention, retention, reproduction and motivation represent four crucial stages in the modelling process, and ways of maximizing each must be considered by the trainer.

Attention

Although attention alone does not guarantee that new behaviours will result it is a necessary condition for modelling to occur. In order to focus attention it is important that the observer is not swamped with learning points. Consequently, it is necessary to minimize any competing stimuli in order to concentrate attention on the focal points to be observed (Griffiths, 1976). It is also important to note that the availability of models who exhibit a certain type of behaviour will influence what is learned. Thus in a one-to-one training situation a trainee will tend to imitate the behaviours of his/her senior colleague, on the basis that there is no other model available. This, of course, poses difficulties in that there is a limited repertoire of behaviours from which to learn, and what will work for one individual may not necessarily work for another because of differences in personality, style, attitudes etc. As a result in any training programme a range of models displaying competent behaviours should be depicted, thus enhancing the likelihood of the trainee identifying with at least one of them (Perry and Furukawa, 1986). It is imperative, though, that multiple models are broadly consistent (Fehrenbach *et al.*, 1979).

The functional value of any behaviour as observed by a trainee will also affect attention. Thus the outcomes of interactions are important in that behaviours which gain, for example, patient confidence, produce new clinical information or enhance therapy are more likely to be attended to and remembered. Linked to this is the idea that if behaviour is rewarded or praised it is observed more closely. In addition the research evidence suggests that the attractiveness of the model to the observer affects attentiveness. Models are more effective when they are similar to the observer in terms of gender, age, class, culture, knowledge and experience (Hargie and Saunders, 1983a). Identification with the model is therefore important, and it is for this reason that students are more likely to identify with newly-qualified practitioners than with more mature ones.

Retention

As well as attending to displayed behaviours, in order for them to be reproduced they must be remembered. Bandura (1977a) has suggested that retention processes contribute to the learning of modelled responses and the accurate reproduction of those responses. Essentially the retention process involves the representation and cognitive organization of behaviours, i.e. they are represented in the memory in either an imaginal or verbal form. With skill elements that are essentially nonverbal, the former system is likely to be particularly important. In addition this process also includes observers visualizing or imagining themselves performing the behaviours which were previously seen performed by another individual. This is termed covert rehearsal (Goldstein and Sorcher, 1974). Overall then, the moves in any sequence of behaviour are labelled and catalogued thereby providing a cognitive base from which performance can ensue. It is therefore important to involve trainees in analysis of modelled behaviour in order to develop more comprehensive frameworks from which interpersonal communication can be understood and self-performance modified to ensure more effective outcomes.

It should, however, be remembered that trainees come to the modelling process with perhaps already established views on interpersonal communication, such that there may be a refusal to accept any alternative other than the cognitive framework from which they already work. This may mean that the retention process is hampered. For example, a doctor may refuse to accept that his interviewing of patients across a surgery desk is in fact 'distancing' him from them, justifying it on the grounds that he has never had any problem with doing it that way, or because it allows him to 'control' consultations.

Reproduction

The reproductive stage of modelling concerns the capacity to perform the behaviours which have been observed. It therefore involves converting symbolic representations into appropriate action. Behavioural enactment can be viewed as comprising three separate but associated phases, namely cognitive organization of responses, their actual initiation and their monitoring and refinement on the basis of informative feedback. Thus an individual moves from a mental organization and rehearsal of behaviour through to a critical appraisal of action whereby flaws in behaviour can be identified, excluded or modified to improve the overall performance. Reinforcement may also be provided for positive behaviours.

At this point it is important to emphasize three points. Firstly, observational learning does not mean that observers can carry out any given behaviour perfectly first time, or that they necessarily become replicas of the model. A combination of practice coupled with feedback may be necessary before performance is perfected, and indeed each person brings something of themselves to each behaviour, such that it is subtly different from the actual model. Secondly, the amount of observational learning exhibited behaviourally partly depends on the availability of component skills. This means that if deficits exist in the basic skills required for complex performances these must first be developed by modelling and practice before moving to more complex routines (Baldwin and Baldwin, 1981). One implication for CST might be that basic skills (e.g. questioning) need to be mastered before introducing trainees to higher-order strategies such as counselling. Thirdly, reproduction will only occur where the observer or trainee is motivated to imitate the modelled behaviour.

Motivation

The motivational process is important to the concept of modelling. Individuals are more likely to adopt modelled behaviour if results are valued rather than if accompanied by unrewarding or punishing effects. Thus greater modelling will tend to occur, for example, where the model controls rewards or resources desired by the trainee, i.e. is of higher recognized status, better paid, has more power, etc. However, Bandura (1977a) has suggested that imitative learning can occur without reinforcement in that people may observe, code and retain patterns of behaviour that can be reproduced at a later time even when not rewarded. Such behaviour is unlikely to emerge though, unless there is sufficient incentive. While reinforcement is not a prerequisite for learning to take place it can have a facilitating effect at each of the stages of the modelling process. Anticipation of reinforcement can influence what is observed and behaviours which have been seen to have positive consequences will be more likely to receive increased attention. The prospect of reinforcement can also promote retention by inducing the observer to implement effective symbolic procedures and engage in rehearsal. In designing models it is therefore important to incorporate motivational features in order to enhance and facilitate the learner.

From the trainer's perspective it is important to guide and support the trainee through each of these stages of the modelling process, in order to maximize the potential for acquiring effective repertoires of behaviour in given situations. Failure of an observer to match the behaviour of a model may result from (a) not observing the relevant behaviour displayed, (b) inadequately coding modelled events for memory representation, (c) failing to retain what was learned, (d) physical inability to perform and (e) experiencing insufficient incentives.

Types of model

As has been indicated (Fig. 8.1) models fall into two broad categories, namely descriptive models and demonstrative models. The essential difference between them is that, while the latter present by means of videotape, audiotape or in written form, the original verbal and nonverbal behaviour to be modelled, descriptive models operate at a more abstract level by presenting an account of that behaviour. As such, descriptive models are one step removed from the communicative performance which they represent (Ellis and Whittington, 1981).

Descriptive models

Descriptive models as the name implies are written or verbal analyses of communication behaviour. They describe or label the behaviours both in terms of what they are and their effects and outcomes in any interaction. Thus, for example, statements which reflect back to a patient in alternative language what they have previously said may be labelled as reflective listening, but also could be described in terms of demonstrating interest, concern or understanding, and also facilitating additional patient expression. To some extent therefore descriptive models are both evaluative and interpretative in their presentation, and by their very nature seek to enhance the trainee's awareness and understanding of communication behaviour in various situations. Fig. 8.2 is an example of a pharmacist-patient interaction (a written demonstration model) coupled with descriptive analysis of the interaction.

Descriptive models may be provided orally during lectures and also by

		Descriptive analysis
	Pharmacist greets patient with a smile and comes around the counter	Pharmacist shows warmth
Pharmacist	'Good morning, Mrs Johnson. That's a nice day isn't it?'	Greeting/conversational lead
Patient	'Hello, Mr Pringle.'	Patient reciprocates
Pharmacist	'Dr McKay has prescribed suppositories for your mother. Did he give you any information on how you should use them?'	Opening statement Questions for needs
Patient	'No I didn't think so. Well he may have but I probably wasn't listening properly. I've so much on my mind with my mother so ill. She's not keeping any food down and she needs constant attention.'	Patient responds by expressing feelings Provides information
Pharmacist	'You've obviously a lot to cope with.'	Reflective listening
Patient	'That's right. It's all quite a strain on the family and the children need a lot of attention.'	Continued patient expression
Pharmacist	'I think you deserve a lot of credit for coping so well[a]. It's obviously a difficult time for you,[b] but hopefully this medicine will ease things for your mother[c].'	(a) Self-disclosure (b) Reflective listening (c) Immediacy and shading the conversation
Patient	'That would be a great help.'	Positive patient response

SUMMARY

In this situation the pharmacist portrayed effective attending skills and allowed Mrs Johnson to express and negotiate her own needs. The pharmacist displayed empathy with Mrs Johnson and understanding of her problems, leading on to discussing how the therapy would help to alleviate her mother's condition.

Fig. 8.2 Simple descriptive model of part of a pharmacist-patient interaction.

means of written handouts, either as prior reading material or summaries of the lecture input. An elaboration of the handout approach is the production of self-instructional packages whereby trainees undertake independent, self-paced learning in communication skills. Such written material can be accompanied by model videotaped sequences thus incorporating demonstrations from the practice situation in a recorded form.

Demonstration models

As indicated in Fig. 8.1 there are two main types of demonstration models, namely live models and recorded models. In both cases, the actual behaviour to be acquired is presented.

Live models In this situation the trainer, a trainee, or a third party enacts the behaviour to be modelled in front of the class. In the health-care context this is likely to be a portrayal of a practitioner-patient consultation designed to sensitize trainees to the behaviour of the professional and the outcomes of such behaviour. It also facilitates an understanding of patient behaviour in such situations. Live models offer flexibility in the sensitization phase and are obviously inexpensive to produce. They do not, however, offer the same degree of control as can be obtained with a recorded scenario where the action can literally be stopped and discussion ensue before proceeding with the remainder of the interaction. In addition live modelling may be less controlled in that responses are totally reactive to a situation, while recorded models do offer the opportunity to script the action in order to more specifically programme learning. Related to the former two is the lack of exact reproduction of live roleplay (Eisler and Frederiksen, 1980). A further factor to consider is the environment in which the modelling takes place, in that a classroom context does not necessarily mimic the actual practice situation and to that extent may not create face validity with trainees, who perhaps are aware of, for example, various forms of distraction occurring in the workplace.

Recorded models Recorded models come in three forms, audio-recordings, video-recordings, or written transcripts. With regard to the former two it is now more common to have video-recordings of modelling behaviour than audio-recordings. Indeed video as a training tool in CST has now become widespread not only to exemplify model behaviour but as a potent form of feedback on skill practice attempts (Hargie and Saunders, 1983a). Moreover, in a review of research into clinical interviewing Carroll and Monroe (1980) reported that standardized presentations of illustrative patient interviews are more effective as teaching aids than live, spontaneous demonstrations of patient consultations. As Morrow (1986) pointed out, 'the use of videotaped exemplars is likely to be more consistent and efficient

- Presenting information for observational learning to trainees.
- Highlighting models of positive and negative interpersonal skill use.
- Stimulating group discussion.
- Giving trainees a common learning experience.
- Illustrating self-instructional modules/units/packages.
- Stimulating trainee self-awareness.
- Stimulating trainee awareness of patients' goals and feelings.

Fig. 8.3 Uses of video exemplars for modelling behaviour

than live unrehearsed interactions designed to illustrate certain skills or concepts' (p.343). The potential uses of video exemplars for modelling are illustrated in Fig. 8.3.

Written dialogues of either real or fictional practitioner-patient consultations can also be provided for trainees thereby allowing skill discrimination to be effected. Here it must be remembered that the nonverbal aspects of communication are substantially excluded such that any learning occurring will be more limited than if a video-recording had been used. Written materials are obviously cheaper to prepare than video-recorded models as well as providing a more permanent record for the trainee to return to for subsequent revision, clarification and consolidation of learning. Exercise 8.1 is an example of how a demonstrative model in the form of a transcription may be used to critically analyse and evaluate the effectiveness of particular practitioner behaviour in a health-care setting.

As has been indicated, recorded models offer more control to the trainer in conducting trainees through the different learning elements. Indeed because of the editing opportunities that video presents it is possible to use visual cueing techniques to label individual behaviours on the TV screen throughout a given scenario for the benefit of trainees (Griffiths, 1976). Furthermore, it is possible to utilize such cues on screen to alert trainees to particular elements in the action. The greater control that video models give also permits trainers the facility to 'freeze' the action to draw attention to some feature of nonverbal communication, to discuss what has gone before or challenge trainees to consider how best the interaction could be continued. Video exemplars allow the trainer to feature a wide range of models that would not easily be possible through live modelling. They also guarantee reproduction of behaviour which is not always possible with live demonstrations.

There are also certain disadvantages of recorded models some of which have been identified by Eisler and Frederiksen (1980). As previously indicated, video films are invariably costly to produce both in financial terms and also in respect of the time commitment that will be required to produce them. However, it should be remembered that in recording either real or simulated practitioner-patient interactions it is possible to largely accept the

Exercise 8.1 Skill discrimination using a written demonstration model

Instructions

The trainer should provide trainees with a written dialogue of an actual practitioner-patient interaction chosen for its portrayal of particular behaviours e.g. interviewing technique. The following questions, aimed at examining questioning behaviour, can be used to guide discussion of the key elements of the interaction.

1. Count the number of questions asked by both the patient and practitioner.
2. Identify and categorize each of the practitioner's questions as being either closed, open, leading, prompting or multiple. Then judge whether the question is also a probe and identify the type of probe.
3. Describe the implications of the various types of question and evaluate their influence upon the consultation.
4. Determine to what extent the consultation focused upon physical or psychosocial issues.
5. Identify how and in what ways the questioning approach of the practitioner could have been modified to improve the consultation.

NB This approach can be expanded to analyse other forms of behaviour within the same interaction e.g. listening. The technique can equally well be applied to the analysis of audio- and video-recorded models.

behaviour enacted, in that the material is typically discussed with the group. This reduces the time-commitment that may be required to produce and film 'perfect' consultations and, as will be discussed later, enhances the face-validity and impact of the whole presentation. A second disadvantage is that in having exemplar material available there may be a tendency for the trainer to rely too heavily on this mode of learning to the extent that trainees become overloaded with taped material and fewer learning points are remembered. Finally, the production and use of audio- or video-recording demands that consent is obtained from those involved. The ethical issues surrounding recorded material have been discussed in Chapter 7 and the reader is referred to that section.

Overall then demonstrative models have a crucial part to play in modelling behaviour. As pointed out in Chapter 5 one picture may be worth a thousand words but a demonstration is worth a thousand pictures. Thus demonstrative models may have greater potential to help long-term retention than descriptive models. They also foster attention and are motivating for trainees and these three factors of retention, attention and motivation contribute to the reproduction of desired behaviour in trainees.

Homework

One further way of consolidating the sensitization phase is the assignment type approach whereby the trainee is given homework to complete prior to the next training session. Here trainees are encouraged to continue the process of skill discrimination through written problems or observational learning. The exercises given to trainees may be structured in such a way as to cause them to think critically of the interactions to be conducted. Observation of actual practitioner-patient interactions may be used to focus attention on specific behaviours of communication and their impact on the consultation. Alternatively, written dialogues of interactions may be presented to trainees for analysis and report back at the next session (see Exercise 8.1). Homework may also involve the trainees writing a short essay on the use of a particular skill in their professional situation, e.g. explaining skills in patient education. A further example of a homework type assignment is indicated in Exercise 8.2. That homework as a form of learning is effective has been demonstrated by Falloon *et al.* (1977) who in a study of social skill training of outpatient groups showed that those who were given structured homework assignments did better on nearly all of the outcome measures.

Exercise 8.2 Questioning technique

Instructions

Each trainee should be asked to identify the type of leading question given below and suggest an alternative wording of the question to eliminate the 'lead'.

'I take it you've found the speech therapy sessions helpful, Mrs Hamilton?'.

'You're not having any pain are you, Mr Sloan?'

'You would, I think, want to give your children fluoride drops to strengthen their teeth, wouldn't you?'

'You know, of course, you're asking me to break the law by asking me to sell you an antibiotic?'

'After your operation for varicose veins did you take regular walks?'

For discussion

Trainees should be asked to submit their re-worded questions to the trainee group for review and analysis. Trainees should seek to identify the problems and implications of the above questions and to what extent the alternative questions overcame these difficulties. The limitations of the suggested alternatives should also be identified.

8.3 USES OF MODEL TAPES

There are a number of ways in which recorded exemplars can be used during CST. It is important for trainers to consider using such material as creatively as possible since to merely show a series of videotaped scenarios may in itself tend to become repetitive and demotivating for trainees, especially if there is little stimulus variation to the presentation. Model tapes can be employed in four main ways.

Self-instructional package

In this instance trainees are provided with self-contained recorded material which can be replayed in their own time, accompanied by written explanatory literature. While this approach may be favoured, particularly in situations where the curriculum is already crowded, it does in fact suffer from serious deficiencies. In the first place, for such an approach to work successfully, sufficient playback facilities are needed. Secondly, in what is a very practical area of training the self-instructional method is primarily directed at the cognitive level at the expense of performative learning. Thirdly, to attempt to develop interpersonal skills in isolation appears to be a peculiar approach to this area of professional competence, in that skills can best be refined and improved through structured feedback in the interpersonal dimensions of practice (Hargie and Morrow, 1986b).

Brief vignettes during lectures

Here a maximum of five minutes of recorded material is shown at any one time, the object being to illustrate a point rather than to explain. Each vignette needs to be closely linked to the elements of the lecture and is specifically chosen to emphasize a particular point or issue or to provoke discussion from trainees. When used in this way it encourages participation by trainees, thereby fostering a wider exploration of the subject under discussion. Thus exemplar material can be used to stimulate and motivate participants to involve themselves fully in the training programme, while at the same time creating a valuable learning experience.

Opening/closing lectures

As well as interspersing taped material throughout a presentation, model exemplars can be used with good effect at the beginning or end of a lecture. For example, showing a tape at the start of a lecture will stimulate attention and provide a focus for the session. Similarly a tape at the end of a lecture can be used to recap and reinforce the points already presented, and to send the trainees away with the topic fresh in their minds. As has already been stated it is important not to overload trainees with taped material such that a number of important points are forgotten, simply because of the volume of material presented.

Roleplay stimuli

Roleplay, as a popular method of skill practice, will be discussed in detail in the following chapter. It is relevant to mention here, however, that an effective technique of introducing a particular roleplay scenario and stimulating participation in it, is through the presentation of appropriate videotaped material to the group.

8.4 SOURCES OF MODEL TAPES

Model tapes are available from a number of sources. In the first instance a wide range of commercial tapes are available to trainers on topics such as interviewing, handling bereavement, dealing with aggression, counselling and negotiating, among others. Some of these are generic in nature in that they do not focus specifically on any professional group (e.g. Ivey's 1976 tapes on counselling). Others are produced to directly address the needs of a particular profession (e.g. Brown's 1983 tapes for social workers; Jessop's 1979 tapes for nurses). Within the health professions the latter type of tape is not yet widely available in the UK although some attempts have been made to present the management of particularly difficult interpersonal situations (e.g. Brown, 1983). (Lists of commercially produced videotaped material can be found in Ivey and Authier (1978), Marshall *et al*. (1982) and Kagan *et al*. (1986).)

Commercial tapes may not always be appropriate for the trainee group in that there may be differences in culture between the people and situations depicted on the recording and the trainees. For example, material produced in the USA may not mirror a European situation, and indeed within countries there may be wide regional variation such that it will be important to present model videos that trainees can easily identify with.

Consequently, we would recommend that trainees give consideration to producing their own tapes in that regional variations in culture, dialect or practice can be depicted so enhancing the face-validity of the recordings for trainees. While it does require a certain level of expertise and time commitment in producing one's own tapes the results are usually well worth the effort.

A third source of practice-related video-recordings is that which results from roleplays which have been video-recorded during training. However, in advocating the use of such material it is imperative that the trainer obtain written permission from those involved in the roleplays before showing them to another audience. Even if permission is given, the trainer, in using these tapes, should always alert other trainees that the performance of the individual recorded was in the context of a training situation, and that it does not necessarily mirror their real practice. This is especially true if the exemplar shown depicts poor communication performance.

Self-produced model tapes

Mention has already been made of the value of the trainer producing his or her own model tapes specifically designed to meet the requirements of a particular trainee group. It is possible to produce these exemplars using a minimum of equipment and certainly does not require the involvement of a professional production team. All that is required is a camera, a video-recorder, two clip-on microphones (or one omni-directional microphone), a spotlight and a television monitor. Of course, given the resources a second camera would allow an alternative perspective of the interaction to be filmed but it also means that the material either needs to be 'mixed' as it is shot or edited at a subsequent date in the studio. The latter procedure is both expensive and time-consuming and is usually employed only if the material is subsequently to be marketed.

   Although such exemplars can be produced with relative ease there are a number of important practical points that any trainer should carefully consider before embarking on filming. The first thing required is a detailed plan of all the interactions to be enacted. At one level it requires the trainer to have prepared 'loose' scripts of all the encounters by way of a guide to roleplay participants as to how the interaction should be developed. At a second level, a timetable needs to be prepared of the order in which scenarios are to be filmed so that a rota can be worked out among the volunteer actors as to when they are required. A second factor that needs to be considered in the planning stage is that all recordings in one area should be completed before moving into another location, e.g. ward situation to office situation. A third factor to address at the planning stage is to identify what props or dress (e.g. uniforms) will be required in order to make the roleplay completely authentic. Failure to do this will inevitably mean that the scenario, no matter how good it may be, will suffer from a lack of credibility and will invariably be criticized accordingly by trainees.

   The selection of actors is also an important factor in preparing model tapes, since the quality of the finished product is dependent upon their acting ability. It is possible to use professional actors in such circumstances but that is usually costly and there may also be difficulties in these people conveying, without considerable rehearsal, real credibility especially in the practitioner's role where technical language and know-how may be in-volved. The use of naturally good performers within the profession or individuals who have undergone CST is perhaps the ideal as far as choice of actors is concerned, in that these people will appreciate the nuances of the communication process and will have a ready understanding of what is required of them. They will also have already experienced roleplay and to that extent will not be camera shy. They should be able to 'get' into roles quickly and adapt any written scenario to fit their own personalities and previous experience in the real practice environment. Furthermore, in contrast to professional actors, these individuals are totally convincing in the practitioner's role in that they are literally 'playing themselves'.

Scripts are useful in determining the overall pattern of any interaction, and the more structured roleplay approach (Hargie and Morrow, 1986b) is likely to produce the best results. Here the nature of the interaction, based on a loose script, is worked out in detail and discussed with all the actors. At the same time spontaneity is encouraged so that as indicated it eliminates 'stiffness' in acting or the 'script-bound' phenomenon, which usually occurs when amateur actors try to use scripts. Total spontaneity can be induced into exemplars by providing the actor practitioner with minimal warning as to how the patient will present, thus producing a more natural response. Similarly, if inter-professional communication is required other professionals can be drawn in to play their 'own' parts.

As far as the technicalities of filming are concerned little detailed knowledge is required to produce tapes of reasonable quality. Obviously, it is important to ensure satisfactory sound levels and also that the cameraman focuses upon the relevant behaviours of those acting. Spotlights are also useful, but with a light-sensitive camera this may not actually be necessary. Finally, the environment in which the recordings are made is quite crucial in order to obtain face-validity for trainees. Although it is often possible to simulate a real environment it usually is extremely costly to do so effectively. Thus, it is usually necessary to film interactions in the real practice context, i.e. the ward, the home, the pharmacy, the consulting room etc. This means that filming on location will demand careful attention to detail at the preparation stage even down to the degree of cabling that will be required for the equipment.

8.5 MODELLING CONSIDERATIONS

In using various forms of model tapes trainers should give consideration to a number of factors. Firstly, mention has been already made to using models which trainees can closely identify with in terms of sex, class, knowledge and experience. Secondly, it is important that models should be seen to cope successfully in the practice situation. Moreover, they should be seen to improve with time rather than being perfect at the outset. The advantage of this approach is that trainees are given realistic behavioural targets to meet, with their own performance progressively improving along with the models. Thirdly, skilled behaviour should be seen to be rewarded in that trainees are more likely to imitate the behaviour of successful people (Baldwin and Baldwin, 1981).

Fourthly, while a positive approach in modelling is important it can be useful for trainees to view scenarios of 'how not to do it' i.e. negative exemplars. The use of negative exemplars is cautioned in that one danger of using this type of model is that the trainee can actually copy negative behaviour (Alssid and Hutchinson, 1977). As Hargie and Morrow (1986b) point out, 'this danger is particularly prevalent where the negative model is not grossly incompetent and the trainee, who is also inexperienced, actually identifies with the weak model. Where negative models are to be employed, therefore, they should be markedly incompetent (p.66).

Fifthly, negative models should never be shown without being counter balanced by positive models. Indeed, positive models should be longer and be shown more often that negative exemplars. Here the object is to highlight and reinforce positive behaviour while illustrating the consequences of inappropriate interpersonal communication. This is best achieved, as will be discussed later, by demonstrating positive and negative approaches to the same situation, thereby visually illustrating some of the strategies that can be used to ensure more successful and satisfactory outcomes. Consequently, positive models will be most successful if they (a) depict a variety of models, (b) are vividly presented and not 'hidden' within a range of other behaviours, (c) are shown frequently, particularly where complex behaviour is involved, (d) are explained by 'cueing' techniques which draw attention to the features of behaviour to be modelled, and (e) terminate in a restatement of the essential learning point.

8.6 OVERVIEW

Sensitization is the initial stage of the training sequence. Its functions are to provide trainees with a broad introduction to CST and the aims, objectives and content of the particular programme which they will follow. More specifically, it is intended to provide them with a theoretical appreciation, and sound working knowledge of each of the skills focused upon. This is achieved through the processes of skill analysis and discrimination. Modelling is a central facet of the latter. It has been defined as the process whereby one person learns behaviour patterns through observing them being performed by another person. The process of modelling has been shown to be a critical feature of social learning. This chapter has sought to explore the dimensions of the sensitization phase with particular emphasis on the conceptual and practical aspects of the modelling process. Moreover, guidelines have been presented for trainers relating to the preparation and utilization of descriptive and demonstrative models in CST, with a special focus on the production and application of recorded videotaped models.

9

The practice phase of training

9.1 INTRODUCTION

Once sensitization has been completed the next phase in the training process is that of practice. Trainees should arrive at this stage with essentially a broad understanding of the CST procedure, a realization of the structure and content of the particular programme which they will follow and an awareness of its relevance in equipping them to meet the demands on their communicative competence which they will experience, or perhaps already have, in their chosen profession. More particularly, they should have a knowledge of the specific skill being concentrated upon at that point in training, its characteristics, components and functions in various apposite interpersonal contexts, together with an appreciation of the principles which govern its use. These are typically derived from the theoretical underpinning of the skill. Some appreciation of the appropriateness of different behaviours in particular situations and standards of performance which pertain will also take place during sensitization. As a result, and in relation to outcome, it would be perfectly reasonable to expect students to be able to talk knowledgeably about the skill, to write an essay on it, to make judgements on the effectiveness of its use by another, indeed to make a good attempt at implementation. To anticipate a full-blown and highly polished performance at the first attempt, however, would normally be un-realistically ambitious. In order to promote such levels of proficiency, opportunities to operationalize the information provided during sensitization are commonly regarded as indispensable. Put another way, sensitization can be thought of as a necessary but not sufficient conditon for the promotion of skilled behaviour. Trainees must be allowed to practice.

In the light of this rationale, it is scarcely surprising that the vast majority of the various training interventions which could readily be subsumed under the rubric of social or communication skills training, and details of which are available, have incorporated some element of practice. This was found to be the case by Kurtz and Marshall (1982) who undertook a survey of publications in this area over a twelve year period. A total of 141 studies were accessed in a variety of fields including medicine, social work and counselling. In a high percentage of cases skill practice played a central role in the instructional sequence. A similar survey conducted by Hargie and Morrow (1986a) in pharmacy schools in the UK and Ireland revealed consistent although less pronounced outcomes. In some 70% of programmes, skill practice formed part of training. Again, when methods employed in teaching communication skills to preclinical and clinical students in Medical Schools in the USA were examined by Kahn *et al.* (1979a), practice featured prominently.

This chapter will consider some of the main functions of providing a practice component in training of this nature together with details of the various methods which are available, such as behaviour rehearsal, covert rehearsal, *in vivo* interaction and roleplay. Advantages and disadvantages of each will be discussed and an outline given of practical procedures involved in their implementation. An important part of the chapter will be devoted to the use of observation and recording procedures, particularly video-recording, and some of the steps which can be taken at this stage to maximize their potential and overcome common difficulties. We will continue, though, by unravelling the different influences which have led to decisions being taken to make use of practice as part of training.

9.2 BASES FOR INCORPORATING PRACTICE INTO TRAINING

Why practice should be thought to be so crucial in this respect provokes some interesting speculation. It would seem that trainers justify their inclusion of this component through arguments drawn from one or more of at least five somewhat disparate sources – intuition, epistemology, perceptual-motor skills literature, social learning theory and empirical evidence from CST research.

Intuition

There is an inescapable feeling of 'rightness' in the logic of the old adage that 'practice makes perfect'. Since the ultimate aim of the business is to produce health professionals who are capable of communicating effectively with those with whom they come in contact, since communicating is essentially an active process, and since effecting improvements in this sphere entails bringing about changes in behaviour, it would seem to be little more than common sense to let trainees put what they have been taught into practice and refine their performance as part of the instructional sequence. The thrust of the argument continues along these lines. However the fact that some programmes don't seem to have a practice element would suggest that this particular intuition lacks universality. When two intuitions lead to diametrically opposed conclusions a reconciliation can seldom be arrived at unless additional sources of evidence are contemplated.

Perceptual-motor skills acquisition

The conceptual relationship between social and perceptual-motor skills proposed by such as Argyle and Kendon (1967) will be recalled from earlier chapters. Accepting that there are certain fundamental commonalities between these two types of activity suggests that similar sorts of procedures are likely to be involved in their acquisition. In the learning of motor skills, the importance of practice has long been acknowledged – or to be more precise the importance of practice allied with instructions and/or feedback. It would be unthinkable to try to teach someone to ride a bicycle, drive a car, or shoot clay pigeons without having that person, at some point, attempt to ride, drive or shoot!

At the more formal level of theories of motor skill acquisition, Fitts (1962) postulated that there were three basic stages involved in the process. The first, labelled 'cognitive', features instruction in the various facets of the activity together with the rules and strategies which apply. The subsequent 'associative' phase requires practice so that new patterns of behaviour may become established and errors eliminated. In the final 'autonomous' stage, these patterns come to be performed in a reflex-like fashion. If social skills are perfected in essentially the same manner then practice would seem to be called for.

Social learning processes

The importance of practice is given further credence by some who have concentrated more specifically, on the processes by means of which social learning takes place. The name most commonly associated with social learning theory is that of Bandura (1977a) who believed that the 'learning' of interpersonal acts, in the form of the creation of corresponding cognitive representations, can take place through observation. These notions of modelling will, of course, be familiar from the preceding chapter. Initial attempts at constituting skilled performance, through the conversion of these mental representations into commensurate action, frequently meet with only limited success, necessitating further practice in order to arrive at an accomplished performance.

Epistemology

Others take a more epistemologically oriented line of argument in their justification for having trainees engage in skill practice. The point is made that knowledge, far from being monolithic in nature, can take a diversity of forms. Attempts by philosophers down the centuries to specify just how many exist and agree upon their discriminating features have, unfortunately, met with little success.

The distinction between 'knowing that' and 'knowing how' was mentioned in Chapter 1. It is possible to know that something is the case e.g. that a patient has diabetes mellitus, without knowing how to treat it. It is equally possible to know how to treat it e.g. administer insulin, while being singularly inept at translating that knowledge into practice e.g. manipulating the syringe. This disjunction between knowing and the implementation of that knowledge in action has been voiced by Bochner and Yerby (1977) when commenting upon the acquisition of communication skills. They differentiated between cognitive and experiential learning. While the former produces a conceptual understanding of the process, the latter expedites successful skill operationalization and is dependent upon specific practice in an interpersonal context. Without it, changes in knowledge and attitude may not be reflected in behaviour.

Communication Skills Training research

Finally, in support of the inclusion of a practice component in CST, reference can be made to the limited research which has addressed this issue. The broad finding has been that the complete CST package, including practice, is more effective than any of its abridged versions (Wallace *et al.*, 1981; Froehle *et al.*, 1983). An interesting outcome of the experiment by Wallace *et al.*, (1981) was that increases in measures of skill comprehension were not accompanied by corresponding improvements in performance when practice and subsequent feedback were omitted. Nevertheless, exceptions to this general finding exist (e.g. Peters *et al.*, 1978). Having reviewed some of the work in this area, Fuqua and Gade (1982) found that the evidence supporting the practice element *per se* was inconclusive.

Few, however, have advocated the use of practice on its own as an effective training medium. Upon closer inspection the importance of its role would appear to depend upon a number of factors including its association with other training components, the nature and complexity of the skill under focus, the ability level of the particular group of trainees, the extent to which they already possess elements of the skill, and the level of proficiency deemed acceptable by the trainer in keeping with the objectives of the programme.

9.3 FUNCTIONS OF PRACTICE

A number of different objectives for having trainees implement skills information in practice have been offered. The more central ones have already been intimated but will be specified more explicitly in the following list. They include to:

1. Facilitate the motoric reproductive element of skill acquisition. By performing the various actions that go to make up the skill and experiencing the consequent kinaesthetic feedback, appropriate patterns of behaviour can be built up in keeping with underlying intentions. Care must be taken though to ensure that such procedures don't degenerate into the mere rote production of stereotypic behaviour to the neglect of the mechanisms which effect the selective application of appropriate skills in context;

2. Enable the outcomes of skill deployment to be realized. One possible reason for failing to make use of already acquired skills may be due to an inaccurate anticipation of negative consequences e.g. the belief that listening to patients' anxieties and encouraging their ventilation will only exacerbate them;

3. Highlight incongruities between what trainees think they do and what is actually done. Only through interacting and being made aware of their involvement in it can discrepancies between trainees' intentions and actions be reduced;

4. Create a more realistic and personally meaningful appreciation of the circumstances which attend skill deployment. It is difficult to create this level of awareness through lectures or observing models – one has to experience it;

5. Effect changes in attitude. By acting in a particular manner in accordance with some skill, more fundamental attitudinal adjustments may be created which will serve to maintain that type of behaviour in future;

6. Enable the professional role for which the student is ultimately being trained to be 'tried out'. The extent to which such opportunities are afforded will depend largely upon the type of practical experience provided;

7. Gain confidence. Promoting feelings of self-confidence is an important but frequently overlooked aspect of CST. Bandura (1977b) pointed out that failure to display appropriate levels of skill in a given situation may be due to the lack of a sense of self-efficacy. In other words, not having sufficient confidence in one's ability to put acquired skill to use;

8. Furnish broad insights into the complexities of certain social situations and the rules and conventions that pertain;

9. Produce more lasting benefits from training. It has been speculated that

the outcomes of programmes lacking practice and feedback components may be transitory;

10. Involve students more fully in the learning experience. It is widely
accepted that learning is more successful under these circumstances and
that students who are playing an active role find it more attractive and
stimulating.

9.4 METHODS OF PRACTICE

There are a variety of techniques from which to choose when considering
how best to provide an appropriate and meaningful practical experience
as part of the training sequence. Among the most common are covert
rehearsal, behaviour rehearsal, roleplay, simulation exercises and games
and *in vivo* practice (e.g. interviews with patients).

Before outlining the possibilities which each has to offer some time may
usefully be spent contemplating the underlying dimensions which discriminate between these options, in an attempt to arrive at a reasonably
organized if not quite exhaustive taxonomy.

Perhaps the most basic distinction is between simulation and *in vivo*
practice. The former seeks to recreate the key operational features of some
actual situation within the classroom, while the latter makes use of the 'real
life' encounter. *In vivo* practice is centred in the work place, perhaps with a
patient or health professional.

There are obvious advantages in maximizing the fidelity of the practical
experience by ensuring that what takes place during it approximates to the
real world equivalent in as many important respects as possible. Trainee
motivation and the extent to which the effects of training carry over to the

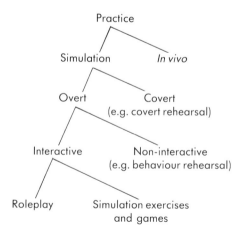

Fig. 9.1 Dimensions of practice.

work-place increase as a result. But this does not mean that the one must mirror the other in every respect. If it did then presumably all skill practice would be best conducted in the ward, the consulting room, the patient's home, etc. In the early stages of training, in particular, the consequences of doing so could be highly counterproductive. There are merits, rather, in representing actual situations which would lend themselves to the use of a certain skill, through simulation.

Flowers and Booraem (1980) define simulation as the imitation of the form of something or someone without the assumption of the reality. Some of the associated advantages have been outlined by Stammers and Patrick (1975). Among these are:

1. Safety. The consequences of making errors are less grave than in the real situation;
2. Overcoming ethical problems. These can arise when inexperienced students deal with patients or clients;
3. Control. The simulated environment is largely free from the vagaries which beset its 'real world' counterpart. No student need, therefore, be faced with demands that outstrip the resources which they have available, at that particular stage of their professional development;
4. Additional instruction. It is much easier to provide supplementary guidance and coaching. Again feedback possibilities are enhanced as will be illustrated in the following chapter;
5. Varying the time span. The ability to manipulate the temporal dimension of the piece of interaction can be a considerable benefit;
6. Costs. Creating practical experience through simulation tends to be a much less expensive option than some of the alternatives including periods of placement in the field.

Simulation practice may be either overt or, by utilizing mental imagery, take a covert form. Overt practice can occur within the context of an extended piece of spontaneous interaction. Perhaps the most common example of this is roleplay. But non-interactive overt practice is another possibility which merely requires that aspects of the targeted skill be produced separately and in isolation as part, for example, of a behaviour rehearsal exercise.

In addition to roleplay, practice may be achieved through the use of various simulation exercises and games. (The use of roleplay and simulation procedures in the *evaluation* of skill performance are considered in Chapter 11. Here they will be discussed as methods of enabling skills to be practised).

Covert rehearsal

At present there is a rejuvenation of scientific interest in the topic of mental imagery. Reviews of therapeutic interventions which directly exploit this phenomenon are provided by, for example, Mahoney (1974) and Goldfried and Goldfried (1980). The use of covert rehearsal in CST belongs to this genre. To date it has featured more extensively in the remedial and developmental spheres, than in the specialized training of health professionals. However it has been put to use, and with some success, in counsellor education (Baker *et al.*, 1985).

Simply put, this technique requires trainees to 'visualize' performing the targeted skill through mental images. They must imagine a specified situation and then go over 'in their mind's eye' the appropriate action. Practice is therefore entirely covert taking the form of an imagined reproduction of the skill or procedure introduced during sensitization. According to Bandura (1977a) the process facilitates the temporal and spatial organization of cognitive elements into a pattern which approximates to that presented in the earlier stages of instruction, prior to behavioural enactment.

Practice through covert rehearsal can be incorporated into either group or individualized training regimes and is carried out in the following stages:

1. A state of physical and mental relaxation is induced by the trainer. (Information on relaxation techniques can be found in Bernstein and Borkovec, 1973; Wolpe, 1973; and Morris, 1980.)
2. The scene in which the skill is to be utilized is depicted as graphically as possible so that it can be readily visualized by trainees.
3. Members of the class are instructed to imagine themselves responding in accordance with the targeted skill. They may be asked to respond 'internally' to a trigger statement made by a significant other in the scene.
4. They should be encouraged to picture the consequences of their covert performance so that judgements may begin to be formed as to the likely effects of really behaving in this way.
5. The scene can be gone through several times to promote the contemplation and imaginal testing out of a variety of coping strategies before attempts are made to identify the one that seems most appropriate. This stage, strongly recommended by Cartledge and Milburn (1986), is more likely to foster an understanding of effective interaction as a process demanding a flexible, decision-making approach rather than the unthinking performance of rigid, stereotypical patterns of behaviour.
6. Experiences are discussed and general outcomes and recommendations established during de-briefing.

Advantages and disadvantages of covert rehearsal

There are various advantages and disadvantages associated with this form of practice which should be appreciated by the trainer before trying it out. Among the latter can be listed:

1. 'High risk' option – it can flop! It tends to be better suited to the more mature, experienced, well-motivated and imaginative student.
2. Can be viewed as silly or boring.
3. Some trainees find it difficult to create and sustain the appropriate imagery.
4. Difficult for the trainer to comment on 'performance'.
5. No guarantee that that which is imagined will be successfully enacted.

Advantages, on the other hand, include:

1. Potential for modifying cognitions and emotions. This may well be where its real value lies. Imagery-based interventions have been found capable of producing changes in, for instance, perceptual sensitivity, self-awareness, self-control, and reduced levels of anxiety (Hazler and Hipple, 1981; Baker *et al.*, 1985).
2. May be extremely useful in cases where other types of practice would be difficult to arrange, for either logistical, safety or ethical reasons e.g. dealing with physical violence on a psychiatric ward, coping with explicit sexual advances, etc.
3. Trainees, once familiarized, can readily use it on their own.
4. Special benefits in helping trainees deal with situations that are anxiety provoking. Given the proper expertise, there is scope for extending these exercises in accordance with systematic desensitization procedures.
5. Some empirical evidence attesting to its efficacy particularly with more advanced trainees learning more complex skills (Baker *et al.*, 1985). It is an interesting speculation that at the level of higher-order operation, competence may essentially involve the development of plans and strategies for using already acquired subskills in original ways. Such reorganization probably takes place, more importantly, at a cognitive rather than a behavioural level and, in consequence, lends itself to rehearsal which is covert in nature.

It is unlikely that covert will ever replace overt rehearsal as a means of providing practice in CST. But the potential which it has to offer, in a complementary capacity, has yet to be fully appreciated. Baker *et al.* (1986), reported that the combination of the two methods resulted in a form of practice which was superior to either alone in the acquisition of counselling skills.

Behaviour rehearsal

In the overwhelming majority of CST programmes, participants have been required to overtly implement the skills information presented. Practice has been explicit and often carried out within the framework of an ongoing spontaneous interaction such as an interview, group discussion, case conference or counselling session, often in simulation.

Behaviour rehearsal techniques are non-interactive in this sense. They don't require the participation of others. Trainees can practise on their own provided that they have a concept of the targeted skill and the criteria governing acceptability of performance. As pointed out by Hargie and McCartan (1986), some behaviours lend themselves more readily to this very focused means of practice. Among these are various facets of non-verbal behaviour. In order to improve active listening and the communication of empathic understanding, for example, students may be given the task of perhaps reading a well known poem, nursery rhyme or story in such a way that different pre-determined emotions are conveyed through paralanguage. Those who might find this material rather childish can be asked instead to be a 'newscaster' by picking a story from the newspaper and reading it in accordance with such underlying states as enthusiasm, boredom, sympathy, sincerity, joy and so on. If an audio-recorder is used (and most students have one) these attempts can be played back, evaluated and, since each shouldn't last long, repeated and improved upon.

Advantages and disadvantages of behaviour rehearsal

Advantages include:

1. Focus upon objective behaviour. Trainees must be able to translate their understanding of the skills material into practice.
2. Trainees can practise on their own. It can therefore be used as homework.
3. Some may feel less inhibited when others are not involved.
4. Easier to devote full attention to a specific aspect of behaviour unhampered by the complexities surrounding ongoing interaction.

Behaviour rehearsal has also disadvantages such as:

1. May be regarded as silly or childish. A thoughtful introduction can often overcome these attitudes.
2. Trainees must have a firm and accurate realization of what constitutes acceptable performance.
3. Opportunities for checking progress by drawing upon the views and comments of others may be lacking.
4. Little appreciation can be gained of the consequences of implementing the skill during interaction.
5. Emphasis is upon the production of a particular behaviour to the possible exclusion of such vitally important matters as the circumstances determining expediency of action.

Some of these drawbacks can be overcome by including other trainees in the process. Thus in the exercise described above, the poem or passage could be read to another, or to a small group, rather than to a taperecorder. They would then have to guess the emotion 'behind the words'. An alternative along these lines, which could also be used in connection with the skill of Reflection of Feeling, is suggested in Exercise 9.1.

Exercise 9.1 Conveying feelings

Aim

This exercise is designed to facilitate the identification of verbally implied feelings and their accurate communication by nonverbal means.

Preparation

Make out sets of about 25 cards, each card with a few sentences on it suggesting, but not explicitly mentioning, some underlying affective state. Some of these may be fairly easy e.g. anger, depression, etc., others more subtle e.g. confidence, attraction, and so on.

Organization

Divide the group into subgroups of 4–5 members. Provide each subgroup with a set of cards. At the end, feedback from each subgroup on the discussion points may be shared.

Instructions

Place the cards face down on the table and have someone pick the first. Having done so this member should decide upon the feeling which underlies the words and then try to convey it to the rest of the group by nonverbal means only. Starting with the member on that person's right, the rest of the group should try to identify this feeling. Once someone succeeds the statement on the card is read out, if the majority of the group decide that the feeling depicted was not really the one on the card the same member has to try again. Members take it in turn, in this way, to select a card. If after each member has had two attempts at guessing, a particular feeling cannot be identified that card should be passed on to the next for that person to try. A tally of guesses required to achieve identification for each card can be recorded and, at the end, an average score arrived at, on this basis, for each member. (This is optional).

Issues for discussion

1. How easy was it to grasp the emotional message on the card? Would the presence of paralinguistic and nonverbal accompaniments have made a difference?
2. Having decided upon the emotion, what were the problems in trying to convey it?
3. Were some feelings much easier than others to depict? If so which ones and why?

Behaviour rehearsal techniques are not limited to non-verbal aspects of performance. Exercise 9.2 outlines a procedure to provide practice in the skill of questioning.

Exercise 9.2 Asking questions

Aim

To facilitate the use of different types of question.

Preparation

1. A set of about 5–6 cards each outlining (a) a particular situation, and (b) some background detail on the individual featured e.g. You are new to the ward. Mrs Brown has been in hospital for almost a week with severe lower back pain. Having introduced yourself you ask . . .
2. A sheet listing a range of types of question e.g. open, closed, leading, extension probe, clarification probe, etc. It is necessary to give some thought to the sequence to ensure that, for instance, probing questions are at the end rather than the beginning.

Organization

Divide the group into subgroups of 5–6 members. Provide each subgroup with a set of cards and a sheet of question types.

Instruction

The exercise commences with a member picking a card and reading it to the rest of the group. This same member then asks an appropriate question in keeping with the first type listed on the sheet e.g. if this happened to be 'open questions' an appropriate response could be 'How are you feeling to-day, Mrs Brown?'. The next member then asks a question, on the same topic, according to the second type on the sheet, and so on until a question of each type has been posed.

The second card is then lifted by the member opposite the one who picked the first and the exercise continues. Throughout, the group has the added task of monitoring to ensure that each question asked is indeed of the specified type and that members don't take an inordinate length of time when having a turn.

A scoring system can be implemented such that each correct response is awarded a mark with a mark being deducted from an individual's total for each mistake.

Discussion

Discussion can focus upon particular examples that proved problematic. Further sensitization may be necessary if it is found that some types of question consistently caused problems.

Group-based methods of behaviour rehearsal, if suitably introduced, can be fully enjoyed by trainees. Group involvement means that feedback from others is available and the individual is not forced to rely solely upon his own, perhaps idiosyncratic notions of propriety. Nevertheless, while these techniques do enable closely targeted and highly concentrated practice to take place what they can provide is necessarily limited due to their inherently restricted nature. For this reason they frequently prelude interactive experiences such as roleplay.

Roleplay

Roleplay has a remarkably wide range of educational applications and, in terms of CST, is probably the most common form of simulated interactive practice. It requires the trainee to take on, and behave in accordance with a role not normally his own, or if his own, one that would not usually be played in that situation. The role may be that of an imaginary person or someone who actually exists and is known to him. The other or others taking part in the interaction may likewise be indulging in roleplay and what transpires can be largely predetermined or completely improvised.

The origins of roleplay tend to be traced back to Moreno (1953), who introduced it as a means of improving the general social skills of a group of delinquent girls in anticipation of their release from the institutional setting in which they had been living. It is eminently suited to this type of intervention for several reasons:

1. It affords the safety and control of simulation;
2. The experience provided of a situation can closely replicate that of the 'real world' equivalent;
3. Trainees find it attractive when properly organized and presented;
4. It offers substantial opportunities for concerted feedback;
5. Situations which occur infrequently in reality, can be arranged as required;
6. Since students are also involved as roleplay partners they gain some insights into what it is like to be in the position of 'the other' in the encounter. Opportunities exist, therefore, for improving awareness and sensitivity;
7. It engages the totality of the learner and changes can be effected not only in behaviour but in beliefs, attitudes and feelings.

This latter point is worth elaborating upon. While the primary objective of roleplay, as a means of CST practice, is to produce improvements in particular pre-established facets of performance, it can make more extensive contributions. According to Milroy (1982), these include:

1. facilitating the integration of theory and practice
2. gaining broad experience of a role

3. promoting greater awareness of self and others
4. furthering problem-solving capacity
5. focusing upon difficult situations and contentious issues.

The objectives which one has in mind, though, will be more or less successfully met depending upon the type of roleplay engaged in.

Types of roleplay

While different labels have been attached to varying roleplay procedures, a dimension which has been the basis of perhaps the most common distinction is that of structure.

Structured roleplays   Here the goals and circumstances of the roleplay are preordained. The general scenario is presented to the students at the outset and key characteristics of the roles involved, such as status, personality, knowledge, disposition, etc., are settled. The relationship which each participant shares with the others is also clarified. The lines along which the roleplay will develop tend to be envisaged beforehand together with the particular issues to be brought forth. The main purposes of the exercise typically revolve around experiencing the inbuilt tensions and influences which emerge and arriving at acceptable solutions.

This type of roleplay tends to be provided by the trainer, especially in more elaborate cases requiring quite detailed information in written form. Trainees, however, may also be given the task of formulating examples perhaps based upon real situations previously encountered.

Distinct similarities exist between structured and what has been referred to by Wohlking and Gill (1980) as *method-centred roleplay*. This approach is particularly suited to skills training when the skill in question is simple, easily broken down into a series of steps, and when the social process involving the skill is quite short and largely ritualistic e.g. admitting a patient, conducting a hearing test, etc.

Unstructured roleplay   Here what takes place is much less premeditated. Although initiated with an explicit aim in mind the unfolding interaction depends largely upon the improvizations of those taking part. While roles and a specific situation are identified prior to commencement, judgements as to how the roles should be played, relationships between them and the progression of the encounter, together with its outcome, are left to be worked out as it develops. Students are frequently involved in devising these exercises based upon their concerns, attitudes and experiences.

The Wohlking and Gill equivalent is termed *developmental roleplay*. In this case a challenging problem is presented and trainees are encouraged to formulate and test various strategies in dealing with it. A special feature of this approach is that it facilitates the scrutiny of feelings and motives underlying action. It can also be used successfully in the training of advanced communication skills which are part of more complex interactive processes such as counselling or negotiating.

Semi-structured roleplay The essential characteristic, as the label implies, has to do with the intermediate level of constraint imposed upon the interaction. In practice this type of roleplay is often trainer-initiated but it permits greater scope for trainee interpretation than the more structured counterpart. Consequently, it often proves more attractive to trainees.

Stages in roleplaying

The likely success of this type of simulated interactive practice depends largely upon the trainer being aware of the various stages involved, the particular requirements of each and how they should be handled.

Preparation A lack of adequate preparation is probably the most frequent cause of those taking part failing to benefit from the experience. A useful starting point is in establishing the learning objectives to be accomplished. These stem from the educational needs of the group and may be quite narrowly focused e.g. specific skill improvement, mastery of a certain technique, etc. or more general and abstract such as effecting a tighter integration of existing knowledge. They need not be mutually exclusive, of course. While several objectives may be pursued in the course of a single roleplay, being overly ambitious in this respect can de-focus the exercise leaving students confused and uncertain.

Having identified appropriate learning objectives, thought has to be given to the type of roleplay best suited to achieving them. Features of the group including maturity, familiarity, motivation and experience must not be overlooked since these will have an important bearing upon what is likely to work. As a crude rule-of-thumb, less structured, developmental roleplays tend to be more successful when:

1. The objectives are to increase awareness, change attitudes, explore feelings or illuminate underlying issues;
2. Trainees are more mature and experienced;
3. Trainees are more familiar with, and trusting of each other;
4. The interactive process featured is highly complex;
5. The programme is well advanced.

In some instances it may be useful, for example, to increase students' awareness of the problems faced in a certain situation being dealt with by having them take part in a developmental roleplay during sensitization.

When these circumstances don't prevail and when the general purpose is, perhaps, to refine skills, especially those which are quite basic, then more structured variants should be contemplated.

In addition to determining the degree of structure there are a variety of other techniques which can be used and which should be considered at this stage. Amongst these are:

1. *Multiple roleplay* This involves dividing the group into subgroups each of which enacts the scenario simultaneously. Everyone is involved and some members may be designated to act as observers recording what takes place for the purposes of feedback. Multiple roleplay is frequently associated with the more structured, method-centred approach.
2. *Fish-bowl technique* In this case several trainees enact the roleplay in the centre of the room with the rest of the group looking on – hence the name. This is arguably the most common variant being particularly suited to exploring the complexities of situations and gaining insights into underlying issues. As a means of skill practice though it is more limited.
3. *Role rotation* Here a number of trainees take it in turn to play the main role, usually the 'health professional'. Other roles may also be rotated although there is an attendant risk of seriously compromising the continuity of the interaction. Role rotation is one method of offering at least some skill practice to a number of trainees in a short space of time.
4. *Role reversal* The essential feature of this technique is that participants have an opportunity, at some point during the interaction, to switch roles so that, for example, 'the GP' now becomes 'the patient' and vice versa. This can be a very effective way of developing self-awareness, changing attitudes and encouraging empathic understanding. By having student nurses play the role of patients with various problems and handicaps, Williams (1978) reasoned that a greater appreciation of the special needs of these groups could be brought about.

Once issues of learning objectives and type of procedure to use have been settled the trainer must give thought to actually providing a suitable roleplay. Here there are three possibilities:

1. Borrow or purchase existing material from sources such as Pfeiffer and Jones (1970) and Clark (1978);
2. Trainees create the roleplay, with proper guidance from the trainer;
3. Trainer creates the roleplay.

Writing roleplays is not difficult and has the advantage of more completely meeting the requirements of the particular training programme. There are benefits, however, in adopting a systematic approach:

1. Identify the background situation or scenario. It should be meaningful to the group and in keeping with the established learning objectives;

2. Write the scenario establishing the location of the action together with the salient events which have led to it. This should be done simply and concisely;
3. Decide upon the roles. It may be imprudent at the beginning to specify roles which differ radically from those familiar to trainees;
4. Write role-briefs. Producing role-brief cards is a useful way at this. These should document the relevant motives, beliefs and abilities of the player together with the major influences to which they are subjected. Again, one has to consider how much each player must know about each of the others and what information should be private;
5. Decide upon a time-frame. This can vary widely depending on the purpose of the exercise but 10–20 minutes is usually adequate for skill practice;
6. Decide upon setting, props, etc. Roleplay is not acting and there is seldom need for an elaborate arrangement of props. Occasionally, though, some may be invaluable. Having a large doll, for instance, is an extremely useful aid when a trainee health visitor is explaining to a 'young mother' how to bath baby!

Some of these points are illustrated in the semi-structured roleplay provided in Exercise 9.3.

Exercise 9.3 Semi-structured roleplay for listening

Aim

1. To give practice in the skill of listening.
2. To create an awareness of some of the circumstances which can get in the way of effective listening.

Preparation

Make copies of roleplay scenario and role-briefs.

Scenario. The Brown family comprises Mr Brown and Mrs Brown (Junior) both in their early forties; the children, Joan (8 years), Samantha (6 years) and Colin (5 years); and Mrs Brown (Senior) who is in her late seventies and moved in following the death, 4 years ago, of her sister with whom she had been living. She has been bedridden for the past year as a result of an extensive stroke and her condition has slowly but steadily deteriorated until she now needs constant attention.

Mr Brown, a primary school teacher, has an elder brother who lives in London but with whom he has little contact and two younger sisters, both married, who live nearby but have little to do with their mother.

Having attended to Mrs Brown's pressure sores, during a visit, the Community Nurse came down stairs to find the daughter-in-law in tears with her husband trying to console her. Mr Brown asks the Community Nurse if she could help to find out what is wrong and Mrs Brown (Junior) begins to explain how she is finding it all too much . . .

Mrs Brown. Recently you have been finding it increasingly difficult to cope with looking after the house, the children, your husband and your mother-in-law. Although your husband cares deeply for you and the children, and you for him, everything seems left to you to deal with. No one seems to recognize how much you are expected to do. While you get on well with your mother-in-law and would hate to have her feel rejected, you find that you can no longer tend her. What about her son and daughters, don't they have any responsibilities . . .?

Mr Brown. You owe your mother a lot and are very fond of her. In spite of the fact that your father died when you were young she was determined that you would not have to leave school to find a job. You simply can't have her dumped in a geriatric ward or nursing home. She was always there when you needed her – you can't let her down now . . . yet there is your wife and children.

   At the time your aunt died, both sisters objected strongly to you taking your mother to live with you and a family quarrel ensued. Although they visited your mother in hospital, at the time of her stroke, they have not done so since she was discharged. You think that, regardless of their feelings toward you and your wife, they should come to see her. But they, like you, have a stubborn streak!

Community Nurse. This has come as something of a surprise. Of course you had been alert to the possibility, but Mrs Brown (Junior) had appeared to be managing without apparent difficulty. Indeed, you had admired her resolve, fully appreciating the demands which this sort of situation can make. When your own mother fell ill you had nursed her at home until she died, giving up work in order to do so. Indeed, in many ways, Mrs Brown (Senior) reminds you of her . . .!

Organization

Divide the group into subgroups of three members each, or 4–5 if observers are used. Roleplays should last about ten minutes and should, if possible, be video-recorded. At the end feedback should be provided within subgroups. The main points to emerge can be raised with the whole group.

Instructions

Introduce the roleplay, establish appropriate climate, allocate roles and re-hearse the major characteristics of the skill of listening.

Discussion

Following the enactment, discussion should involve feedback from video-recordings and/or observers, and should centre upon:

1. The extent to which both the husband and wife were listened to and the verbal and nonverbal bases of those judgements;

2. Characteristics of the situation which made listening difficult;
3. Factors which, in general, detract from accurate listening and how these can be overcome.

Introduction This involves orienting trainees, both procedurally and affectively, to the technique. The latter can, on occasion, be much more difficult but unless an accommodating disposition can be created the exercise is doomed to failure from the beginning.

Depending upon the group, roleplay may be introduced either directly or indirectly. The former involves presenting the notion, explaining what it entails and dealing with any misgivings or resistances which may arise e.g. belief that it requires acting ability, too artificial to be useful, etc. With the indirect alternative, 'roleplay' is not mentioned as such. Rather the group is gradually brought to a stage where they are doing it without being aware of the fact e.g. moving from discussing what should have been done in some situation to inviting a student to demonstrate it.

Regardless of the strategy invoked it is imperative that a facilitative climate be created. This is typified by a freedom from anxiety, an openness to change and the confidence to experiment while accepting that mistakes may happen. This may be more difficult to create with trainees who are subject to mild levels of communication apprehension. The role of the trainer is crucial in this respect. His approach should be open, honest and sensitive. Perhaps above all the overriding purpose of the enterprise as a structured learning experience rather than a form of assessment should be stressed.

The procedural aspect of the introductory stage has several facets encompassing:

1. The allocation of roles to trainees. This can be done by asking for volunteers although there may be merit in having particular members play certain roles. Doing so on a counter-to-type basis can be a valuable way of changing attitudes and promoting interpersonal sensitivity e.g. having a rather assertive member play the relatively powerless role of patient.
2. Establishing and briefing observers. This is especially important if the interaction is not being video- or audio-recorded. Observers should be in no doubt as to what exactly it is that they are required to focus upon. Various types of recording schedule, some of which will be reviewed in the next chapter, and in Chapter 11, can help in this respect and make the procedure more thorough and systematic.
3. Recapping on the major features of the targeted skill, when the roleplay is designed to facilitate skill practice. This need not take long and indeed may be omitted when the practical follows on directly from the sensitization phase.

Videotaped material can also be used as a means of effectively introducing trainees to roleplay. Several strategies may be adopted. A short segment of an interaction can be played and trainees asked to demonstrate how they think the interaction should proceed. This can be a particularly successful way of 'triggering' a piece of developmental roleplay.

Alternatively, a quite short but complete practitioner-patient interaction may be presented where the interpersonal performance of the practitioner is rather poor. Trainees can then be asked to roleplay the same scenario, demonstrating improved performance on the part of the health professional. Exemplars should be carefully chosen to reflect the training needs of the group and to present situations which they will find challenging. The resulting roleplays are, of course, much more structured in this case. Students tend to find this approach highly motivating. Moreover, trainers can have a positive model of the same situation prepared in advance thereby allowing the group the opportunity to compare their efforts against alternative strategies during feedback.

Interaction Participants should now be ready to commence. Once the roleplay gets under way the instructor's job (assuming he is not directly involved) is largely one of monitoring. The temptation to constantly intervene to ensure that things happen exactly as was intended should be curbed. It spoils the coherence of the enactment, makes it difficult for roles to be played convincingly and is generally de-motivating. Van Ments (1983) has, however, identified a number of occasions when intervention is warranted, such as:

1. One or more player persistently dropping out of role. This may be due to an inadequate introduction to the exercise;
2. Roles being excessively overacted. This can stem from inexperience or, more insidiously, be a deliberate attempt at sabotage!
3. Stultified performance. A common cause is anxiety or insufficient time to get into role;
4. Over-involvement of players. The trainer should be on hand to defuse the situation;
5. A player in difficulty. Here a tactful rescue is called for. The trainer should always be mindful of the embarrassment which can result from this situation and try to minimise it;
6. Roleplay deviating markedly from what was envisaged. If it appears unlikely that any useful learning points will accrue from its continuation the enactment should be aborted;
7. Providing feedback. The trainer may feel justified in occasionally interrupting to draw attention to some important happening.

The trainer also acts as a director, during the enactment, ensuring that a time schedule is adhered to and that things happen when they should.

Feedback and discussion   In many respects this is the most valuable stage of the roleplay process and typically requires from two to three times as long to complete as the interaction itself. During it, the events of the interaction are analysed and clarified, underlying causes of what happened are identified and general principles governing interpersonal communication arrived at. Since these issues more properly fall within the ambit of the following chapter, which deals with the feedback phase of training, they will not be further elaborated upon at this point.

One further function of this final part of the roleplay exercise has to do with 'de-roling' or easing participants out of the roles played. Its salience increases in relation to the depth of immersion achieved – especially in roles demanding a strong emotional involvement. This can be done by facilitating the ventilation of residual feelings and progressively relating to these individuals more obviously as students rather than the characters of the roles. If need be, participants may be asked to repeat their names, proper roles, true circumstances, etc. It is not always necessary to go to these lengths though, and indeed, some find this quite superfluous.

Roleplay is probably the most common method of practice in CST. Through it a reasonable fascimile of the sort of situation with which the trainee will have to cope can be created in the safety of the classroom. It does have limitations, however, including:

1. Some trainees find it difficult to accept;
2. Some trainees, while acknowledging its value as a learning technique, experience difficulty in taking on and sustaining a role;
3. Outcomes may not carry over from the training environment to the real world.

Simulation exercises and games

The relationship between roleplay and simulation exercises and games is complex and the dividing line between them tenuous. For a start, all of the practice methods already covered in this chapter rely upon simulation to some extent. In this broad sense, simulation can be thought of as a simplified 'representation of a real-life dynamic situation' (Milroy, 1982, p.178). It provides a rubric which subsumes a variety of techniques each with features which enable loose distinctions to be made. Some of these take the form of games and exercises.

Simulation exercises are structured affairs which depict the salient parameters and vectors of some real or hypothetical event and require the student to operate in accordance with them in reaching a decision or completing a task. Although they may involve an element of roleplay they tend to be distinguished from it on a number of counts. These have been neatly encapsulated by Jones (1985, p.5) in the following statement:

'Although simulations have roles, they do not have play, but are concerned with a job and a function not a new personality'.

Simulation exercises are often group-based. They are incorporated into training to create an awareness of, for instance, role relationships and conflicts, the various constraints and influences which can impinge upon different positions within a social structure, and to provide the individual with an experience of how an organization or system works. It is possible, on the other hand, for these exercises to be carried out in dyads. (Exercise 9.4.) A central objective in this case, is to provide a skill practice opportunity within a context that can frequently be remarkably similar to 'the real thing'.

Exercise 9.4 Obtaining a medical history

Aim

To offer practice in conducting a medical history-type interview.

Preparation

1. A content sheet. This should outline the various areas of content to be covered during the interview. A copy should be provided for each student.
2. A process sheet. Here the different skills and processes of the interview which are being practised should be included.

Organization

Divide the group into dyads, or if it is necessary to use observers, triads.

Instructions

Identify interviewers, interviewees, and observers. While interviewers and observers are being briefed, interviewees can have a coffee-break. Distribute content and process sheets and familiarize interviewers with them. Interviewers should be given some time to plan and prepare, realizing that a complete history, which will probably necessitate note-taking, is required. Observers should be clear what they are to look for and how it is to be recorded.

While interviewers and observers are getting ready, interviewees can be briefed. This should be minimal. All they need to know is that they will be required to give their medical history to date. If there are facets of it which they would rather not disclose these can be withheld, but they should try to make it as genuine as possible.

Interviews should last about fifteen minutes. Given time, each student can have the opportunity to interview.

Discussion

Discussion can focus upon the following issues:

1. How effectively were the pre-established skills and procedures implemented?
2. How complete was the history? Were there areas ignored?
3. Were some areas easier to explore than others?
4. What did it feel like to be interviewed in this way?

The distinguishing feature of *simulation games* is the element of competition which is inbuilt. Here participants have goals which they strive to achieve. There is frequently the possibility of some being able to facilitate or thwart others in their quest. In any case it is important that, at the end, there is a winner, clearly identified through pre-established criteria. If the optional scoring procedures provided are incorporated, Exercises 9.1 and 9.2 take on distinct features of gaming, albeit games with an uncharacteristically restricted ambit and narrowly focused objectives.

The trainer should approach simulation exercises and games with the same four stages in mind as those which typify roleplay, namely:

1. Preparation. Here aims and objectives are often quite broad such as illuminating a concept, providing initial experience of a novel situation or insights into how some complex system operates. But they can also be quite specific and personally oriented e.g. increasing awareness of personal involvement in a given situation or improving levels of skill in it.

   When it comes to getting hold of games and exercises of this type, the two main alternatives are either to use ones already developed or design your own. Those intending to pursue the former option may find useful sources in Dukes and Seidner (1978) and Flowers and Booraem (1980). Trainers who prefer to construct their own should consult, for instance, Jones (1985).
2. Introduction
3. Interaction
4. Feedback and discussion

Much of what was discussed, under these points, in relation to roleplay is of relevance here and will not be repeated.

Advantages and disadvantages of simulation exercises and games

Again many of the advantages and disadvantages of this method of practice have already been mentioned, particularly in relation to the comments made about simulation in general as an approach to practice. Advantages include:

1. Little of consequence hangs upon mistakes being made;
2. What takes place can be largely pre-determined and is capable of being closely controlled by the trainer;
3. The intention, in using simulation exercises and games, is frequently to reduce the complexity of the actual situation by extracting only the salient features or influences from it;
4. The possibility of ethical issues being raised as a result of having trainees practise in the real situation are eliminated;
5. Additional instruction during the interaction is easier to give although the trainer must recognize the dangers of violating the integrity of the simulation in so doing;
6. There are extensive opportunities for providing detailed information on what took place during the interaction;
7. Simulation exercises and particularly games, if properly prepared, carefully chosen, and adequately introduced, can prove extremely popular with trainees who often find them less threatening than roleplays. This is particularly the case with exercises which have as the major focus, the operation of systems rather than the performance of a particular individual.

Nevertheless, drawbacks also exist among which can be cited:

1. Some trainees, failing to appreciate the benefits to be derived from this technique, may see it as grown-ups 'playing games' and therefore regard it as ridiculously childish;
2. In order for it to succeed, considerable thought and careful planning must go into the design of the simulation. Even so it is often impossible to anticipate all weaknesses at this stage. These often surface, for the first time, during the enactment and can spoil it;
3. These techniques, especially when group-based, can take up considerable time which, in turn, can create practical problems of two sorts. Firstly, they may require a disproportionate amount of the total time given over to this part of the course. Secondly, it may be difficult to find a suitably large slot on the students' timetable to accommodate them. It is often necessary, therefore, to spread the exercise over several sessions, although the enactment should be completed in a single one;
4. Compared with roleplay, simulation exercises and games tend not to lend themselves to in-depth analysis of particular relationships; the illumination of the intra-personal factors, including feelings and attitudes, which subtend social behaviour; or the promotion of profound levels of self-awareness;
5. There is always the possibility that learning which takes place in the simulated environment will fail to be applied in the situation for which trainees are being prepared.

In vivo practice

It will be recalled from Fig. 9.1 that simulation and *in vivo* practice are the two basic alternatives when it comes to devising some sort of practical exercise which will permit trainees to attempt to operationalize their knowledge of the targeted skill. The majority of practice techniques available in CST, including those already discussed, rely upon simulation in some form. On the other hand there are exceptions which are not premised upon the essential 'as if' requirement of this approach, where 'make believe' is not a condition and where uncontrived interaction is engaged in. It is to *in vivo* methods that attention will now be directed.

This procedure necessitates, firstly, participants acting in accordance with the roles which they would typically play in those situations in which they are located – in other words 'being themselves'; secondly, that which transpires between them being natural rather than contrived; and, thirdly, this interaction being grounded in an appropriate situational context. *In vivo* practice is overt rather than covert, with the skill being implemented during the course of an ongoing interpersonal encounter. Thus the student operates in the normal work setting, whether that be a ward, pharmacy, health clinic or client's home, with an actual patient, client, relative or health practitioner, about some genuine concern in order to meet a real need or achieve a proper goal. The much greater demands placed upon trainees as a result will be readily appreciated. Not only do they have to perform the skill or procedure focused upon but there is often a more general, but very real, expectation that they 'be a member' of the profession to which they aspire. Great care must, therefore, be taken to ensure that the individual is adequately prepared for what, potentially, can be a tremendously beneficial learning experience.

In the training procedure described by Maguire (1984b) for instructing medical students in interviewing procedures, this type of practice was given. Having been introduced, through videotapes, handouts and discussion, to the different stages of the case-history interview, the skills required, the areas which should be explored and difficult situations which may be encountered, each member of the group carried out an interview with a patient. This component was part of a clerkship in psychiatry and patients were recovering from an affective disorder, psychoneurosis or alcoholism. Interviews lasted fifteen minutes during which students had to find out about the patients' present problems, being sensitive to those that were physical and social as well as psychiatric. Students were told that they could take notes if they wished and afterwards were required to produce a written history. Apart from the fact that patients were, to some extent, hand-picked on the basis of their willingness to co-operate and the likelihood that they would not prove too difficult to deal with, this exercise was, to all intents and purposes, what these students would be required to carry out as part of their routine duties if, once qualified, they chose to work on that ward.

Advantages and disadvantages of in vivo *practice*

Some of the strengths and weaknesses of this method have already been attended to in other contexts. Due to the nature of their relationship, the disadvantages of simulation techniques often coincide with the advantages of *in vivo* procedures and vice versa. Risking repetition in the interests of completeness, the advantages can be itemized as including:

1. Greater realism. There can be no motivational difficulties due to charges that the exercise is false or artificial if trainees are adequately prepared to undertake it and are made aware of what they are trying to accomplish;
2. Problems of transfer of training, which bedevil simulation practice are removed;
3. More general experience of the work environment is gained, in addition to practising aspects of communication;
4. Trainee self-confidence can be promoted through the successful accomplishment of an exercise of this sort;
5. It affords a strong locus of integration for the many elements that comprise the health professionals' training course.

Disadvantages which should be recognized are:

1. Reduced control over what takes place. It is always difficult to anticipate and legislate for the many problems, even crises, which can occur in the real situation;
2. Students who perform badly due either to lack of preparation, or perhaps a rather difficult patient, can find the experience quite traumatic and confidence can suffer as a result;
3. Ethical considerations. Patients may have their confidence in the level of care which they are receiving shaken following an unsatisfactory encounter with a weak trainee;
4. The exercise may become defocused. There is a greater possibility that, in the added complexity of the real situation, where predicting what may take place is much more hazardous, trainees may lose sight of the specific objectives of the exercise;
5. Difficulties in providing detailed levels of feedback;
6. Organizing *in vivo* practical experience may be much more difficult than any of the alternative forms of practice already outlined and may incur greater financial cost.

Summary

By this stage, two points should be obvious about choosing methods of practice to include in training. The first is that there is no 'best' one in any absolute sense of the word. All have strengths and weaknesses which must be appreciated and taken into account. Given such factors as the level of ability, competence, experience and confidence of the group, the facet of the communication process under consideration, and the specific learning objectives, some of these characteristics will weigh more heavily than others in reaching a decision.

The second point is that any choice made should not be arrived at on an 'either – or' basis. It is seldom a case of selecting one to the exclusion of the rest. Rather, different combinations and sequences of exercises can be put into effect, some serving as preparation for others. *In vivo* practice is often used at the culmination of a programme whereas behaviour rehearsal exercises are incorporated in the earlier stages. Taking a more cross-sectional perspective, some methods may build upon others. With a difficult skill to master, covert rehearsal may precede roleplay, for instance, during the practice phase.

9.5 OBSERVATION AND RECORDING OF PRACTICE

It should be realized, before proceeding, that observing and recording the skill practice exercise does little to further what takes place during it. Indeed it may even have a detrimental effect if mishandled. The benefits which do undoubtedly accrue are experienced at the subsequent stage of feedback and analysis in terms of increased information which can be made available for discussion.

There are several techniques which can be exploited when obtaining a permanent record of what transpired during the practical. These make use of observers, audio- or video-recordings. The discussion of these options in the present section will be restricted to the recording implications which they pose for the practical session *per se*. Other aspects will be raised in the following chapter and in Chapter 12.

Observers

The possibility of involving one or more of the group as observers of the interaction has already been mooted. With multiple roleplay methods requiring trainees to work in triads, a 'round robin' procedure can be followed in which each takes it in turn to act as an observer for the other two. It may be advisable to have a plurality of observers involved when the exercise is more extensive in number of participants, duration, and learning points. Regardless of the particular method of practice, before commencing, observers should be thoroughly briefed in what to attend to and how to record it. They may be physically present while observing, although watching from behind a one-way screen or via a CCTV link is often less intrusive.

Audio-recording

It is now common practice to replace the observer with an audio-recorder or video-recorder. Although the latter has all but rendered the former obsolete in this form of training, an audio-recording of an interaction can represent an invaluable source of material upon which to base analysis and discussion. This is especially true when the focus is upon the verbal domain of communication with a skill which is essentially verbal in nature, such as questioning or reflecting, being practised.

Video-recording

Without doubt this has become the most popular method of providing a permanent record of the practice stage of training. Indeed there is a tendency, among the less well-informed, to mistakenly equate CST with the use of video. Video-recording is neither a necessary nor sufficient condition of this form of training but merely a means of detailing what took place during practice. While it has the potential to be of tremendous benefit in this regard it can also have a detrimental influence in the hands of an insensitive, over-zealous trainer. Considerations which should be acknowledged can be grouped under two headings; firstly, those that precede recording proper and have to do with introducing trainees to it, and secondly, recording procedures themselves.

Introducing video

The trainer must contemplate how best to expose trainees to being video-recorded. Trainees react to the prospect differently. Some positively relish the opportunity. These tend, in general, to be young, attractive, confident extroverts with high levels of self-esteem. At the other extreme distress may be engendered among a small minority who are typically older (late middle-age), female, less attractive, introverted, anxious and with poor self-concepts. The majority frequently experience various levels of apprehension at the thought of having their practice attempts observed and recorded in this way. The trainer should be aware of this concern and take steps to deal with it so that the training process is not impaired. Barnes (1983) advocates delaying the video-recording until students have become familiar with role-play on its own, especially when a relationship hasn't been established with the group.

According to Berger (1978), there are four strategies which can be pursued when introducing video. The first is simply to have the equipment present when the group arrives. Any queries or misgivings elicited can then be addressed. If none are forthcoming, members may be asked for their reactions. A second possibility is to present a *fait accompli* by having the equipment running before the trainees come and briefly explaining that it is being used before beginning. Thirdly, the notion is floated prior to the practice session, the value of this device stressed and commitment sought to take part in recording. Any negative reactions should, of course, be explored further and, if possible, defused. Finally, a more seductive approach can be followed in which videotaping is casually mentioned well in advance of the practical and then increasingly more frequently leading up to it. It has been our experience that the third mentioned strategy works best with most groups.

As has been stressed by Renne *et al.* (1983), participants must be informed at the outset, as to what is involved. Attempting to make a recording without the trainee's knowledge or consent raises serious ethical issues and should be desisted. (Ethical issues of this type were discussed in Chapter 7, it will be recalled). Reassuring participants of the prospective audience and demonstrating concern with matters of confidentiality are methods of alleviating initial hesitancies. Tackling the possibility of feelings of disquiet head-on is another. It is premised on the assumption that when opportunities to disclose and discuss negative emotions in a setting of acceptance and understanding isn't given, those feelings are frequently exacerbated. By mentioning that people often experience a certain degree of nervousness when confronted with a novel situation such as being 'in the eye of the video camera', members will often admit to similar affective states. Having been acknowledged these can then be discussed openly and frankly. Reminding trainees of the limited purpose of being recorded and construing the exercise as an opportunity to try out new ways of interacting, accepting that mistakes may be made, rather than as a form of assessment, can also help to reduce anxieties. There is a danger, however, in making an undue issue of initial misgivings and by so doing promoting rather than assuaging them.

Several advantages stem from demonstrating the video equipment to students before their first practice session and training them in its use. Being able to operate it helps, in many cases, to overcome any lingering feelings of threat, especially among those who habitually react in this way when confronted with modern technology. Discovering how simple the camera and recorder are to work can be very reassuring for such individuals and encourage a sense of being 'in control' rather than, in some mysterious way, 'being controlled'. But apart from helping students adjust to the prospect of performing in front of the camera, there is a further benefit to be gained from such instruction. It opens up the possibility of the group itself being given the responsibility of making the recordings under the guidance of the trainer. All members may thus be more completely involved in the total exercise.

We have found that students prefer to be recorded for the first time in a group rather than in a dyad, or on their own. The old adage that there is safety in numbers would seem to pertain. No doubt the fact that there are others present means that no one feels too individually exposed or responsible for sustaining the interaction. It is possible to move in and out of the conversation as confidence ebbs and flows. The purpose of this initial encounter is merely to ease the group into the business of being videotaped and give them a chance to see themselves 'on television' afterwards. They should be made aware that there will be no attempt to systematically analyse what took place, during playback, and the trainer should take all necessary steps to ensure that the experience is as non-threatening, indeed enjoyable, as possible.

While the content of the discussion is immaterial, the group should have some topic in mind before the recording starts. This tends to reduce awkwardness and embarrassment at the beginning caused by members being unable to think of 'what to say'. Time is not critical but the discussion shouldn't last too long; ten to fifteen minutes should suffice in most instances and provide adequate opportunities for each member to participate to some extent.

Using video

Making the video-recording is invariably governed by the necessity to achieve a balance between two frequently conflicting requirements. One is to produce as accurate a representation of as much of what took place during the encounter as can be achieved: the other to distort that encounter as little as possible in the process. The former can be best carried out in a studio which lends itself to multi-camera arrangements and where levels of light and sound can be carefully controlled in order to optimize technical quality. Unfortunately, this environment tends to be maximally reactive. Trainees typically complain that it makes practice seem artificial and unnatural. What takes place during interaction is distorted as a result and is regarded, rightly or wrongly by those taking part, as being entirely unrepresentative of how they would normally behave in a more familiar setting.

When such recordings are being made for feedback purposes only, rather than for demonstration, it is best to resolve this dilemma in favour of making the recording process as unintrusive as possible. Most of the pertinent detail can usually be obtained from productions that fall far short of the high levels of technical excellence required when, for example, broadcasting. Such a reduction in quality is, therefore, an acceptable price to pay if it means that participants can, during the subsequent stage of the training procedure, readily identify with and 'own' their performances. A corollary is that video equipment can be effectively employed in CST even though the trainer may not have access to the rather specialized facilities of a recording studio.

When a recording is being made, the trainer must be alert to any possible signs of distress by the participants being taped. Sometimes an interactor will 'dry-up'. If it isn't possible to prompt and if it seems unlikely that they will readily resume, the recording should be brought to a premature end rather than subject the individual concerned to further stress or embarrassment. While remaining sensitive to the need of someone to whom this has happened to talk about the experience, such incidents should be largely played down. Time permitting, the opportunity to carry on and finish should be given once a more composed state has been regained.

9.6 OVERVIEW

The opportunity for trainees to put the material covered in the preceding phase of sensitization into practice is seen as a central feature of CST. Indeed this particular focus is probably the reason why the process has come to be referred to as 'training' rather than 'education' or 'instruction'. Its distinctiveness is derived from this more than any other single component. Why practice should be thought to be of such importance can be attributed to a plurality of sources. However, evidence deriving from empirical studies carried out within the ambit of CST is, perhaps surprisingly, controvertible. While some researchers have reported the effects of skill practice, in isolation, to be positive, others have failed in corroboration. When considered in combination with complementary techniques which typically go to make up a CST package, the outcomes have been more favourable.

Survey data has certainly demonstrated the ubiquity of the practical element in programmes which have been implemented to improve levels of communication within the health professions. Some of the objectives which trainers have had in mind when requiring trainees to practise have been quite narrow and specific while others have been much broader. Perhaps the most common has had to do with furthering the behavioural reproduction aspects of skill performance. Others include enabling consequences of performance to be experienced; highlighting discrepancies between what is thought to be done and what actually is done by students; providing practical knowledge of the interpersonal complexities of situations and the operation of different social structures; facilitating the restructuring of beliefs and attitudes; creating a greater awareness of self and others; and permitting new roles to be tested.

These can be accomplished by means of one or more of a range of options, some of which make use of simulation. They include covert rehearsal; behaviour rehearsal; roleplay and simulation exercises and games. Alternatively, *in vivo* practice can be provided. The choice will largely depend upon a complex of considerations the most important of which have to do with the learning objectives specified; characteristics of the group and the particular point that the programme has reached. These points will be further considered in Chapter 12.

Although observing and recording performance during practice can be potentially disruptive, and steps must be taken to minimize this possibility, it is typically carried out in order to facilitate subsequent feedback and discussion. This can be done by members of the group who have been designated to act as observers and briefed accordingly. More frequently audio- or video-recordings of the interaction are made, the latter being the most popular. The instructor must always be mindful that videotaping can cause some trainees varying degrees of unease, especially in the early stages, and should be used with sensitivity.

10

The feedback
phase of training

Sensitization is necessary but not sufficient for effective training to take place – the same could be said of practice. Practising is unlikely to produce any significant improvement in communicative ability if it merely consists of blindly repeating some piece of behaviour devoid of any real appreciation of its enactment, the extent to which it approximates pre-established standards of propriety, or the consequences which it may engender. Under these circumstances it is just as probable that some wholly inappropriate response will be perpetuated. For progress to take place there must be an awareness, on the part of the performer, of the characteristics and consequences of action enabling judgements on appropriateness to be reached and adaptations effected, as required. In other words, as intimated in the preceding chapter, practice must be accompanied by resulting feedback to enable increased levels of skill to be attained. This phase is, therefore, crucial to the success of the whole training sequence.

One of the most commonly cited of the early experiments in support of the role of feedback in learning was conducted by Thorndike (1927). Such findings led Bartlett (1948, p.86) to declare that, 'The common belief that "practice makes perfect" is not true. It is practice *the results of which are known* that makes perfect'. Little has happened in the intervening years to confound this dictum. It is echoed in the conclusion reached by Salmoni *et al.* (1984, p.361) having conducted a wide-ranging review of the motor skills literature, when they failed to unearth any, 'evidence that convincingly contradicts the fundamental idea that some form of information feedback (about errors or the movement goal) is critical for learning'. As a consequence of assertions such as these the belief that feedback is conducive to heightened achievement is now regarded as essentially axiomatic. Indeed, it has been held by some as the single most important element in the inculcation of skill (Fitts, 1964).

As a component of the CST procedure, feedback has been the subject of some empirical investigation. While a comprehensive review of the work that has been carried out will not be attempted, the general finding to emerge, with some exceptions (e.g. Peters *et al.*, 1978), has been broadly positive. The benefits to be derived from furnishing trainees with details of the consequences of their practice efforts have been documented by Wallace *et al.* (1975); Speas (1979); Twentyman and Zimering (1979); and Sanders (1982). Correspondingly, it would appear that the vast majority of pro-grammes which have been reported have incorporated a feedback element. Indeed, Kurtz and Marshall (1982) found it to be the most commonly used training technique. Similarly Carroll and Monroe (1979), when deriving instructional principles based upon the results of their survey of communi-cation skills training provision in US medical schools, stipulated that, 'a crucial variable is the provision for direct observation and feedback on students' interviewing behaviour. The feedback principle is so fundamental to the design of instruction that it may often be regarded as merely an educational platitude' (p.498).

The bulk of this chapter will outline the major functions served by this phase of the training regime together with a range of possible modalities and sources which can be exploited in providing performance-related detail for trainees. This will include discussions of the features and use of audio, video, written and oral feedback provided by trainers, trainees, or indeed those who have partnered trainees during the practice interaction. Consider-ation must also be given to organizing and conducting the feedback tutorial including practical advice on how to avoid some of the problems and pitfalls which can confound this stage of the training procedure. We will continue, though, by considering alternative conceptualizations of feedback and the differing forms which it can take.

10.2 THE OPERATION OF FEEDBACK

In the CST literature it is common to find terms such as 'reinforcement' or 'knowledge of results' used instead of 'feedback'. While these, for the most part, are used interchangeably, they do have slightly different connotations that are reflections of contrasting views of the *modus operandi* of this aspect of instruction. The fact that feedback has the potential to facilitate learning and improve performance is commonly accepted – how it functions to effect these outcomes is open to several interpretations.

As mentioned in Chapter 3 there are broadly three theoretical interpreta-tions of feedback. These have been identified and dicussed by, among others, Annett (1969) and Adams (1987). Let us imagine a situation where the Sister in a medical ward has just observed a student nurse cope with a life-threatening crisis, involving one of the patients, in a very accomplished manner. She takes the student aside and praises her for dealing with the situation calmly, quickly and efficiently. On a subsequent occasion, under similar circumstances, the nurse displays even greater aplomb. Assuming that this was due, at least in part, to the feedback given by the Sister, we can attribute its effects either to the fact that she gave the student certain information, that she increased her motivation, or that she reinforced certain aspects of the student's behavioural repertoire. The effects of feedback can, therefore, be accounted for in terms of motivation, information or reinforcement.

Those who regard feedback as a means of influencing the level of motivation of the recipient point to the fact that individuals are typically more interested in the task which they are doing, are prepared to invest greater effort and make a better job of it, when it leads to a recognized and accepted positive outcome. Such feedback has energizing properties serving as an incentive to strive even more determinedly. Perhaps this resulted in the improved performance of the student nurse in the example above! Conversely, lethargy and low morale leading to reduced effort and poor quality output frequently results from insufficient incentive. Viewed in this way, feedback produces direct changes in performance rather than in learning and consequently its impact tends to be comparatively transient. This is not to deny, however, that it can indirectly promote learning by increasing the amount of practice which the trainee is prepared to undergo.

Alternatively, feedback can be looked upon as a means of reinforcement, acting to increase the frequency of occurrence of that behaviour which produced it and perhaps even doing so in a completely reflexive manner. Cairns (1986), has argued that 'the feedback concept described in most communication theory is equivalent to the reinforcement concept of operant conditioning . . .' (p.129). Here strong parallels are drawn between systematically modifying some targeted behaviour of an animal in a laboratory experiment by providing food, or some other reward, each time it appears and praising the trainee for displaying high levels of a particular skill during a practical. Did the praise lavished upon the student nurse in the example have the effect of strengthening the behaviour which she had just displayed, making it more probable that she would act even more calmly, quickly and efficiently when faced with a similar situation? Presumably those who talk of providing reinforcement rather than feedback as part of CST have, at least implicitly, a model of this sort in mind.

Contrasting with the previous two theories is the notion of feedback as information, operating very much at a cognitive rather than an affective level. By making the learner more aware of what he did and the extent to which it approximates some recognized standard, data which can be assimilated and acted upon is produced. If this information about the response and its outcome is accurately interpreted and implemented a new response can be generated, on the next occasion, which is more appropriate than the previous attempt. Here skill acquisition is very much thought of in terms of effective information processing. Perhaps it was the result of knowing that the way she behaved matched the Sister's requirements for effective nursing, that produced the improvement in the student's crisis-handling ability! When 'knowledge of results' is the chosen term, feedback is often thought to operate in this fashion.

While it is relatively easy to theoretically distinguish between these three operations of the process, the practical problems of doing so in any specific instance will, no doubt, have been realized by now. The feedback given by the Sister, in our example, could well have served to motivate, inform and reinforce at one and the same time. This probability is readily accepted by Salmoni *et al.* (1984) when they concluded their discussion of the elusive functional mechanism of feedback by suggesting that perhaps, 'It acts in many ways simultaneously' (p.382). Most CST trainers would probably accept this eclecticism. While much of what takes place during this stage is concerned with making additional information available to the performer, the common dictum that feedback should be essentially positive rather than negative has more to do, it would seem, with motivating and reinforcing.

10.3 TYPES OF FEEDBACK

In order to appreciate the possibilities which exist when, following practice, trainees are made more fully aware of how they performed, a more analytical approach to the concept of feedback must be taken. There are a number of distinctions which can be drawn, each with significance for CST. These include intrinsic versus extrinsic feedback, knowledge of results versus knowledge of performance, concurrent versus terminal feedback and immediate versus delayed feedback (Holding, 1965; Stammers and Patrick, 1975).

Intrinsic versus extrinsic feedback

This is one of the most fundamental discriminations that can be made. Intrinsic feedback is available as a natural consequence of performing a task. Indeed it has already been discussed at length in Chapter 3 as a component of the model of interpersonal communication developed there. The notion will be recalled of behaviour being responded to by the other involved in the encounter thus providing feedback which can be acted upon in order to achieve the specified goal. This feedback is intrinsic to the task.

It is with *extrinsic* feedback, however, that the present chapter is concerned. Extrinsic feedback refers to supplementary information which, while not forming an integral part of the task, enables decisions to be reached about its accomplishment. It can be supplied by observers in the form of verbal comments or by a variety of mechanical devices such as buzzers, lights or other visual displays, together with audio- and video-recordings. Most commonly in CST it has taken the form of trainer and peer comments together with videotaped replays of practice.

A general finding would seem to be that extrinsic feedback is an effective means of facilitating skill acquisition but, frequently, performance can suffer once it is removed. It is, therefore, important that it should not distract the trainee from attending to the salient cues residing within the interaction and upon which reliance will ultimately have to be made, but rather serve to highlight them. Towards the end of training, Stammers and Patrick (1975) recommend that feedback which is extrinsic be gradually removed as levels of performance improve.

Knowledge of results versus knowledge of performance

Strictly speaking, knowledge of results conveys information on the extent to which the outcome of action matches some standard or achieves a desired goal. The trainee will have been made aware of that standard during the sensitization phase by, for example, viewing a model tape depicting the communicative element under focus. Indeed it has been speculated that the most important role of the trainer in the feedback tutorial may be to facilitate comparison, by students, between their own attempts and the performance of the model (Ellis and Whittington, 1981). The goal striven for may have been suggested to the student prior to practice in the context of, for instance, a structured roleplay. With less structured forms of practice greater opportunities exist for students to formulate their own goals for the interaction. Either way the trainer who helps the student appreciate the extent to which such goals were actualized, makes knowledge of results available.

Where the trainee has little recollection of action or does not know how to best modify it to approximate the standard or goal more fully, knowledge of results may be of little advantage. What is required is knowledge of performance or *kinematic* feedback which deals with the sequence of action producing the particular outcome, rather than with the outcome itself. Salmoni *et al.* (1984), pointed out that videotape replays of what took place are one method of furnishing this type of information which, potentially, can be extremely effective. Showing students the sequence of behaviours carried out so that they can appreciate what took place and how it relates to the eventual outcome of performance has been recommended by Adams (1987), as a way of giving knowledge of performance.

During CST, making both knowledge of results and of performance available is, of course, important.

Concurrent versus terminal feedback

This distinction concerns the point in the performance of the task at which the feedback intervention begins. Concurrent feedback is made available during the enactment while, as the title suggests, terminal feedback is delivered upon its completion. In the vast majority of CST programmes it is the latter type of *extrinsic* feedback that is employed. Thus the business of analysing and discussing what took place awaits the termination of practice. It may be felt beneficial, especially in the absence of audio or video replay facilities, to intervene during the enactment to draw attention to some highly significant feature, but this happens infrequently.

A more thoroughgoing form of concurrent feedback which has been reported is the 'bug-in-the-ear' technique (Salvendy, 1984). This consists of an ear-piece worn by the trainee while interacting which can be used by the trainer, watching from behind a one-way mirror, to relay information on how the encounter is being handled. Although some research has attested to the effectiveness of this procedure (Mader, 1974; Nyquist and Wulff, 1982), disadvantages have also been documented (Salvendy, 1984).

Immediate versus delayed feedback

The length of time between the termination of practice and the commencement of terminal feedback is the key factor in this case. The general consensus of opinion would seem to favour immediate feedback (Hargie and McCartan, 1986), although Pope (1986) suggested that it could be delayed for up to twenty-four hours, in the absence of other intervening responses, and still be effective. Certainly this period of delay should be kept to a minimum if the trainer intends, during the feedback tutorial, to draw upon trainee recollections of perceptions, feelings and intentions operative in the course of the interaction. On the other hand, there may be advantage in having a break following a long or particularly intense roleplay before beginning to examine what took place. If it is felt that de-roling is necessary then such a break is essential to enable this to be undertaken.

One of the proposed advantages of video replay is that it serves to reinstate what happened during practice. Watching what took place not only re-establishes the verbal and nonverbal content of performance, but may also create a vivid awareness of cognitions and affective states experienced at particular points in the interaction. As a consequence, the length of the intervening period prior to feedback may be less critical.

In sum, extrinsic feedback on skill performance during CST is typically immediate (or relatively so), terminal, and should provide knowledge of performance as well as of results.

10.4 FUNCTIONS OF THE FEEDBACK PHASE

In the broadest terms, and at a theoretical level, the major functions of this part of training have, of course, been already discussed. They are, it will be recalled, to motivate, reinforce and/or inform. Beyond that, however, and from a more fine-grained, practical perspective a range of less immediately obvious functions can be identified. Some of these have been noted by van Ments (1983). They include to:

1. *Promote reflection upon what took place during practice* In addition to the more immediate advantages associated with a specific practice session there are long-term benefits in encouraging trainees to reflect upon situations encountered. By analysing what transpired they can begin to form general conclusions about interpersonal interaction in health contexts and how it operates. They can also consider how they can go about producing a more favourable outcome when confronted with similar situations in the future. Apart from improving their handling of such situations, this approach promotes positive feelings of control over outcomes; a belief that they have the capacity to be more effective communicators; and a responsibility for continued skill development.

2. *Clarify what ensued during the practice interaction* Once the attempt at skill practice has come to an end, there may be differences of opinion as to what happened. These may be at different levels. But before embarking upon more profound analysis and discussion, it is imperative that all concerned are in agreement on the facts of the exchange.

3. *Establish why things happened as they did* The feedback tutorial presents splendid opportunities for isolating and examining, in a very practical manner, the complex of situational, personal and interpersonal factors that impinge upon the communicative process.

4. *Re-affirm standards of performance* During feedback, the standards of performance should be re-affirmed so that trainees have a firm appreciation of the extent to which they deviated in their attempts at practice.

5. *Identify ways in which improvements can be effected* This function is an extension of the previous in that suggestions as to how performance can be altered to more nearly match what is expected should be offered.

6. *Facilitate self-awareness* One of the central objectives of CST is to, sensitively and non-threateningly, make students more fully aware of their needs, attitudes, feelings, beliefs, etc., together with their characteristic styles of interacting; how these may be construed by others; and the consequences which can result. Such knowledge forms the basis of the sort of skill with which this book is concerned. The feedback process affords unique opportunities for bringing such awareness about.

7. *Inspire confidence* One of the overriding principles governing the provision of feedback is that the trainer be always mindful of the influence which it can have upon feelings of self-esteem and self-efficacy. Part of the skill of the trainer lies in ensuring that, perhaps despite a somewhat indifferent attempt at skill practice, trainees never leave the session with their confidence deflated. (On the other hand the smugly

overconfident can be tactfully alerted to the limitations of their performance.)

8. *Develop observation skills* Effective communication, as outlined in Chapter 3, depends not only upon what we say and do but upon our perceptions of events taking place around us. We must be astute in observing and interpreting the actions of others. This requires sensitivity to social cues and the attachment of appropriate meaning and significances to them. Certain communication difficulties may stem from a lack of competence in this regard (Trower, *et al.*, 1978).

   Observation skills, like skills in general, can be sharpened (Boice, 1983) and the feedback stage is particularly well-suited to this objective. With the aid of video replays of their own and others interactions trainees' attention can be drawn to the subtleties of exchange which can easily go unnoticed. By discussing and comparing their perceptions of events, invalid meanings placed upon them can be detected and rectified.

9. *Draw conclusions about interpersonal behaviour and facilitate the generalization of learning* It is important that the lessons to be learned from the session do not get lost amid a welter of detailed analysis. These should be summarized, in the form of conclusions, before the session is terminated and trainees encouraged to contemplate their implications in the wider, extra-training context.

10. *Locate learning outcomes in the broader ambit of training* Links should be forged between what happened in prior sessions and how the present one will be developed, to prevent the training sequence becoming a fragmented experience and to facilitate integration of learning. Feedback is an occasion when such connections can be highlighted although it should not be thought of as the only one.

11. *Establish action consequences* This is a prospective aspect of feedback. Based upon conclusions reached following analysis and discussion, and in accordance with suggestions and advice proffered, trainees, either individually or collectively, should commit themselves to some future action. This may be general (e.g. try to talk less when interviewing) or specific (e.g. be more patient with Mrs Brown), to be undertaken within or without the training programme, and feature behaviour, knowledge, perceptions or some other aspect of the skills process.

10.5 MODALITIES OF FEEDBACK

Attention will now be turned to the various media which are typically utilized in CST programmes to provide information for feedback purposes. The most common are videotape, audiotape, written material and oral comments. While each can be used independently, some combination is more often the case in actual practice. Thus oral comments tend to accompany whichever of the other modalities is selected.

Videotape

This is undoubtedly the method of feedback that is more popularly associated with CST than any of the others. Since it is now highly unusual to come across a CST programme that doesn't feature self-viewing, this is understandable. It would seem that an almost inextricable bond has been forged between the two. As a consequence it has been assumed, in some quarters, first that any exercise which involves trainees watching how they behaved in some recorded social encounter can be rightfully labelled CST and, secondly, that it is not possible to conduct CST without video replay. Neither is the case. Video, as a feedback modality, is merely an adjunct to this form of training, not a defining characteristic of it. Having said that, though, it is a particularly useful means of providing trainees with insights into their performance – hence its popularity.

Among the features of video playback which have attracted it to trainers can be listed the following:

1. It is potentially the most complete form of feedback encompassing verbal, nonverbal and paralinguistic aspects of performance (Twentyman and Zimering, 1979). As expressed by Hirsh and Freed (1978, p.120), 'To read is not as effective as to be told. To be told is not as effective as to be shown. But to see for ourselves is perhaps the most insightful method of learning. VTR and replay lend themselves to this best way of learning.'
2. It is available once skill practice is completed thus enabling immediate feedback to be provided.
3. It constitutes a permanent record of what took place which, if necessary, can be reviewed on different occasions over a period of time. Possibilities of slow-motion playback and 'freeze-frame' options to facilitate the in-depth analysis of some element of nonverbal behaviour should not be overlooked.
4. It is an objective modality. The record of what took place, while subject to minimal technical distortion, is free from the sorts of subjective bias which can taint, for instance, oral and written feedback. This does not mean, however, that the *perception* of what is depicted on tape is unaffected by the vagaries of individual representational processes (Trower and Kiely, 1983).
5. Perhaps the most attractive feature of video replay is that it presents feedback in pictorial form. This eliminates the difficulty and frustration of searching for the proper expressions to adequately describe, in sufficiently graphic detail, the important nuances of some nonverbal action.
6. Video seems to have an intrinsic appeal for trainees who, for the most part, react positively to it (White and Clemens, 1971; Brook, 1985).

No doubt positive features such as these are responsible for many of the exaggerated claims and unrealistic expectations which pervade discussions of the effectiveness of video feedback and have gone largely unchallenged until recently. There has been a tendency to regard this element as the *sine qua non* of successful training outcome. Recent reviews of the available research have arrived at a more guarded conclusion (Hung and Rosenthal, 1978; Fichten and Wright, 1983). Indeed Sorenson and Pickett (1986, p.13) go so far as to say that, 'When videotaped feedback is used by itself, ... students make no greater gains in competency than control groups.'

In order to maximize the potential of this modality, it would appear that the following circumstances should prevail:

1. Trainees' attention must be directed to the pertinent features of playback. The need for feedback to be focused in this way is widely recognized (Carroll and Munroe, 1980). It could be to this end that students prefer to have tutors present during playback sessions.
2. Video feedback should be provided within the context of a structured training sequence. There is evidence attesting to the contribution which this component can make when complementing sensitization and practice procedures (Wallace *et al.*, 1975; Speas 1979; Sanders, 1982).
3. Extent of exposure to self-viewing would seem to be important (Hung and Rosenthal, 1978). Unless the recording lasts long enough for trainees to be exposed to sufficient instances of the targeted feature of performance, training effects may be limited. Allowances must also be made for the 'cosmetic effect' i.e. trainees' initial preoccupation with physical features of appearance rather than the subtleties of skilled communication, when seeing themselves on tape for the first time (Hargie and Saunders, 1983a).
4. Trainees should be in a receptive frame of mind. Heightened states of anxiety or feelings of threat will lessen the benefits to be derived.
5. With regard to content, it has been suggested that concentrating upon positive rather than negative features of the recording, during replay, may be more efficacious (Hung and Rosenthal, 1978). Self-modelling procedures are a promising extension of this principle (Hosford, 1981). This involves editing the videotape to remove segments where trainees are displaying inappropriate behaviour so that they only see themselves behaving competently.

    The additional time required to undertake editing may, however, be prohibitive with large groups of students. Again this practice reduces the extend to which the recording is representative of the actual performance. In editing, the trainer may also strongly imply negative criticism of that performance.
6. There is some limited evidence that video feedback may be more effective when carried out in small, rather than large groups of twelve or more members (Decker, 1983).

It is likely that the more of these conditions the trainer can implement the more beneficial this form of feedback will be. Nevertheless, one must always be mindful of the fact that self-viewing isn't invariably a constructive experience. It may be hurtful and damaging in certain cases and can be mishandled. The trainer has to be constantly alert to this possibility and always ready to quickly intervene, if need be, to prevent it happening. While many experience mild anxiety when first exposed to video, which soon dissipates, for a small minority this reaction may be more extreme, as mentioned in Chapter 9. Distress may be caused by 'self-confrontation'. This has been described by Hargie and Morrow (1986c, p.362) as occurring, 'when the ideal self-image of the individual is challenged by the public image as portrayed on the TV screen'. It is more likely to be experienced by what Fuller and Manning (1973) termed the HOUND type (i.e. homely, old, unattractive, nonverbal, dumb) rather than the YAVIS type of trainee (i.e. young, attractive, verbal, intelligent and successful). Such a disaffected student should be treated sympathetically and given support and informal 'counselling'.

Sometimes a systematic desensitization-type procedure works with less extreme cases, depending upon the personal feature causing the problem. This involves moving the camera back from the interaction or using a wide-angle lens during recording so that, initially, the student's image is small and at a distance rather than close-up. Gradually it can be increased. Failing that, the trainer may consider employing an alternative feedback modality. The possibility of such a student requiring professional help from a counsellor or psychiatrist should not be overlooked in some extreme cases.

Audiotape

The use of audiotape as a feedback modality has been largely eclipsed by video, due largely it would appear, to its neglect of the very important nonverbal dimension of communication. However, just as the potency of video has tended, on occasion, to be overstated the merits of audio have largely gone unsung. The contribution which it can make, at this stage of training, has been underestimated to some extent. While sharing a number of the positive features of video playback just listed, audio feedback, in comparison, has several additional advantages including:

1. Less information being carried to confuse and distract the trainee from the targeted (verbal) skill;
2. Less threatening for some (Niland *et al.*, 1971);
3. Greater availability. Audio cassette recorders can be bought quite cheaply and most young people seem to own one.

Considerations such as these spurred some researchers to determine the relative effectiveness of these two feedback modalities. Reviewing studies into the acquisition of teaching skills, Griffiths (1974, p.17) concluded that, 'the evidence provided does show that audiotape feedback can be as effective and sometimes more effective than videotape feedback within the verbal domain'. Maguire (1986) also reported that, 'feedback of performance by audiotape replay or television was worthwhile, but audiotape alone was almost as good as television at the basic level of the skills being taught' (p.155). Again these skills were exclusively verbal in nature. Where measures of outcome have been more wide-ranging and have included non-verbal criteria, the results of audio replay have been less impressive (Mulac, 1974). This serves to underscore the one big drawback of this type of feed-back – its confinement to the verbal and paralinguistic domains of com-munication.

Written material

As an alternative to video- and audiotapes, or indeed as an adjunct, feedback can be delivered by means of written comments. (For reviews of research see Fichten and Wright, 1983; Brook, 1985.) These may be made by selected observers during the course of the interaction or based upon a recording of it. The importance of giving focused feedback has already been stressed, in like fashion the attention of observers should be channelled to the relevant features of performance. Some form of observation schedule is often provided for this purpose and to assist in the task of recording the appropriate detail. But schedules vary greatly in the extent to which they structure these activities, with some being much more analytical than others.

An example of one which is quite global and can be used for giving feed-back on the skill of explaining is presented in Fig. 10.1. Here the observer is merely presented with several headings corresponding to the key facets of the skill under consideration. It is left entirely to the users to decide how best to express their perceptions and judgements in written form. Consequently, there may be considerable variability in, for example, the quantity, specifi-city and content of information included. Some may be primarily descriptive in their comments, others essentially evaluative.

Reports of molecular and analytical schedules being employed effectively as feedback devices, can also be found (MacLeod, 1977). An example, again designed with the skill of explaining in mind, is presented in Fig. 10.2. Students often find these instruments furnish increased information and are

Coverage of topic

Sequence of key elements

Pace of delivery

Clarity of presentation

Feedback obtained

Fig. 10.1 Global schedule for explaining.

	Very well done	Well done	Fair	Could be better	Could be much better	Comments
Introduction						
Suitable vocabulary						
Vagueness avoided						
Adequate concrete examples						
Within listener's experience						
Fluent verbal style						
Verbal emphasis						
Nonverbal emphasis						
Use of pauses						
Appropriately paced use of audiovisual aids						
Stimulating delivery						
Suitable structure						
Main ideas clarified						
Parts linked to each other						
Concise summary						
Understanding checked						
Feedback acted upon						

Fig. 10.2 Analytical schedule for explaining.

more helpful than their less analytical counterparts. Feedback provided is both systematic and structured. As can be seen, the skill is represented by a larger number of more precise items and the system for recording observations, in this case a rating procedure, promotes greater consistency. Supplementary comments can also be added. This type of schedule is particularly useful because it outlines, for the benefit of the trainee receiving feedback, a profile of performance which readily highlights areas of stength and weakness. (Further information on skill assessment can be found in the following chapter.)

Benefits would also seem to accrue for the *trainee* from using such a schedule. Thus Sorenson and Pickett (1986) reported that those who were involved in conducting ratings of the interviews of other students subsequently evinced substantial improvements in their *own* interviewing skill!

Oral comments

This is probably the most frequently employed feedback modality. It is extremely unusual, with the possible exception of individually based self-instructional packages, not to have a feedback tutorial in CST where those involved share the responsibility of commenting upon skill practice and, by so doing, provide the performer with a fuller appreciation of what took place and, hopefully, how it could be bettered. This discussion may be based upon a recollection of the just-completed practice interaction, but more typically is grounded in the contents of video-recordings, audio-recordings or observation schedules. To suggest that its role is supplemental to these is, however, to misrepresent its importance. It is probably more appropriate to regard the other modalities as making additional material available for discussion.

Unfortunately there is no guarantee that the outcome of such discussion will be necessarily advantageous. Rather than fostering insight and understanding it can produce resentment, rejection and recalcitrance if improperly conducted. Oral feedback can be positive and constructive or, even if well intentioned, negative and destructive (Phillips and Fraser, 1982). Several writers including Rackham and Morgan (1977), Turock (1980) and Pendleton *et al.* (1984) have suggested ways of maximizing the former. The following guidelines draw upon their recommendations.

Oral feedback is most effective when it:

1. Deals only with what the trainee is capable of changing;
2. Concentrates on the performance rather than the person. It is not the individual who is under scrutiny but rather what they did during the practice session;
3. Is geared to the learner's needs. Feedback should be at a level and couched in terms that the learner can readily relate to. It should also, for the most part, be restricted to those particular aspects of the communicative process under focus rather than attempt to be all-embracing. Overwhelming the trainee with detail is one of the most common abuses of feedback;
4. Is specific rather than general. Commenting in vague generalities does not create the detailed knowledge upon which subsequent improvement depends;
5. Clarifies what took place;
6. Is mainly positive rather than negative. Another common abuse of feedback is to dwell upon the weaknesses. Being over-critical often leads to defensiveness and can be de-motivating and confidence-sapping especially in the early stages of the training programme. But of course it may be necessary to draw the learner's attention to mistakes or omissions. This is best done after the strengths of the performance have been outlined and should be followed by further praise of these positive elements;
7. Provides positive alternatives. Merely pointing out inappropriate acts may not necessarily help the trainee to improve upon them next time;
8. Considers links with the causes and consequences of behaviour. Outlining what the learner did is important but a full appreciation of the

performance requires the causes and consequences of it to be considered. By doing so intrinsic feedback within the interaction can be highlighted and a debilitating reliance upon extrinsic sources avoided;

9. Is generalizable. It is crucial that information on a specific performance be such that its wider relevance to future encounters is recognized. The trainer should always strive to ensure that there is an awareness of the application, to the job, of what takes place in training.

10.6 SOURCES OF FEEDBACK

With the written and oral variants, the distinction between modalities and sources of feedback is much clearer than with video- and audiotape. Written and oral comments on performance and outcome are given mostly by tutors, peers, and participants in the practice interaction.

Tutors

A common finding is that students prefer to have a tutor present during the post-practice critique session and react more favourably to CST programmes when this happens. This is partly due to the instructor being recognized as having a valuable knowledge-base together with expertise in analysing interaction and drawing comparisons with accepted standards of proficiency (Turock, 1980). Indeed some trainees have a tendency to bestow almost mystical powers of understanding and insight in this respect! This can have both advantages and disadvantages. On the positive side, it legitimizes the right of the tutor to pass comment and increases the likelihood that feedback given will be accepted and implemented. The views of fellow students may not be as readily accepted, especially in the early stages of the programme. A disadvantage is that the tutor may be pressured into a more directive style than would be wished.

In spite of student preferences there seems to be no consistent evidence that tutor presence *per se* leads to more effective outcomes in terms of increased levels of skill (Dickson, 1981). It may be that feedback from this source is more influential with less experienced trainees, especially those who, following the sensitization phase, have failed to fully grasp the nuances of the communication skill under consideration and the standards of performance which pertain.

In should be recognized, though, that tutors' involvement during the critique session is much more than as a source of feedback. Additional roles will be discussed in the following section.

Peers

As already intimated there may be an initial reluctance on the part of trainees to accept comment from a fellow student, especially if it is negatively evaluative, and indeed there may be a hesitancy on the part of some peers to offer it. But having all the members of the tutorial group contributing their observations and opinions on what took place, if properly handled, can make an invaluable contribution to feedback. According to Turock (1980), the instructor can take steps to maximize the potential of this source by:

1. Clarifying with trainees, before viewing the interation, what exactly it is that they are meant to be observing;
2. Reminding trainees that feedback should be based, not on personal preference, but on the material presented during sensitization
3. Encouraging trainees to document their observations;
4. Reinforcing feedback that is accurate, specific, constructive and concise;
5. Serving as a model for trainees to emulate.

In the process of providing feedback, trainees must exercise their perceptual capabilities. The feedback tutorial is therefore a setting within which much worthwhile work can be done in the development of observation skills. It will be recalled from Chapter 3 that the ability to search out, identify and accurately interpret salient cues is central to effective communication. Such skills are not intuitive but can be worked at and improved. One teaching technique advocated by Hogstel (1987), makes use of videotape analysis and is remarkably similar to what takes place during the post-practice critique session.

Participants

Those who participated in the skill practice exercise can comment upon what transpired from the unique perspective of having been part of the interaction – others can only 'look in from the outside'. In addition to the individual practising, they may be peers, patients or others (e.g. drama students) providing a particular practical experience. The special insights into the dynamics of the encounter afforded by their involvement in it should not be overlooked since it makes possible an additional dimension of feedback which takes account of intrapersonal considerations such as intentions, beliefs, feelings, etc.

One way of tapping this source of information is by using process recording techniques. A process recording is basically 'a detailed reconstruction of what is going on/happening/occurring in the interpersonal relationship between [the professional] and patient. It is a verbatim serial account of the interaction between two individuals' (Jones, 1984, p.114). Different formats for recording this type of analysis exist. The one presented in Fig. 10.3 requires both interactors to separately record their verbal and nonverbal behaviour together with that of the other, to note what meanings they attached to the other's behaviour, to state their intended consequent reaction and to make critical evaluation of what they actually did. Although the procedure can be time-consuming and it may not be possible to analyse all of a lengthy interaction or to provide this form of feedback for each student's skill practice, it is a useful way of gaining access to some of the processes that subtend communication. The instructor, however, must be alert to the possibility of trainees 'inventing' perceptions and intentions in the interests of consistency and with the benefit of hindsight, rather than basing those parts of the recording upon recollections of what took place.

An alternative method of uncovering this type of detail is by means of Interpersonal Process Recall (IPR) (Kagan, 1980). Here the objective is to develop specific skills and promote interpersonal awareness through facilitating the systematic recall of thoughts, feelings, intentions, etc. that occur during the course of interaction. The procedure requires interview participants to watch a video-recording of their interaction and through recall to share an understanding of their moment-to-moment influence on each other. A third party, called an inquirer, serves as a catalyst in this enterprise. Gershen (1983) has discussed IPR as an approach to developing the interpersonal skills of dental students, while McQuellon (1982) has reviewed its successful application in the training of a range of health professionals including dentists, nurses, dietitians and pharmacists.

Where the trainee has taken part in *in vivo* practice, for instance carrying out a patient interview, the benefits to be derived from having the patient contribute feedback has been recognized (Maguire, 1986). Some reports of this being implemented can also be located although there is little by way of

Place:
Significant situational factors:
Goals (long-term and short-term):
Description of the other:
Preconceptions:

Other's behaviour (verbal and nonverbal)	Interpretation of other's behaviour	Intended response to other	Own behaviour (verbal and nonverbal)	Critical evaluation of own behaviour

Fig. 10.3 Process recording format.

formal evaluation of the outcome. Thus Kent *et al.* (1981) described how patients who had volunteered to give medical students further practice in interviewing were subsequently invited to join the feedback tutorial and offer their comments on how the interaction had been conducted from their point of view.

10.7 ORGANIZING AND CONDUCTING THE FEEDBACK PHASE

It is convenient to think of this taking place at two levels: firstly, at the broad level of the complete session, and secondly, with regard to the review of the specific skill performance.

The feedback session

A useful way of structuring the feedback tutorial is to view it in terms of three major processes. These are firstly, briefing the trainees and establishing a facilitative climate; secondly, reviewing performances; and thirdly, drawing conclusions and establishing commitments. While these processes roughly correspond to sequential stages there may be some overlap e.g. conclusions and commitments may take place during practice review as well as at the end of the session.

Briefing trainees and creating a facilitative climate

Trainees should be informed, at the outset, how the tutorial will operate, what they can expect to happen as it unfolds and what will be required of them. A more demanding task for the trainer, and one to which special attention must be paid in the very first session, is the creation of a group syntality conducive to the mutually beneficial process of giving and taking feedback. It is not an overstatement to say that the success of the entire CST programme may well depend upon how successful the instructor is in this respect. Failing to recognize this typically leads to a number of problems encountered at this juncture, such as:

1. *Defensiveness* Kipper and Ginot (1979) have shown how defence mechanisms can cause distortions in the accuracy of feedback from self-viewing. Overly defensive students may react to comments by, for example, denying that the featured incident took place or construing it in such a way as to make it more personally acceptable e.g. attributing the event to the presence of the camera. (It may be recalled, from Chapter 3, that such bias is quite common in the attributional process.)
2. *Hostility* The session degenerates into a spiral of accusation and counter-accusation – attack and counter-attack.
3. *Reticence* Trainees are extremely reluctant to offer comment and when they do, do so briefly and in very general terms.

4. *Collusion* An implicit norm is established which requires all feedback to be positive – regardless of accuracy.

In a group that is relaxed and where there is acceptance, trust and genuineness so that members feel sufficiently confident and safe to set aside defensive barriers and display an openness to the views and suggestions of others, such problems are unlikely to occur. But bringing this spirit about can be difficult. While the seeds must be sown in the first session, it is something that takes time to mature as the group evolves. The instructor can do a lot to nurture it, however, by for instance:

1. Reminding students that the programme is essentially about learning and development rather than personal evaluation and assessment;
2. Being open, accepting, genuine, etc. himself;
3. Working hard to foster a positive relationship with the students;
4. Presenting feedback as a means rather than an end;
5. Being primarily positive especially in the early stages;
6. Discussing the provision of feedback, including negative emotions that can arise, in order to promote sensitivity, denote understanding of the situation and improve the quality of detail offered.

Reviewing performances

When this is undertaken within the small group setting, as it normally is, rather than on a one-to-one basis with a student, there are two main organizational options. One is to review each performance before the next trainee practises. This alternative tends to be followed when mechanical modalities are not available. It has all the advantages of immediate over more delayed feedback in these circumstances. Again those students practising later have the benefit of being privy to the feedback offered to those at the start. Such advantage may, however, be more illusory than real according to Brook (1985) who documented evidence suggesting that those still to practise may be adversely affected. As far as contributing feedback is concerned, these students are often more preoccupied with their own interview than with the one currently being reviewed. The quality of the tutorial can deteriorate as a consequence.

Video-recordings afford the possibility of replaying and analysing the performances of those in the group one after the other. This is probably the more commonly implemented alternative.

Drawing conclusions and establishing commitments

As already mentioned, this can take place in relation to each individual performance following the critique. An important contribution of the tutor lies in synthesizing the multi-source feedback, distilling the salient themes and presenting these to the individual concerned in summary form. This, of course, is accompanied by the appropriate reinforcement of positive facets of the performance, identification of areas for improvement and the re-capping of suggestions as to how these could be effected, together with expressions of support and encouragement. Some commitment to the implementation of these agreed proposals should also be sought and the trainee encouraged to consider the wider relevance of the learning experience to the field.

At the end of the tutorial it is worthwhile for more general learning points to be reiterated and consequences for action reaffirmed. This is also an opportunity for making connections with what has been established in prior sessions together with anticipated future extensions.

The practice critique

Concentrating more singlemindedly upon reviewing the performances of individual students, several approaches can be identified in terms of the style of tutoring adopted. Such style is a reflection of a multiplicity of con-siderations including the way in which the trainer views his role in the process and the relative weighting given to its various facets.

The role of the tutor

We have already discussed the part played by the tutor as a powerful source of feedback. Providing insights into what took place during the practice interaction, in this direct fashion, is only one of a number of functions performed. The trainer is also, at different junctures:

1. a facilitator – eliciting feedback from group members and promoting contributions;
2. a chairperson – organizing and conducting the discussion, preventing monopoly, digression, overtalk etc;
3. an arbiter – intervening in cases of irreconcilable disagreement;
4. a protector – preventing harm from over-zealous negative criticism;
5. a counsellor – being an ever-listening ear for students and their concerns;
6. a supporter – providing reinforcement and encouragement;
7. a judge – making sure that everyone has an opportunity to have their say, synthesizing the discussion and formulating an agreed conclusion.

How the tutor goes about the task of conducting the critique will depend upon the importance attached to each of these sub-roles.

The style of the tutor

Perhaps the most fundamental feature of the characteristic way in which the tutor carries out the practice review has to do with the degree of direction and prescription offered. These qualities form the basis of a distinction drawn by Bailey and Butcher (1983) between what they label the *directive* and the *casual-analytic* styles of supervision in CST. The former is likely to be chosen by those who emphasize the tutor's contribution as an information resource. Here he is very much seen as an expert who describes and interprets what took place, identifies instances of good and bad practice, explains happenings, establishes the extent to which intended outcomes were actualized, and stipulates changes to bring about improvements in skill performance. He controls and dominates the tutorial with the other members obliged to listen passively. Although it does have some merits, this style is perhaps more frequently associated with shortcomings. McGarvey and Swallow (1986) discovered that supervisors who manifested it were reacted to less favourably by students than counterparts whose approach was more learner-centred.

With the casual-analytic style, 'the trainer explores interview events with observers and the interviewer by seeking a description of interview behaviour and interviewee reactions, eliciting suggestions for alternative behaviours and exploring the likely effectiveness of these ...' (Bailey and Butcher, 1983, p.110). In this case the roles of facilitator and chairperson are much more prominent. Rather than giving information the tutor strives to elicit it from the members of the group in analysis, evaluation and collaborative group discussion. Self-monitoring and observation skills, together with a heightened commitment to change, tend to be promoted as a result.

Although the latter is often favoured, it would be an unwarranted oversimplification to present it as the best way of making feedback available. Qualifying factors must be acknowledged including time available for feedback, the thoroughness and success of the sensitization phase, the level of sophistication, experience and perspicacity of the trainees and ultimately, the trainer's own conceptualizations of professional interaction and the training process. Being able to implement different styles based upon an awareness of such considerations and a commitment to rational decision-making would seem to be the hallmark of success (Bailey and Butcher, 1983). Accordingly, Hargie and McCartan (1986) advocate a compromise 'Listen → Tell' style with the tutor changing, towards the end of the critique, to become more directive in order to raise points and present information that would not otherwise be forthcoming.

Stages in the critique

The way in which the trainer considers his role and the particular style of tutoring adopted has structural implications for the critique and how it unfolds. Writers have presented different scenarios of the stages through which it develops. Most, however, would seem to acknowledge two underlying principles:

1. Establish the facts before undertaking a more profound analysis;
2. Discuss positive before negative features.

For those who favour a less direct, more student-centred approach, a third principle can be added;

3. Let the performer have first say.

These precepts are influential in the identification and sequencing of the following stages of the critique, based upon the proposals of Pendleton *et al.* (1984).

1. Observe and analyse. The whole interaction may be observed before discussion commences. With longer practices, however, it may be more expedient to stop at various points for this purpose.
2. Clarify what took place at the factual level.
3. The individual who practised comments upon standards of performance and goals achieved concentrating upon positive features.
4. Other group members comment upon such positive features.
5. The trainee who practised comments upon standards of performance and goals achieved concentrating upon negative aspects.
6. Other group members comment upon such negative features.
7. Differences of opinion are reconciled and consistencies formulated.
8. Reasons for what happened are discussed. Again those who took part in the practice session have a major contribution to make.
9. Positive alternatives to improve performance are offered.
10. Main conclusions are summarized and generalized together with the establishment of action consequences.

Content of analysis

Interpersonal communication is a multifaceted and enormously complex phenomenon. Even when a limited aspect is isolated for the purposes of training, and regardless of the style of tutoring adopted, analysis and feedback can be directed at one of several levels ranging from the familiar to the profound, the descriptive to the interpretive, and from the surface features of behaviour to the underlying dynamics of action.

Level 1 At its least sophisticated, discussion can focus upon a descriptive analysis of the readily observable aspects of behaviour. In terms of the model of skilled communication, presented in Chapter 3, attention here is largely centred on the 'Response' component. Early CST programmes tended to be pitched at this level and were often founded upon the behaviour modification paradigm with feedback regarded as a means of changing behaviour through the operation of selective reinforcement.

Level 2 In this case the typical content of the previous stratum is extended by taking the personal significance of behaviour and the intentions of the actors into account. Thus individuals' perceptions of events and meanings attached to them, together with the plans and strategies underlying action, are recognized and their significance evaluated. By so doing the attention of trainees is directed via the contribution of goals, perceptions and mediating factors, to the process of skilled interaction (see Fig. 3.2). The insights to be derived from analysis at this level are very much in keeping with the recent, more cognitively oriented developments in social skills training (Trower, 1984).

Level 3 The focus of analysis here is more concertedly on those psychological sub-structures encompassing beliefs, attitudes, values, motives, etc. that have a bearing on the perceptions and intentions already referred to above. In addition, 'Personal' and 'Situational factors' are incorporated and the possible ways in which these could have influenced what took place during practice discussed. While this can be extremely illuminating, resulting in a deep understanding of self and social situations, it can also be threatening and stressful. The trainer must always be mindful of the dangers and the distress which self-examination can cause. With short programmes run by inexperienced instructors, it may be best avoided.

Level 4 A further and still more profound level of inquiry can be countenanced which is directed at unearthing and identifying those forces and influences which serve to sustain the individuals' beliefs, attitudes, values, etc. This level of analysis should only be contemplated by well-trained and experienced instructors. The general ambience of the feedback session and the self-exploration encouraged becomes more redolent of some of the more psychodynamically oriented approaches to training in interpersonal communication.

10.8 OVERVIEW

There is general agreement that the learning and performance of skill is dependent upon information on attempts at practice being made available for the benefit of the learner. Feedback is consequently indispensable to the successful acquisition and refinement of communication skills. Its facilitative influence can be specified in terms of motivating and energizing trainees, reinforcing specific elements of performance and therefore increasing their likelihood of being retained, or furnishing data which can be used in reducing errors and improving outcome. It most probably operates in all three ways to varying degrees.

This chapter has been exclusively concerned with extrinsic feedback i.e. feedback which is over and above that present in the doing of the task itself. It may be provided by means of videotape or audiotape replays of what took place. Additionally, written or oral comment on appropriate facets of the performance can be supplied by trainers, peers or indeed participants in the practice interaction including, perhaps, patients. A typical group-based feedback tutorial combines videotape replay with written and oral comments from peers, participants and the instructor. It is important, in organizing this tutorial, that time be spent, especially at the start of the programme, creating a facilitative climate within which students can begin to feel relaxed, open, accepting and trusting, before undertaking reviews of what transpired during the practice phase. This review can be pitched at different levels of complexity from a description of the behaviour witnessed to a more in-depth exploration of those factors identified in Chapter 3 as constituting skilled interpersonal performance. Feedback should, at least, strive to encompass the personal meanings attached to behaviour by trainees and the intentions, plans and strategies which were operationalized to effect the skilled communication under study.

11

Evaluation of Communication Skills Training

11.1 INTRODUCTION

This chapter is devoted to the third main stage of CST – evaluation. Evaluation is an integral part of the general educational system. Indeed it is difficult to conceive the system functioning effectively without applying evaluative procedures, since success in almost every phase of the education process is based upon evaluation. At the same time it should be remembered that evaluation at the continuing education (CE) level, in particular, is comparatively weak, with perhaps a reason being that continuing education deals with adults whose mere presence indicates a motivation towards learning (Ryan, 1978). This latter observation is important in that CST programmes, certainly within the UK, are being offered to established health professionals who have never previously had the opportunity to engage in communication skills training, unlike those more recently qualified practitioners who are much more likely to have undergone some form of CST prior to accreditation. However, at any level it is increasingly important to demonstrate the effectiveness of the programme being offered in that further financial resources are unlikely to be committed to a training course where positive benefits cannot be established.

While the need for evaluation is clear the assessment of CST is particularly difficult. Certainly, many claims have been made for the success of this type of training yet they suffer from a fundamental weakness in that the reliability and validity of most social skill assessment procedures are uncertain. As Bellack (1979) has stated 'it is unclear whether the predominant assessment strategies are adequate, whether specific instruments are sound, or whether the most appropriate aspects of interpersonal functioning are being targeted' (p.158). Thus for the trainer considering evaluation two basic questions must be addressed – *what* should be measured and *how* should it be measured?

Evaluation of any programme of training must be carried out against the background of previously defined objectives, since it is not possible to measure the results obtained from an educational system when the objectives have not been explicitly stated. Reference has been made in previous chapters to what constitutes communication skills and the behavioural repertoires and underlying cognitions that go together to make up effective performance. These provide the basis of what is to be measured.

11.2 THE NATURE AND PROCESS OF EVALUATION

Various definitions have been offered to describe the nature of evaluation. Guilbert (1981) has defined it as a continuous process, based upon criteria that have been co-operatively developed and concerned with measurement of the performance of learners, the effectiveness of teachers and the quality of the programme. It is continuous in that it may lead to a revision of educational objectives, or continuous in a formative sense by providing the learner with information on his progress. The criteria refer to the acceptable levels of performance that have been established, while the co-operative aspect of evaluation involves a team approach from teachers and collaboration between teachers and students in implementing the evaluation programme. Educational evaluation has also been defined as 'the process of delineating, obtaining and providing useful information for judging decision alternatives' (Beggs and Lewis, 1975, p.6). Evaluation is therefore the process of gathering information as well as the process of making decisions based upon this information.

Gallego (1987) has further suggested that the definitions of evaluation fall into two main categories, namely qualitative and quantitative. The former largely reflects subjective judgements while the latter is best understood in terms of objective measurement. In making such a distinction it is perhaps better to think in terms of an evaluation continuum spanning between these two pole positions.

In general, evaluative judgements are used to contribute to planning, improve present practices or products, or justify a practice or programme. Walsh and Green (1982) have defined various types of evaluation. Evaluations which contribute to planning are termed 'needs assessments'. Those which are performed to improve present practice or products are called 'formative evaluations'. This latter term is also used to describe continuous assessment of students where information is systematically provided on an individual's progress during a course of study or training. This is distinct from 'certifying evaluation' which is used traditionally to position students in order of merit or qualify for some form of accreditation. Essentially, it is designed to protect society by preventing incompetent personnel from practising. 'Impact evaluations' refer to those processes which are carried out to justify a practice or programme.

A number of specific criteria are indicators of impact. Within the health-care field these include participant satisfaction with the programme, changes in practitioner knowledge, changes in practitioner performance, and changes in patient health-care status (Walsh and Green, 1982; Young and Willie, 1984). These may be viewed as ascending rungs of a ladder of which patient outcomes and health status are the most important. However, because of the multiplicity of variables affecting improvement in medical care it is important to attempt to assess the impact of training on practitioner satisfaction, knowledge and performance in order to document their links to patient health status.

In relation to student evaluation the assessment process should follow four main stages. These concern (a) the criteria or the acceptable levels of performance that the student must attain, (b) the development of measuring instruments, (c) the interpretation of the measurement data and (d) the formulation of judgements as a basis for future decisions or actions. Reference has already been made to the fact that any evaluative test procedure must be directly related to educational objectives. Moreover, any testing system must be realistic and practical and concentrate on those issues which are both important and relevant. In addition, it should be comprehensive but brief and marked with precision and clarity (Guilbert, 1981).

Crisp (1986) has outlined a number of communication objectives in relation to the medical consultation which may be adapted to suit other contexts of interpersonal communication within the health fields. Furthermore, Exercise 11.1 is designed to assist trainers to begin to analyse and define their objectives in planning and implementing CST. Based on what the trainer's expectations of trainees are following such a course, it will be possible to begin to develop test instruments which are relevant to the training process and which have the capacity to fulfil the qualities of tests discussed later in this chapter.

Exercise 11.1 Establishing the basis of a test instrument

Consider the CST programme that you are about to introduce. Against the background of the objectives you have established (a) list the contents of the course that you expect trainees to know and understand, (b) list a set of behaviours which you expect trainees to recognize and accurately interpret, and (c) list a set of behaviours which you expect trainees to adopt and integrate into their interpersonal communication performance. These may be set out under the following headings:

Knowledge and Understanding

Recognition and Interpretation

Application and Assimilation

11.3 SOME PROBLEMS IN EVALUATION

There are a myriad of problems that surround the evaluation of CST of which the following are both important and frequently encountered. Firstly, there is the problem of deciding what is to be evaluated. Education evaluation has a two-fold purpose. One is concerned with the operational objectives of evaluation which include such features as the programme planning process, structure, decision-making procedures, personnel, physical facilities, finances, recruitment, training, public relations and administrative management. The other is concerned with the educational objectives dealing with aspects such as programme objectives, trainees, methods and techniques, materials and quality of learning outcomes (Knowles, 1980).

Secondly, there is the cost of undertaking assessment procedures, both in terms of finance and time. Both these factors can mean that severe restrictions are placed upon the type of evaluation that can be carried out and its essential worth. Thirdly, there is a possible lack of expertise on the part of course tutors in designing evaluative systems allied to CST that go beyond measuring mere intellectual skills to assess professional performance and patient outcomes. Fourthly, and linked to the previous factor, is the degree of difficulty in actually measuring practitioner performance in the work situation or patient health outcomes. Fifthly, there is the problem of designing test instruments which fulfil the criteria of validity, reliability, objectivity and practicability. As Oetting (1976) has pointed out:

> Once goals have been established, it would be ideal to find a previously validated instrument in the literature that would measure these variables. Unfortunately they are usually not available. Evaluation goals, if well established, are often too specific to warrant using standardised instruments. The evaluator must construct new instruments or measurement methods (p.13).

Such factors play an important part in the evaluation process at all levels of education. However, at the continuing education (CE) level other issues emerge linked to assessment. The fact that there is a lack of objective evaluation of CE courses may reflect the thinking that the provision of CE opportunities is a service to the profession and, as long as there is uptake of such courses, that is sufficient evidence of their usefulness and effectiveness. There is also the concern that practitioners who voluntarily participate in CE programmes may consider formal evaluation an infringement of their professional rights and freedom, and may either refuse to take part in evaluation procedures or withdraw from participating in CE.

In the overall context of CE, Knowles (1980) has pointed out that there are four universal problems related to evaluation:

1. The complexity of human behaviour and the myriad of variables affecting it make it impossible for us ever to be able to 'prove' that it is 'our programme' alone that has produced the desired changes.

2. To date the social sciences have not developed the rigorous research procedures and measurement instruments for producing the hard data required for evaluating many of the subtle and more important outcomes of a CE programme. It should however be pointed out that considerable gains have been made in this area over the last fifteen years.
3. Intensive evaluation procedures require substantial time and financial resources, which are not prepared to be committed by planners and participants, simply to document the value of training which they already see.
4. CE is, unlike youth education, an open system in which participation is voluntary so that the worth of a programme is more readily tested by the degree of persistence and satisfaction of its participants.

These observations only serve to illustrate the complexity of the task facing a trainer at whatever level of training in respect of initiating evaluation. However, it is to the methodological strategies that we now turn in an attempt to provide practical advice on how testing can be implemented even in situations where the constraints are considerable.

11.4 QUALITIES OF THE ASSESSMENT PROCEDURE

As has been alluded to, the two main desirable qualities of any test are those of validity and reliability. A brief outline of these concepts is presented firstly, to alert trainers of the issues that require to be considered in the design of any evaluative test procedure in respect of CST, and secondly, to provide some background information that will foster a better understanding and critical assessment of evaluative reports on the outcomes of training programmes.

Validity

Validity is concerned with the question: To what extent does the test instrument measure what it is intended to measure? Unfortunately, in designing tests often the emphasis is on answering factually orientated questions, yet the teaching objectives have included the application of principles coupled with the trainee's ability to develop problem-solving skills. Thus for tests to be valid they must be designed to cover all the aspects of instruction, including behavioural dimensions as well as factual knowledge.

Consider the example where a clinical nurse tutor wishes to design a test to determine if a student can effectively counsel a patient on the use of stoma care products. In writing the test items she includes only questions about the types of product, their unique features and the clinical situations where they are indicated. Here then is a situation where the test measures knowledge about stoma care products but does not measure what the tutor intended, i.e. it is not a valid measure of the counselling skills of the student.

It is perhaps obvious that a test may be valid for one purpose but not for another. However, the same test can have degrees of validity depending on its construction so that the notion of validity is in fact a very relative one (Kimberlin, 1985).

It must also be remembered that the concept of validity is multidimensional in that there are different types of validity, namely content, criterion related and construct validity. Table 11.1 differentiates between these classifications. Content validity is of primary concern to tutors who wish to develop knowledge-based tests of a particular subject data. Criterion validity is concerned with comparing test scores to some external variable or variables (criteria) which measure the same trait. With criterion-referenced tests trainees are expected to reach a certain level of mastery (criterion level) of the material being studied before proceeding further. Tutors may use criterion-referenced pre-tests to predict which students will master the training or indeed where the mastery level should be set. In order to support both these decisions such pre-tests will require some estimate of criterion-related validity.

Faulkner (1985) has suggested that criteria-referenced measurement is an appropriate method for judging nurses' ability to interact with their patients. In a study of nurses' assessment skills, Faulkner and Maguire (1984) developed an instrument which scored individual behaviours or techniques on a 0–4 scale where 0 equalled total omission of the technique and 4 equalled very good use of the technique with no omissions. The techniques considered were adapted from the medical context and included for example, avoidance of jargon, encouraging precision, handling emotionally loaded material and controlling interviews. In this evaluation pre- and post scores were measured to determine any changes in performance.

Finally, construct validity is designed to assess how well a test measures more abstract concepts such as 'problem-solving ability', 'awareness of patient needs', 'perceptions', 'anxiety' etc. Gronlund (1976) has defined a construct as a 'psychological quality which we assume exists in order to

Table 11.1 Types of validity (after Gronlund, 1976)

Content validity	The degree to which the test measures the subject matter content and behaviours under consideration.
Criterion-related validity	The extent to which test performance predicts future performance or estimates current performance on some valued measure other than the test itself.
Construct validity	The way in which performance can be described in psychological terms.

explain some aspect of behaviour. Reasoning ability is a construct. When we interpret test scores as measures of reasoning ability we are implying that there is a quality that can be properly called reasoning ability and that it can account to some degree for performance in the test. Verifying such implications is the task of construct validity' (p.81).

Reliability

Reliability may be defined as the consistency with which a given test measures a specific variable. Thus it is concerned with the reproducibility of test scores on different occasions given the same testing conditions. It must however be recognized that valid results are by necessity reliable, but reliable results are not necessarily valid. While validity is a relative term, reliability is a strictly statistical concept and is expressed in terms of a reliability coefficient or through the standard error of the measurements made. For further consideration of the statistical aspects of this feature see Speedie (1985) and Page and Fielding (1985).

In considering reliability as a fundamental quality within a test it must also be recognized that the concept of reliability extends to those who administer the test, in the sense that observation-type tests require the observer to be reliable. Thus, while it is possible to construct a specific categorization system of behaviours or actions to be assessed the rater must be consistent in his attention to and interpretation of the specific facets of these behaviours. This will mean that in any form of interaction analysis the propensity to be unstructured, ill-defined or highly subjective will be minimized by clearly defining the criterion to be assessed and providing precise instructions on the methods of scoring to be adopted. Maguire *et al.* (1978) and Faulkner and Maguire (1984) have described specific criterion-referenced behaviours or techniques used for measuring interpersonal skills, their application being matched with high levels of inter-rater reliability.

Other characteristics of tests

In addition to validity and reliability, a number of other qualities are important to the test instrument. Firstly, it should be objective in that independent examiners agree on what constitutes a 'good' response to a particular question or task. Secondly, it should be practical in that it can be carried out with limited expense and within a reasonable time frame. Ideally it should be easy to administer, yet the complexity of evaluating communication skills militates against achieving this goal. Thirdly, against the background of the objectives set for training any assessment procedure should reflect the weight of teaching in any particular area. Thus, assessment of trainees following a course on patient interviewing skills should seek to provide the correct balance in the evaluation procedure in terms of measuring questioning skills, listening skills, explaining skills etc. Fourthly, any test procedure should also be discriminatory in that it should be possible to distinguish between good performance and poor performance of trainees in relation to a given variable. Within the health field such assessments have led to the recognition that doctors and nurses in particular tend to avoid dealing with psycho-social aspects of patient care, concentrating on the physical aspects of disease (Maguire *et al.*, 1980b; Rosser and Maguire, 1982; Maguire, 1985).

11.5 METHODS OF EVALUATION

A wide variety of methods have been employed to evaluate education and training programmes. Interviews with participants, programme advisory councils, questionnaires and instructional group feedback are all examples of methods that have been used to measure the operational objectives of a programme (Ryan, 1978). Substantially, these reflect the degree of satisfaction of participants with the programme, but also provide some insight into processes, attitudes or behavioural changes.

The competency of practitioners relates to their knowledge, skills, attitudes and behaviours following a training programme, and their ability to apply these in the patient care setting. Examples of the methods used to evaluate these criteria include real or simulated practical tests, execution of a project, observational rating scales and tests, short open-answer questions, multiple choice questions and programmed examination (Guilbert, 1981). Some of these primarily relate to assessment of cognitively based skills.

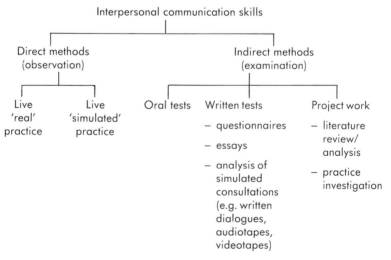

Fig. 11.1 Evaluative methodologies to assess the outcomes of CST.

However, real or simulated tests and observational recording go much further to chart actual performance. The use of 'patient simulators' (trained patient instructors) to teach and evaluate diagnostic, clinical and interpersonal skills is a good example of a performance indicator. In addition, the use of video to record and subsequently analyse performance is an increasingly used evaluative tool. Fig. 11.1 sets out the types of methodologies that may be used to evaluate the competency of practitioners.

As far as evaluation of patient health is concerned this, as would be expected, is much more difficult. In this situation the criteria for evaluation would focus upon monitoring, for example, compliance with drug therapy, disease control, death rates, discharge times from hospital, referral rates, surgery rates and the like.

Advantages and disadvantages of test procedures

Obviously in conducting CST there is the underlying assumption that communication skill can be learned and developed. Thus it is at the performance level that the trainer needs to direct his evaluative efforts in order to assess the trainee's communicative ability, accepting of course that patient outcome measures are the ultimate test of effective communication. Against this background, indirect methods such as multiple-choice questionnaires, essay examinations, and written analyses of patient-practitioner dialogues only serve to measure the cognitive abilities to the trainee along with, to some extent, writing skills. Oral examinations again tend to measure cognitive ability but do offer some insight into an individual's capacity to express himself clearly. However, the degree to which this could be generalized to the work situation is clearly dubious. Furthermore, oral examinations lack standardization, objectivity and reproducibility of results.

Direct evaluations do offer distinct advantages in the assessment of interpersonal skills. First, they permit examination of the candidate in a real or simulated situation through observation and analysis of performance. Secondly, they provide an opportunity to confront the trainee with specific situations that have not been illustrated during training, thereby assessing problem-solving and adaptive or applicative abilities. Furthermore, they indicate the degree to which generalization has occurred over tasks and persons. In this respect, as indicated in Chapter 2, Maguire *et al.* (1986) have shown that within the medical discipline interviewing skills trained in a psychiatric setting were successfully applied to interviews with physically ill patients.

Thirdly, and connected to the previous issue, they also allow for attitudes to be observed and tested, as well as assessment of and responsiveness to a situation where there is a high degree of complexity. In considering practitioner attitudes it is important to point out that these can and do have an important bearing on the outcomes of performance. For example,

Morrow and Hargie (1987a) have indicated that the more positive a trainee's attitude to training the greater will be the degree of positive influence in communication behaviour. Furthermore, Mason and Svarstad (1984) have shown that in relation to involvement by community pharmacists in patient counselling, those pharmacists who had the most positive attitude to counselling were also more involved in actual counselling activities. That attitudes appear strong determinants of practice behaviour means that it will be important in any training strategy to seek to develop constructive attitudes as well as verbal and nonverbal skills. Fourthly, direct evaluations allow for the assessment of communicative ability when under pressure and to distinguish between the important and trivial aspects of the encounter and respond accordingly.

The disadvantages of such direct tests tend to centre on the difficulties in standardizing the conditions in the same way as it is possible in a bench experiment. With actual patients, their responses cannot be controlled to obtain exactly the same behaviour with each trainee being assessed. Furthermore, such situations may suffer from intrusions of one kind or another and they may lack true objectivity in respect of the observer. One way of overcoming the problem of reproducibility of patient responses is to use patient simulators who have been trained to act in specific but standardized ways from one trainee to another. However, this poses difficulties in terms of the time and expense involved in training simulations, and where a range of patient situations are being simulated, ensuring equivalency of difficulty between them. One further disadvantage of direct tests is that they pose more logistical problems especially when dealing with a large number of trainees.

11.6 APPLICATION OF EVALUATIVE METHODS

A distinction has already been made between direct and indirect evaluations which serve to identify or measure the outcomes of CST, and evaluations made by students or others of the actual programme of training, the tutors and the training techniques employed. It is important to give some consideration to these latter issues at the outset, the results of which will be of considerable value to the course designer in implementing future training.

CST process evaluation

Guilbert (1981) has stated that 'many psychometric studies have revealed the validity and the accuracy of student opinions as well as their close correlation with objective measurements of the instructor's effectiveness' (p.415). Given this observation it is therefore both convenient and meaningful for the trainer to receive feedback from trainees. Unfortunately, some trainers see this as a threatening procedure which is damaging to their confidence and status as a teacher. Yet anyone who genuinely wants to develop and improve his teaching performance will seek his students' opinions.

There are two main ways of conducting this form of evaluation feedback, namely verbal or written. Verbal feedback can either be carried out in a group context or at an individual level. It can range from being completely open whereby participants are encouraged to make any comments on any aspects of the training, to being more structured in that comments are invited on specific aspects of the course. One simple technique that provides very valuable feedback is to ask the group individually to cite what was for them the most positive aspect of the training and also what was the most negative.

Written feedback may or may not accompany verbal feedback. In this situation various forms of questionnaire technique are used to gather information that will ultimately lead to the improvement of the training process. With simple evaluation questionnaires the purpose is to elicit a response to a statement. Here the statements should consist of a single component thought and specify clearly what is required to be measured. The statement should be presented in such terms that the trainee is required to express a favourable, neutral or unfavourable opinion. Ideally, equal numbers of the statements should be phrased positively and negatively to eliminate any suggestion of overall bias in the questionnaire. As far as provision of alternative responses is concerned 'Yes'/'No' answers serve only to give limited information. Instead a scaled answer is preferable and allows a greater appreciation of the students' opinions. Exercise 11.2 illustrates an example of part of a simple questionnaire of this type designed to gather feedback from a trainee group following completion of a CST course.

Exercise 11.2 Designing an evaluative questionnaire for trainee assessment of a CST course

Below are three examples of statements designed to obtain feedback from trainees in respect of their responses to a CST course. With your own training programme in mind design a questionnaire to permit trainee evaluation of the programme, the tutor and the training techniques used.

In the following questions circle only ONE of the choices using the following code:

> VSA = Very strongly agree
> SA = Strongly agree
> A = Agree
> N = Neither agree nor disagree

D = Disagree
SD = Strongly disagree
VSD = Very strongly disagree

1. This CST course has helped me to identify my own strengths and weaknesses in
   interacting with patients.

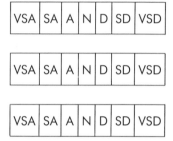

2. The analysis of my own performance
   on the videoreplays was counter-
   productive.

3. This CST course did not really stimulate
   my interest in the processes involved in
   patient interactions.

For tabulation purposes the answers may be accorded a numerical value
e.g. 1–7. In doing so it should be remembered that the intervals between the
integers 1–7 have been assigned the same value. However, in reality that is
not actually the case, so that in any statistical analysis non-parametric stat-
istics will need to be employed. A final point in assigning numerical values
to the range of answers is that on the phraseology of the questions, either
positive or negative, will dictate whether the continuum is ordered 1–7
or 7–1. Furthermore, the timing of the questionnaire will have a bearing
on results in that questionnaires administered immediately after training
produce different results from those administered some time later (Morrow
and Hargie, 1987a).

More complex questionnaires may be devised to not only identify the
students' perceptions of reality in respect of the course of training but also
their levels of expectation. In this type of question the item to be measured is
clearly specified and a scale of answers offered with a qualitative expression
of each degree. Two questions are then asked, one dealing with trainee
perception of the course, the other with trainee expectations of the course
(see Table 11.2).

In relation to analysing and interpreting this type of questionnaire the
deviance between the means of the responses to question A and B gives a
measure of the degree of dissatisfaction or satisfaction of the students in
relation to that item. It should be remembered that dissatisfaction may be
expressed in terms of lack or excess. Also by adding the deviation scores
across the whole range of items in the questionnaire it is possible to get an
overall measure of satisfaction or dissatisfaction among trainees.

Many examples of this type of trainee-feedback evaluation methodology
are described in the literature. For example, Rodenhauser and Sayer (1987)
have described very positive responses from medical students undertaking
an intensive CST course on an elective basis. These responses highlighted

Table 11.2 Complex questionnaire: test item

Item: **Relevance of videotaped exemplars**

What is required to measure is the degree of relevancy of the exemplar material shown on the course by way of illustration of the skills in action.

Never relevant exemplars	1
Rarely relevant exemplars	2
Occasionally relevant exemplars	3
Frequently relevant exemplars	4
Always relevant exemplars	5

Question A   Where would you place this CST course on this evaluation scale? ☐

Question B   Where would it be in order to satisfy you? ☐

---

the value of the course in providing new knowledge and skills required for practice, the need for further training, and the requirement of such training for future students.

Evaluation of teaching techniques and tutors

It is not possible within the scope of this chapter to offer a comprehensive review of the research that has focused on the evaluation of the training techniques used to teach interpersonal communication. However, it is of value to consider some of the findings related to their implications for training practice, since such findings are formative in producing changes in teaching strategies (Menikheim and Ryden, 1985). Some of this research has already been mentioned in preceding chapters.

Teaching techniques

In a review of 73 studies in the teaching of medical interviewing, Carroll and Monroe (1980) indicated that structured feedback to the trainees in respect of their communication performance was a crucial variable in relation to gains in interviewing skills. Where only self analysis was undertaken, via for example individual review of a videotaped recording of their practice, trainees tended to concentrate on their own physical appearance, mannerisms and voice with consequent failure to gain any insight into the more complex interpersonal processes of the interview. In another report, not covered in this review, Maguire *et al.* (1978) clearly demonstrated the benefits of structured feedback over non-feedback orientated teaching allied to patient interviewing. Feedback was given by tutors who used television or audio replays or ratings of practice interviews conducted by students. Television and audio feedback proved the most effective form of instruction and although the differences between the individual groups of students subjected to these two methods was not significant, they all favoured the television group. Additional studies on feedback effects were reported in Chapter 10.

The second feature to emerge from Carroll and Monroe's review suggested that standardized exemplars of patient interviews may be more effective than live, spontaneous demonstrations in that the latter may not be comprehensive of the behaviours desired to be illustrated. A third factor concerned the level of specificity of instruction on particular skills in that those programmes where individual skills were identified, demonstrated, practised and evaluated tended to be more effective than less structured programmes.

Tutors

Surveys of communication skills teaching in various health domains have clearly demonstrated the wide range of individuals involved in CST (Kahn *et al.*, 1979b; Sparks *et al.*, 1980; Hargie and Morrow, 1986a). Moreover, teachers include those who confess to being ignorant of the whole subject of communication skills (Eastwood, 1985). Hargie and Morrow (1987a) have argued that because of the current lack of expert staff within the health professions in respect of skilled trainers of communication skills an interdisciplinary approach is essential. Ideally, a behavioural scientist should be involved in the design, implementation and evaluation of CST in conjunction with a tutor representing the professional background of trainees. This type of work necessitates the marriage of two separate bodies of knowledge and if either is not adequately represented then the training experience may be impaired. The behavioural scientist will ensure that training focuses upon the communication issues without paying too much attention to professional contents, while the practitioner-tutor can ensure that any discussion of communication takes place within the realities of the actual practice situation. Thus, a fine balance between 'process' and 'product' can be obtained. Evidence of trainee endorsement of this approach has been reported (Morrow and Hargie, 1986a).

In addition, the feedback regarding tutors of CST would suggest that, as mentioned in the preceding chapter, there is a valuable role to be played by adjunct instructors, for example patients, patient simulators and student preceptors (Carroll and Monroe, 1980; Knox and Bouchier, 1985). This issue will be considered more fully later in relation to observation tests of trainee communication performance.

Trainee self-evaluation of outcomes

Trainee self-evaluation of outcomes is one step removed from observer-based practical tests. It is an attempt to obtain feedback from trainees regarding their behaviours following training, especially in situations where time and financial constraints make it impossible to go beyond this type of assessment. It must of course be recognized that this is an inherent limitation within this methodology, in that the reflections of the individuals concerned will be highly subjective. However, Hanson (1981) has pointed out that 'the limits of a self-reporting methodology must be weighed against the potential costs of a methodology using onsite observations' (p.58).

Menikheim and Ryden (1985) have used a self-reporting technique to assess the perceived competencies of nurses related to interpersonal skills before and at two stages following training. The results demonstrated significant gains in perceived competency across the areas assessed, gains which were maintained 8–11 months following training in a sample of nurses representing 20% of the original training group.

Morrow and Hargie (1987a) have also used a trainee-report technique to evaluate a continuing education course for pharmacists on developing communication skills. The participants were asked to complete a questionnaire stating the degree of influence the course had on them across a range of itemized behaviours consistent with the content of the course. The continuum of available responses for each item ranged from −3 to +3, minus values indicating a negative influence and plus values a positive influence with 0 equalling no influence. The questionnaire was administered immediately following the training and three months after training. At both stages of evaluation pharmacists rated the influence of the course as being highly positive. Nevertheless, comparison of individual responses to this questionnaire showed a significant difference between the degree of influence at the end of the course and at the follow-up stage. This was predicted on the basis that the effects of continuing education and training decrease with time (Deets and Blume, 1977). This finding, however, does have several important implications, not only in respect of the type of training employed but for the understanding and interpretation of this type of evaluative approach.

Firstly, the fact that some courses may be for relatively short duration means that if more time had been available to deal with each course component more lasting impressions may be expected to be made. Secondly, the decreased level of influence reported may also be attributed to the difference in levels of sensitivity and awareness provided in a training environment where behavioural consciousness was continually being stimulated, relative to the actual practice situation where the same structured stimulation is not available. Thirdly, practitioners who incorporate new behaviours into their performance, to the extent that they become habituated or automated, may underestimate the contribution of previous influential factors. Fourthly, practitioners, subsequent to training, may experience particularly difficult interpersonal situations which call for skills outside the scope of a given course. Because such interactions may have had unsatisfactory outcomes the course of training may be judged to be less effective. Allied to this is the fact that a short course cannot hope to cover all possible practice situations such that trainees may not be able to generalize the skills to other kinds of patient consultations. A final factor concerns the possibility that some desired behavioural change may not be easily possible. One good example of this identified by Morrow and Hargie (1987a) is the inability to provide a private area for patient counselling in a community pharmacy, despite the fact that within the course of training it was seen as a highly important factor in contributing to effective communication.

This latter factor does begin to raise the issue of the internal consistency of the test items in the questionnaire. This relates to the degree to which they are a product or a consequence of the course, or to influences entirely outside of the training itself. Statistically it is possible to measure the internal consistency or correlation between items in a questionnaire from the results obtained from the surveyed group. By so doing items of dubious relevance can be omitted from the questionnaire. Oppenheim (1966) has discussed these issues and the reader is referred to this text for detailed information on questionnaire design and analysis.

Indirect methods of trainee evaluation

Indirect methods of CST evaluation are largely pencil-and-paper type tests although they do vary considerably from the straightforward traditional examination questions to written analysis of simulations or responses to videotaped vignettes. Guilbert (1981) has described a number of these techniques within the health context allied to evaluations in general and the reader is referred to this text for an in-depth appraisal of these methodologies. The application of some of these procedures to the evaluation of CST can be illustrated by reference to a number of selected reports.

Firstly, the modified essay question (MEQ) which is a set of short, open answer questions preceded by a case history has been used to test the cognitive skills of trainees following CST (Knox and Bouchier, 1985; Weinman, 1984). Using both pre- and post-test results or control versus test group results these studies demonstrated clear gains in student knowledge following training. Moreover, they also tended to indicate increased student awareness and acceptance of the psychosocial dimensions of the case presentations, a feature which may underline the behavioural and affective changes found in other studies.

Secondly, Lezberg and Fedo (1980) have described the use of (a) weekly written exercises requiring the demonstration by students of a knowledge of the practical application of specific communication principles,

(b) evaluation summaries of assigned articles dealing with practice-orientated communication situations and issues, (c) participation in interviews and (d) final examinations comprised of multiple-choice questions and essay questions. Within this latter written assessment students were expected to create and analyse a dialogue between a patient and a pharmacist relevant to the practice situation.

Thirdly, an extension and refinement of this latter procedure has perhaps been the basis of the most meaningful forms of written or oral assessments, that is the response to videotaped scenarios of practitioner-patient consultations and audiotaped or written transcriptions of interviews (CINE, 1986). Such techniques are in essence similar to the discrimination phase of CST described in Chapter 8. They largely assess the cognitive and problem solving skills of trainees and allow some indication as to their attitudes to any given situation. While such evaluations may be predictive of what may happen in the practice context this is by no means guaranteed such that observation of trainees in practice will be the only clear indicator of the effects of training.

Olson and Iwasiw (1987) have used the Behavioural Test of Interpersonal Skills for Health Professionals (BTIS) to evaluate the effects of training on listening skills with a group of registered nurses. This test is comprised of twenty-eight videotaped vignettes of common patient-practitioner situations to each one of which trainees are required to respond. In this programme pre-training testing of nurses was carried out with the first fourteen situations of the BTIS. Here the nurses recorded their responses on audiotape. Following training they were similarly tested with the second fourteen situations. A control group of nurses, who received no training was also evaluated using the twenty-eight item BTIS instrument to ensure that the second half of the BTIS did not of itself elicit higher scores than the first half of the test. The audiotaped responses were subsequently scored by trained raters to measure any differences in listening behaviour. The results of the study demonstrated clear gains in nurses' listening skills following training.

A similar technique has been reported by Winefield (1982) among medical students whereby the empathy skills of students were assessed on their written responses to ten two-line trigger statements before and after CST. In matched pre- and post-training measures there was a significant overall increase in empathic responding by students. McPherson *et al.* (1984) have reported on the use of modified forms of Carkhuff's Standard Index of Discrimination (Carkhuff, 1969) and the Helping Relationship Inventory (Jones, 1973) to determine the effect of CST on counselling and interviewing skills of medical students. Forty-eight students comprised the training group and were tested prior to and after training. The results indicated significant changes in their communication performance as evaluated through these instruments.

Within the dental setting, Ter Horst *et al.* (1984) have used the videotaped vignette approach to evaluate the effects of CST by dental students. Here students were divided into a control group who did not receive training and an experimental group receiving CST. Following the course, students in both groups were asked to write down their reactions to a series of videotaped fragments of dentist-patient interactions. These written responses were analysed independently by two raters against a pre-defined communication category checklist. Although there was some evidence of enhancement of performance of the training group over the non-training group on some of the categories assessed, the poor inter-rater reliability levels found in this evaluation meant that the validity of the findings was questionable. Such a study serves to demonstrate the complexity of tests to produce valid and reliable results.

In consideration of these indirect methods of assessment various advantages can be identified:

(a) In general terms these tests are relatively easy to prepare and pose few logistical problems in organization;
(b) Prepared materials, unlike real practice, can also be uniquely constructed to test key abilities on the part of the trainee;
(c) Indirect evaluations are usually convenient to administer both in relation to time and are also applicable where large numbers of trainees are involved;
(d) Because they are largely cognitive evaluations, judgement of the responses is made easier by virtue of being right or wrong, appropriate or inappropriate; and
(e) Such tests are comparatively cheap to administer.

As far as disadvantages are concerned these focus on the fact that such evaluations substantially measure cognitive skills rather than communication skills *per se*, i.e. they indicate a trainee's knowledge and problem solving ability but they don't say how these abilities are applied or what behaviours actually result in the work situation. Further, by virtue of the convenience of these methods and their other advantages trainers may be reluctant to initiate more rigorous evaluation procedures. Reluctance to undertake more direct evaluation may also stem from the fact that within such a system standards for competent communication performance in practice, which cannot be compromised no matter how good a trainee is in other areas of patient care, need to be decided.

At a more specific level, in addition to the above, there are a number of other considerations to be made. This mainly concerns the use of videotaped triggers or vignettes. Here, the very nature of these recorded incidents is such as to only reflect parts of an interaction. They therefore suffer from the disadvantages that their interpretation and any responses to them are isolated and not set within the context of the overall interaction. Video-recordings, audiotapes and written dialogues of complete consultations overcome this difficulty, although the latter two largely omit nonverbal communication. However, video-recordings are more costly to prepare and this cost may be recurrent if different situations are required from one assessment situation to another. The other value of complete consultations is that they can be structured to provide a programmed form of evaluation by conducting the trainee through the interaction and posing questions at strategic points in the process. Obviously by using this form of evaluation some of the above advantages are diminished in that it can be, for example, much more time-consuming to undertake.

Direct methods of trainee evaluation

Since interpersonal skill is manifested by overt behaviours observation of these actions is the most logical evaluation strategy. As indicated in Fig. 11.1 two direct methods of observation have been used to assess interpersonal skills, namely live 'real' practice and live 'simulated' practice. Real practice evaluation refers to those situations where trainees are assessed during actual patient consultations. Simulated situations describe interactions where the consultation is staged either by employing trained patient simulators or through roleplay. Because the former is difficult to implement, simulated encounters are most frequently used for assessment procedures. It should also be realized that direct methods of evaluation are potentially most threatening to trainees such that this form of assessment tends to be utilized among students prior to qualification rather than qualified practitioners.

Simulated practice assessment

Patient simulators are individuals who are carefully trained to consistently present a patient problem to the trainee, with the encounter being carried out in a carefully controlled situation, such that meaningful evaluation of student performance is possible.

The advantages of simulations as an assessment technique are:

1. They can identify specific patient health-care issues or behavioural problems thereby emphasizing the skill areas to be evaluated;
2. Patient simulators can describe symptoms and behavioural problems in specific ways;
3. Patient simulators can provide structured feedback to trainers and also to trainees in respect of the learner's performance;
4. Different trainees can be exposed to the same patient stimuli and comparative assessment can be carried out using the same criteria; and
5. The trainee is not committed to the actual care of the patient such that the problems of obtaining true presentations, if these were real patients being observed, are obviated.

The main disadvantage of this technique is that the physical conditions of a health problem cannot always be easily simulated apart from using individuals who also actually suffer from the particular complaints. Also, training these individuals can be a costly and time-consuming procedure.

The use of this technique among pharmacy students has been reported by Gardner and Burpeau-DiGregorio (1985). Following instruction on interviewing skills with roleplay demonstrations, students were assigned to interview either of two patient simulators. Following the interviews each patient simulator discussed with each student their performance and assigned content and process scores to the interviewer based on previously established checklists. This educational feedback constituted the 'treatment' phase of the course. Following a 10–15 week interval the students 'crossed over' to interview the other patient simulator and assessment was carried out as before. An analysis of the pre- and post-test scores showed that only one student failed to improve on both control and process scores between pre- and post-interviewing. Overall, there was a significant improvement of approximately 20% in both content and process skills.

Evens and Curtis (1983) have also described the use of the patient simulators to teach and evaluate telephone communication skills to health professionals. In this situation audiotaped recordings of interactions between the trainee and standardized simulated calls were evaluated against prepared communication checklists. No firm data was reported on the outcomes of such assessments although the overall result of the training was positive.

An alternative to the use of trained patient simulators is the employment of roleplay situations to evaluate interpersonal skills. Here either other trainees or trainers play the patient role and the individual being assessed is observed for their communication behaviour. Davis and Ternuff-Nyhlin (1982) have described the use of roleplay patients to assess the communication competence of nurses involved in CST. In this training initiative nurses were assessed using a fifteen item behavioural checklist before and after training when interviewing the same roleplayed patient. Each interview was video-recorded. Compared to a control group of nurses not subject to training and assessed similarly, the training group showed gains in communication performance in some areas of the interviewing process. More impressive gains in interpersonal skills following training have been demonstrated among nurses using roleplay-based evaluation (CINE, 1986). Roleplay-based assessment has also been used to evaluate the communication performance of trainee health visitors (Crute, 1986). In this work trainees were perceived to be significantly more competent following training based upon behavioural rating assessments made by independent judges.

As indicated above, observation evaluation methodologies largely depend upon established behavioural checklists from which raters can, in a structured, standardized form, appraise the performance of the trainee.

It must be remembered that with a single rater the objectivity of the assessment is questionable such that a multiplicity of raters is preferable. However, for the results to be meaningful inter-rater reliability must be demonstrated. In Exercise 11.3 an assessment schedule is illustrated allied to interpersonal performance. A wide variety of such checklists have been reported (Davis and Ternuff-Nyhlin, 1982; Maguire *et al.*, 1986; Irwin and Bamber, 1984).

Exercise 11.3 Direct assessment of trainee communication performance

Instructions

Videotape a real or simulated trainee-patient encounter. Replay the interaction and score it across the fourteen items listed according to the nine point scale below.

Scale of Assessment

8 = Excellent; 7 = Very good; 6 = Good; 5 = Satisfactory; 4 = Average; 3 = Unsatisfactory; 2 = Bad; 1 = Very bad; 0 = Appalling.

Communication skills   *Score*

Communication skills	0	1	2	3	4	5	6	7	8
1. Skill in establishing rapport									
2. Listening ability									
3. Self-presentation									
4. Skill in obtaining information									
5. Relevancy of information									
6. Adequacy of information									
7. Allows sufficient time for response									
8. Appropriate use of reinforcement									
9. Ability to monitor situation									
10. Use of appropriate speech									
11. Use of appropriate language									
12. Skill in explaining material/ information									
13. Adaptability									
14. Skill in terminating session									

Total score
% score

Exercise 11.4 Devising a behavioural checklist for interpersonal performance

Instructions

Firstly, the trainer should decide what are the target behaviours to be assessed in the communication skills evaluation. Secondly, choose an actual practitioner-patient situation where these target behaviours apply. Thirdly, outline a continuum of actions along each target behaviour. An example is given below for the trainer to practise with before devising his/her own scale. The trainer should fill in the blank squares appropriately.

Task

To instruct a newly diagnosed diabetic patient on her use of insulin therapy.

Sample target behaviours

			Continua of action		
	−2	−1	0	1	2
When speaking with the patient the language used	often includes medical terms without explaining their meaning	often includes medical terms and sometimes explains their meaning	seldom uses medical terms but does not always explain their meaning	seldom uses medical terms but always explains their meaning	only uses terms that patient can understand
When questioned by the patient about psychosocial matters	always avoids any involvement	frequently avoids involvement but acknowledges existence of such problems			
In trying to promote understanding	never resorts to the use of illustrations or analogies				
When explaining administration technique					

More complex forms of skills checklists can be prepared that seek to itemize more precisely how an individual performs. Exercise 11.4 is designed to illustrate how trainers can devise more complex evaluative procedures to assess interpersonal skill. Moreover, the design of this checklist gives more specific guidelines for the raters and in that respect has the potential for greater consistency and reproductivity of results.

Real practice assessment

This is the most difficult form of evaluation to carry out, particularly because of the organizational and ethical problems it presents, together with possible clinical effects of subjecting patients to such encounters. These latter two issues have been discussed previously in Chapter 7. Although it poses such difficulties several reports have been made regarding the use of this technique.

Within the medical field these evaluations have included both undergraduate students and qualified doctors. The observation techniques involved were primarily videotaped trainee-patient encounters rated against a predetermined behavioural criteria. For example, Wakeford (1983) reported a study with twenty-two first year medical students into the effects of CST. The students were randomly assigned to either an experimental group or control group. Each student was videotaped during a patient consultation at the beginning of the clinical medical course and the experimental group went on to receive CST in contrast to the control group who received the normal training in taking medical histories and in conducting physical examinations. After this period each student was again videotaped and the videotapes were assessed by independent raters on a set of pre-determined criteria. A highly significant improvement occurred with the experimental group with improvements in questioning and listening skills being most marked.

More recently the positive outcomes of CST have been reported by other trainers in the medical field. Omololu (1984) compared pre- to post-training scores of medical students' interviews with patients. In this study significant improvements occurred across the range of behaviours assessed, e.g. positive reinforcement, eye contact and encouraging patient involvement. In a more elaborate evaluation of medical student communication behaviours, Irwin and Bamber (1984) assessed 475 videotaped student-patient interviews equally divided between two practical teaching sessions in the consultation room situation. Their analyses of these encounters demonstrated two distinct features namely, skills which could have been acquired through normal social learning and more technical or professional skills not usually employed in normal social interaction including for example use of confrontation, covering psychosocial issues, clarification and exposition skills. This latter set of skills were shown to be more evident among students at the second practice training stage.

Finally, in a unique follow-up study of the communication skills of young doctors who had received CST during their undergraduate education, Maguire *et al.* (1986) demonstrated the sustained effects of training where video feedback was employed. In this investigation thirty-six young doctors who as medical students had been randomly allocated to either video feedback training or conventional teaching in interviewing skills during a psychiatry clerkship were reassessed five years later. Of these thirty six, half had received feedback training and half had received conventional teaching on interviewing. The groups were matched for their pre-training interviewing skills and time after training. Each doctor was asked to obtain a history of the problems of three patients, two of whom were simulated patients and one real, representing psychiatric, life threatening and chronic disabling categories of illness. Each interview was video-recorded and subsequently assessed by a trained psychologist against a pre-determined interview rating scale. The results demonstrated that while both groups had improved their interviewing skills score after initial training the superiority of the feedback training group at that stage had been maintained over the subsequent four to six years. This was consistent across the range of skills examined with the exception of avoidance of jargon where both groups performed equally well. The control group scored particularly poorly on clarification, open questioning and covering psychosocial problems. Both groups scored poorly on opening and closing interactions but overall the trained group were viewed as being more competent, empathic, warmer and self-assured than the control group. Moreover, the results indicated that the effects of training in a psychiatric setting were generalized to other types of patients.

Such findings certainly justify the implementation of CST to enhance the effectiveness of practitioner-patient consultations. Furthermore, they also highlight the areas of performance that are weakest and which are by implication prime targets for skills training intervention.

11.7 OVERVIEW

Evaluation of CST presents a formidable range of challenges to the trainer. Notwithstanding, evaluation cannot be considered an optional extra following training but must be viewed as an integral part within it. This chapter has therefore sought to identify and discuss a number of the central issues pertaining to assessment procedures. These have included the nature and process of evaluation, the problems inherent in evaluation, the qualities of tests and the variety of methods of evaluation applied within the context of health professional training. Practical guidance has also been offered by way of facilitating meaningful implementation of these procedures within the resources available to the trainer.

PART FOUR

Towards formulating a communication skills training programme

In this final Part a more integrated perspective will be brought to bear upon features of CST which were introduced separately in previous parts of the book. Chapter 12 is devoted to a detailed exposition of the major considerations which a tutor must take into account in designing a particular programme for a specific group of trainees. Constraining influences upon decisions reached will be discussed in respect of, for instance, the identification, organization and integration of content; choice of practical activities; disposition of sessions; integration of the programme in a wider curriculum; and evaluation procedures to implement. Determining factors in each of these areas will include the needs and characteristics of the trainees, the objectives of the programme, available resources, size of the group and the period of time which can be given over to training. The resulting instructional sequence must, of necessity, reflect such idiosyncracies.

While the progressive application of sensitization, practice and feedback techniques can be thought of as the training mechanism at the heart of CST, it would be a mistake to assume that there is a single and immutable template of the archetypal programme which all others must replicate. Neither is it the case that all trainers slavishly adhere to a commonly acknowledged, clearly articulated and rigidly enforced set of design principles. It can't even be claimed that existing programmes bear a striking similarity. One of the most interesting outcomes of the comprehensive survey of interpersonal skills provision undertaken by Kurtz *et al.* (1985) was not the fairly substantial and perhaps predictable area of commonality located but the idiosyncracies attending each of the programmes scrutinized. They concluded that, '. . . interpersonal skills training is marked by a diversity in what is taught, how it is taught and how learning outcomes are assessed . . .' (p.254). Such diversity is arguably much more pronounced in the process than the content of training. It would seem that tutors have been quite prepared to sacrifice the convenience of a reflexive implementation of a standardized package in the interests of more fully catering for the unique needs of particular groups within the constraints of distinct contexts.

This sentiment is one which we would wholeheartedly endorse. It can be traced back to the original philosophy of the approach. As conceptualized by Ivey and Authier (1978, p.299), this technique, '. . . represents an open system, an approach to interviewing training which allows for alternatives and variations . . . Trainers who take the microtraining model and mould it to their own unique setting and trainee population will find that this results in the most powerful and enjoyable learning experience'. A consequence has been the embellishment of the core procedure to produce programmes that, across the piece, differ in almost every identifiable characteristic including length of training, scheduling of sessions, identification and sequencing of skills, deployment of resources and evaluation procedures, to name but a few.

One of the central features of CST has been the practice of focusing upon a single skill at a time. But even this should not be considered inviolable. Authier and Gustafson (1982, p.101) stress that, '. . . with some trainees it is possible to teach more than one skill at a time whereas, with others, it is desirable to break the skills into even smaller components'. It is with decision-making at this level that Chapter 12 is concerned.

Chapter 13 takes a much broader look at CST and its role in improving the quality of communication entered into by health professionals during the course of their duties, and brings the book to a conclusion.

12

Designing and implementing the programme

12.1 INTRODUCTION

Communication skills training is a technique the flexible use of which has resulted in the emergence of a plethora of specific programmes specially tailored to meet population requirements and circumstantial dictates. Its enormous potential can be more completely exploited by pursuing this versatility. In keeping with this ethos, and ever mindful of the enormous range of trainee groups and settings within which training might be conducted under the broad rubric of 'the health professions', we don't intend, in this chapter, to attempt to develop some sort of generic 'model' programme. We don't see this as a particularly sensible or useful exercise. The strategy is rather to concentrate upon the process of planning and designing rather than on the end product. As a result the prospective trainer will, hopefully, be better prepared to tackle the job of formulating an instructional sequence best suited to a specific group under a unique set of circumstances. We will identify and examine the major constraining factors which ultimately determine the alternatives presented in respect of a range of features of the programme. The bases upon which these options are weighed and the practical implications of decisions taken will also be outlined. Throughout, the emphasis will be placed upon practical issues and consequences.

The task just sketched is far from easy. When it comes to answering many of the procedural questions that a likely tutor would probably want addressed, such as when best to introduce CST or the most effective sequencing of content, there is, unfortunately, only limited hard empirical evidence upon which to attempt definitive answers. Until such times as more extensive research is conducted we must make decisions based upon the best sources of knowledge available. In many cases these range from formal theories and principles of curriculum planning and instruction to informal conclusions distilled from personal experiences with this method of training. There will be occasions in this chapter when we will draw heavily upon the thirty-odd years of experience which, collectively, we have now accumulated administering to the communicative needs of the health professions!

12.2 DETERMINING INFLUENCES ON PROGRAMME DESIGN

The distinguishing features of the form and substance of a programme essentially derive from decisions taken in relation to a number of crucial areas of consideration (see Fig. 12.1 in Section 12.3). Each resolution adopted is determined by one or more of several immediate sources of influence such as the needs and characteristics of the group, the objectives of the programme, resources available, the size of the group and the time available for training. In addition, what the trainer elects to do in one area can have a constraining effect upon the options available in another. To add a further dimension of complexity, influencing factors are to varying degrees interdependent so that the impact of one may modify the significance of another in the decision-making process. Group size, for instance, can have a considerable impact upon the salience of the resources available. Group needs and characteristics should relate very obviously and directly to identified training objectives, etc.

Needs and characteristics of the group

A crucial starting point in the planning of any educational intervention is with the needs and characteristics of the group for which it is intended. While many such interventions have their origins in the felt and expressed needs of those for whom they are designed, it is more likely that the necessity for training will have been perceived by some third party, be it manager, administrator, educationalist or researcher. But felt needs should not be overlooked in the process of curriculum design (Knowles, 1980). The advantages are obvious of having a highly motivated and committed group of trainees who acknowledge that further training is required and accept that the procedures being advocated will meet those objectives. Establishing this perspective was an important preliminary to the programme offered by Morrow and Hargie (1985a) to in-service pharmacists and by Kagan (1985) to nurses undergoing post-basic training. Apart from influencing the specific instructional objectives it will help determine the content of training.

Those undertaking CST can be, both individually and collectively, enormously varied. Differences in academic ability, motivation, personality, gender, maturity, communicative competence, professional experience, to name but a few characteristics, may exist and influence the design and operation of the programme.

Associations between certain trainee personality traits and attitude to this type of instruction have been reported. Crute (1986), in a study involving student health visitors, discovered a positive relationship between 'stability' as measured by Cattell's (1970) 16 PF Inventory and attitude to micro-training. A similar finding emerged from work undertaken by Hargie and Saunders (1983b) with a range of both undergraduate and postgraduate trainees. Furthermore, they identified a significant negative correlation between 'anxiety' and attitudes to training. 'Socially precise' trainees (Crute, 1986) and 'extroverts' (Hargie and Morrow, 1988) also seem to be more favourably disposed to CST. The latter discovery is consistent with the conclusion drawn by Morrow (1986) that introverted students react less positively to instructional procedures incorporating elements of CCTV recording and feedback.

The relationship between personality of trainees and performance during training has also been explored. Crute (1986) reported that 'venturesome' students improved more as a consequence of training than those who were 'shy', and the 'self-assured' improved more than those who were 'apprehensive' as measured by Cattell's personality inventory. Edwards (1974) found that individuals displaying high levels of 'autonomy' and 'aggression' on the Edwards Personal Preference Schedule responded more favourably to self- as opposed to tutor-supervision during training.

While it isn't proposed that prospective trainees undertake a battery of personality tests prior to commencing CST, it is important for tutors to be aware of the influence which personality differences can exert on attitudes to, and performance during training. Where possible, modifications to the instructional process should be made to accommodate them.

Gender may also be a further factor associated with reactions to elements of this form of training. Thus Norris (1986), produced some evidence to suggest that male students may find roleplay a more effective learning method than traditional lecture-based instruction, while the opposite is true for females.

As far as professional experience is concerned, students could be, on the one hand, just embarking upon training with no practical experience of the job. Indeed their appreciation of the significance of communication and the relevance of instruction in this sphere may be quite limited. On the other hand they may be practising professionals of many years standing, taking part in CST within the context of continuing education. The requirements of these contrasting groups will evidently differ and must be acknowledged in their respective programmes.

The characteristics of the group should be accounted for in how the instructor generally orients to training. In-service trainees, unlike their inexperienced counterparts, possess decided views on such matters as professional practice. They typically arrive with already established styles and strategies for dealing with different interpersonal situations which presumably, as far as they are concerned, have served them more or less well in the past. Accordingly, they may not be readily predisposed to openly examine and modify what they do and ultimately they have potentially much more to lose in the process. Training will consequently represent more of a threat if it is construed as a situation where the instructor has 'all the answers'. Alternatively the group may resist such as attempt at self-aggrandizement and become alienated. But this rather bleak scenario need not happen if the trainer is sensitive to the particular characteristic of the group and organizes training to utilize the wealth of practical experience possessed by members.

The objectives of the programme

Following on from the general needs of the group the focused attention given to meeting particular objectives has a strong influence upon decisions taken during programme planning. What takes place, and the experiences to which trainees are subjected, will be deemed to best achieve these outcomes. In keeping with what has already been said about the importance of taking the felt needs of students into account, the possibility of having training objectives emerge from a process of joint negotiation between the tutor and trainees may be contemplated, especially with the type of more mature and experienced group already referred to. The point is made by Beattie (1987) that, 'Often, perhaps mostly, the subjects and skills studied will turn out to be those that would have been 'prescribed' by a knowledgeable expert anyway, but it is the process of negotiation and debate that is valued and that changes the whole nature of the teaching/learning enterprise' (p.31).

Within the overriding aim of improving communicative competence, the primary objective which has traditionally typified the sort of training process featured in this book has been essentially behavioural. The intention has been to directly change what trainees *do* when they communicate. More recent trends also acknowledge and take account of the role which internal phenomena such as knowledge, beliefs, attitudes and values have to play in the communicative process (Trower, 1984). Training objectives now tend to be more catholic with those which address behaviour being complemented by others having more to do with:

1. Cognitions e.g. appropriate schemata concerning self, others, roles, interpersonal processes, etc.
2. Perceptions e.g. sensitivity to relevant social cues
3. Attitudes e.g. warmth, acceptance, genuineness, respect for the patient as a person, etc.

4. Beliefs e.g. irrationality of beliefs such as one must always 'grin and bear it', be right, be liked by everyone, etc.
5. Feelings e.g. loss, anger, resentment, confidence, etc.

The relative emphasis placed upon these additional outcomes has quite profound implications at the stage of design. It will determine the salience attached to each of the phases of sensitization, practice and feedback. If bringing about changes in cognitions is prioritized then it is likely that more attention will be devoted to those sorts of activities forming sensitization training, than to practice or feedback. On the other hand, attitudes may be more successfully modified through greater involvement in some experiential task. Again the incorporation of practical exercises must be based upon what the trainer is striving to achieve. Simulation exercises and games are often better suited to increasing familiarity with a procedure or system, method-centred roleplay with training in fairly simple skills, while less structured developmental roleplays are a more useful vehicle for coming to terms with complex processes including counselling, and examining the feelings and personal issues which emerge. The content of training will also, of course, be in keeping with the goals of the module.

Objectives have a further implication for programme design which has to do with maximizing the generalizability of changes which accrue. Unless the effects of training persist over time and transfer beyond the confines of the training environment one could scarcely be satisfied with what was accomplished. Unfortunately many CST interventions have been less than impressive in this respect (Mullan, 1986). It would seem that particular steps must be taken at the design stage to ensure that generalization is achieved. Following the stipulations of Annett (1974) these should include:

1. Making sure that trainees comprehend the principles informing action rather than encouraging responding by rote;
2. Matching the conditions of training to those which pertain in the environment where training will be implemented;
3. Training to consistently high levels of success. It has been found that training beyond the point of initial acquisition produces more enduring effects;
4. Providing trainees with adequate levels of feedback on their performance.

This list has been extended by Stokes and Baer (1977), Morton and Kurtz (1982) and Mullan (1986) as follows:

5. Ensuring the ecological validity of the content of training i.e. the skills should be effective in the natural environment;
6. Providing sufficient exemplars of the skill in use;
7. Practising in different settings e.g. trainees may practise the skill in extra-classroom locations as part of a homework task;

8. Practising with different partners;
9. Gradually altering the focus of feedback from external to internal sources;
10. Arranging for performance to be reinforced in the field. This can be done, in part, by carefully selecting patients for involvement in *in vivo* practice to increase the likelihood of success.
11. Encouraging self-reinforcement;
12. Organizing training according to the principles of spaced practice (This point will be developed later in the chapter.);
13. Planning follow-up and refresher training.

The practical applications of these considerations will be evidenced in the discussions and suggestions throughout the remainder of the chapter.

Resources available for training

The CST programme presented is frequently a compromise between what the trainer would like to do (and feels should be done) and what can, in fact, be accomplished. The resources which can be utilized must be taken into account. Some of these will already be recognized from earlier chapters. They include staffing, accommodation, hardware and software and finance.

Staffing

The advantages to be gained from harnessing the distinct bodies of knowledge and expertise of a behavioural scientist with a background in CST and a tutor from the health professions were mentioned in Chapter 11. This co-operative arrangement has been explicitly advocated by those writing from within the professional domains of dentistry (Jackson and Katz, 1983), medicine (Pendleton *et al.*, 1984), pharmacy (Hargie and Morrow, 1987a) and nursing (Kagan, 1985). Both should be involved in planning as well as teaching. It may also be necessary, especially with large groups of students, to enlist the help of additional tutors to assist with practicals. Suitable staffing is probably the single most important resource which the trainer can have at his disposal. The likely success or failure of the enterprise will rely heavily upon this factor. If need be though, it is preferable to operate with fewer staff than accept tutors who are ill-suited to this form of training. Tutors should:

1. Have a knowledge of CST procedures. If not, students will invariably sense their uncertainty and become demotivated. Again tutors of this ilk, through force of circumstance, tend to 'do their own thing'. This commonly means seeking out familiar terrain and surreptitiously re-focusing the exercise by concentrating, during feedback, on trainees'

professional knowledge rather than interpersonal skill. Students find this both confusing and frustrating. It may, therefore, be necessary, and indeed desirable, for tutors expressing interest to be provided with initial training by the CST member of the team.

2. Be familiar with the experiential approach to teaching. Many teachers feel deficient in this respect. Faulkner (1986) reported that, in a survey of nurse tutors in Britain, only 3–5% felt that they had been adequately prepared to employ these techniques. Little wonder that many teachers are decidedly uncomfortable with them, favouring more traditional didactic alternatives.

3. Possess the skills being trained. This is relevant for three reasons. Firstly, it lends credence to the programme. Secondly, tutors inevitably serve as models and, thirdly, such skills together with corresponding personal attributes like sensitivity, openness, respect and genuineness, help create the supportive climate within which trainees can feel secure enough to take risks.

4. Be committed to this form of communication skills training. Assumptions and values held about education should be consonant with this approach. If students sense that the tutor is less than committed the high levels of motivation which they require to undertake this frequently demanding venture will be difficult to generate.

5. Be knowledgeable of the profession. The behavioural scientist in the partnership should have a sufficient working knowledge of the professional service provided to enable comment to be made about the skills in context. This can be readily provided by the professional tutor.

Accommodation

The most desirable accommodation is that which is custom-built for work of this nature and a number of institutions can now boast communication skills training centres (Ellis and Whittington, 1981). The one at the University of Ulster will be described for illustrative purposes. It presently comprises six CCTV labs. There is also access to a studio equipped to professional standards for recording and editing model tapes. Units are completely autonomous and consist of a recording room (300 sq. ft.) and a playback room (150 sq. ft.) where feedback tutorials are held. Playback rooms each contain a U-matic video-cassette recorder, a colour TV monitor, an intercom, a system of cue lights which are used for relaying messages to the adjacent recording room and a wall-mounted remotely controlled video-camera together with control panel. This camera records through a window in the adjoining wall. Each recording room has two suspended omnidirectional microphones and various pieces of furniture which can be used to create a variety of settings from a lounge to a consulting room. The tremendous advantage of this type of accommodation is that it enables a large number of students, working in separate subgroups, to undertake practicals, including video feedback provision, at the same time.

But CST can be attempted under more spartan conditions. These may, nevertheless, make the task of creating a facilitative group atmosphere more or less difficult. This should not be discounted. The minimum requirement is probably a room large enough to give sub-groups sufficient space to take part in practical activities without distracting each other. It should be warm, well ventilated, pleasant, comfortable and in a location which minimizes the likelihood of external noise or disturbance. Fixed furniture causes problems so chairs, desks, etc. should be movable.

Hardware

Here one tends to think primarily of CCTV and video-recording equipment comprising video-recorder, video-camera, microphone and TV monitor. While not essential, as already stressed, it does offer a powerful instructional tool in the hands of a knowledgeable trainer. Many of the positive features which it affords in relation to modelling (Chapter 8) and as a feedback modality (Chapter 10) have already been discussed. Others are identified by McSweeney (1986) and Cartwright (1986).

Video-recording equipment is now becoming widely available in institutions engaged in the education and training of health professionals (Brown, 1985). For the benefit of the unfamiliar reader, or indeed the more fortunate who has the luxury of choice, it would appear that the most popular formats are U-matic (developed by Sony) and VHS (by JVC) (Cartwright, 1986). Both are well-suited to CST. Compared with U-matic, VHS tends to:

1. be cheaper
2. be smaller and lighter
3. accommodate tapes which are cheaper and offer a longer playing time
4. be the type of machine the trainee is much more likely to have at home. This compatibility means not only increased familiarity but opens up the possibility of tape analysis taking place outside the classroom as homework.

On the other hand U-matic tends to provide:

1. a better quality of visual reproduction. This may not be readily noticeable at the stage of initial recording but can become quite marked if this original is edited and copied in the production, for instance, of a model tape;
2. a VCR machine which is more robust.

Significant developments in video-camera technology have taken place over the last few years. Modern cameras are extremely light-sensitive enabling them to operate quite successfully under normal room lighting. Indeed even in poor conditions, a quite acceptable, even if slightly 'grainy' picture with reduced colour definition, is often possible. Better pictures will be obtained, of course, with special lighting effects.

In addition to being light-sensitive present cameras are now incredibly compact. This is epitomized by the 'camcorder' which combines camera and video-recorder in a single, highly portable unit. The major advantages are appreciated especially in the field where it permits recording to take place with the minimum of fuss and disruption.

Having a camera with a zoom lens attached is a decidedly useful feature in CST, making it possible for the operator to zoom in on one of the participants during recording without having to physically move the camera closer.

There are also benefits to be gained from incorporating a remote control unit enabling the camera to be positioned inconspicuously and operated from a distance, thereby reducing reactivity.

Many of the new generation of cameras have built-in microphones. Unfortunately these only work well when placed close to the interactors. Indeed recording good quality sound can be much more difficult than with vision and generally requires one or more extension microphones. These may either be stationary or of the levalier (or 'collar') variety. The latter, being attached to the clothes of the interactors, permits high quality recordings to be made but may be intrusive. The attached cables can also get in the way and cause difficulties, although replacing these with portable transmitters is a possibility. There are different types of stationary microphone each with distinct characteristics. some are uni-directional and designed for recording a single speaker while others are omni-directional and cope better with group situations. Technical details are provided by Wallbott (1983) and are not dealt with here.

The final component of the video set-up is the TV monitor. Here little need be said apart from the fact that it should be technically compatible with the recorder. It should preferably be colour although, in truth, there is little evidence to suggest that black and white has a detrimental effect on training outcomes (Reich and Meisner, 1976).

If at all possible, and given suitable accommodation, the trainer should try to commission several video-recording set-ups so that sub-groups can practise simultaneously.

The potential of the audiotape medium as a cheap and readily available alternative, or complement, to video in providing feedback was mentioned in Chapter 10. It is also a means of modelling skills which are fundamentally verbal in nature. Audio-cassette recorders can be a useful resource when video facilities are limited, student numbers are large, or for students to record their extra-classroom encounters.

Software

Items which can be listed under this sub-heading include books, handouts or manuals, skill assessment schedules, taped material on communication and communication skills, and blank video/audio tapes. There is an ever-increasing publication of books on communication skills and communication skills training, a considerable number of which are of relevance to the health professions. Some of these have already been extensively referred to (See Table 8.1). These books prove an invaluable source of lecture content, if lectures are intended to be used as part of the process of skill sensitization. They may also be drawn upon if skill handouts or manuals are put together by the trainer for distribution to trainees. Furthermore, students can be referred to them for further reading.

An alternative to compiling manuals, although one which reduces the flexibility of training, is to adopt those which have been prepared on a commercial basis by, for example, Ivey and his colleagues at the University of Massachusetts (Ivey and Gluckstern, 1974, 1976; Jessop, 1979). These often incorporate skill assessment schedules. However, such schedules can quite easily be constructed by the trainer and, since this option takes into account the nuances of the particular programme, are frequently accepted as being more directly relevant and beneficial.

Commercially produced audio- and videotapes, often part of instructional packages on various aspects of the communicative process, are available to be used either instead of or together with model tapes which the trainer may make (see Chapter 8).

As well as pre-recorded tapes, blank tapes for recording skill practice are needed. This is usually one of the more easily met resource demands, especially in the case of the cheaper VHS variety. For the most part a single tape will be used and re-used, following feedback, during the next practical. There may be advantages, though, in keeping recordings (with students' permission) until the end of the programme so that students can re-play and discuss them in their own time between sessions. By comparing later with earlier attempts, levels of improvement can (as a rule) be readily appreciated thereby increasing motivation.

Finance

Most of the resources for training already mentioned ultimately depend upon the size of the budget which can be drawn upon. With sufficient funding, adequate software and hardware can readily be made available, suitable accommodation obtained and optimal levels of staffing countenanced! Indeed it is possible to improve the quality of staffing given sufficient finances to operate training for tutors in CST procedures.

The funding of the programme has further implications for decision making in respect of procedures to follow in identifying the skills content of training and evaluating learning outcomes. This factor may place severe restrictions on the degree of sophistication which can be entertained in both of these endeavours.

Group size

Strictly speaking the number of trainees *per se* has little bearing upon how the trainer may wish to organize and conduct the programme. It is the relationship between programme objectives, group size and available resources which is the telling factor. Given adequate space, staff and video-recording facilities, even the largest group can be comfortably handled. Real practical difficulties arise when, with limited resources, programme objectives require every trainee to practise during each practical session devoted to a separate skill. While these problems may begin to manifest themselves during sensitization, if students are engaged in experiential exercises, it is principally at the stages of practice and feedback that they become chronic. Here they are exacerbated by the necessity for this part of training, if it is to be meaningful, to be conducted in small groups of ideally less than ten students. The resolution of this dilemma will require decisions to be taken in respect of the utilization of resources, constitution of sub-groups and allocation of time to different training components each of which will be discussed later in the chapter.

Time

The final constraining influence upon programme design is the amount of time which has been allocated to it. The feeling of never having quite enough time to incorporate all of the facets of the communication process that seem relevant, nor do all the things that one would ideally like, is no doubt one shared by others charged with providing inputs into the curriculum. It is perhaps amplified by the quintessentially experiential nature of CST. While this approach to teaching has much to commend it, it does tend to be time-consuming. One is sometimes faced with the decision of covering only core features thoroughly or incoporating additional material by, for instance, focusing upon several skills per session or reducing the amount of time devoted to practice and feedback.

If CST is added to an already crowded curriculum, as is frequently the case, the time which can be given to it is often meagre being squeezed into the few hours grudgingly relinquished by someone else or culled from students' private study. Present estimates would consequently suggest that in dentistry the proportion of the curriculum set aside for this purpose could be as little as 2% (American Dental Association, 1977), in nursing less than 5% (MacLeod Clark and Faulkner, 1987), while in pharmacy the modal figure would appear to be less than 7 hours per student (Hargie and Morrow, 1986a). It is to be hoped that with an ever increasing acceptance of the role of effective interpersonal interaction in the health professions, these figures will gradually be revised upwards. Meanwhile programmes have to be devised to account for them.

12.3 PROGRAMME CHARACTERISTICS

The practical consequences which the various sources of influence just reviewed have for decisions which shape the programme and give it identity will now be examined. These are outlined in Fig. 12.1.

Duration of programme

There is no definitive answer to the question of how long the programme should last. The most obvious determining factor is of course the amount of time available. Group size and available resources can also play a part. If subgroups have to practise consecutively rather than concurrently the total hours devoted to training (although not necessarily to each student) will be increased.

Programme objectives are relevant in addition. Dickson *et al.* (1984)

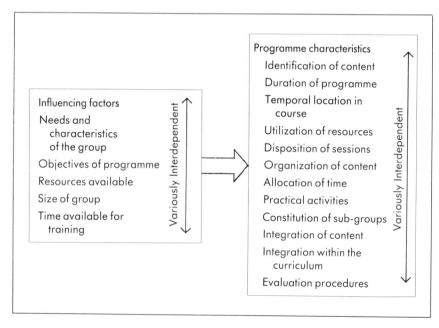

Fig. 12.1 A decision-making framework.

distinguished between time and competency-based programmes. The former take place within a fixed temporal framework with a pre-determined number of sessions being devoted to different content areas. With competency-based programmes the overall length and speed of progression through the sequence is determined by the systematic satisfaction of pre-ordained criterion levels governing performance. While this learning format is probably the more effective instructional approach, allowing for individual pacing and competency attainment as a basis for advancement to more complex communicative processes or situations, its flexibility can create massive logistical problems. This is undoubtedly one of the reasons why CST in the health professions is invariably time-based.

The length of programmes differ enormously ranging, for example, from a mere three hours in the case of undergraduate medical students (Omololu, 1984) to 115 hours for health visiting students (Ellis and Whittington, 1981). Indeed it would seem that there is a general tendency for programmes to be either quite short (less than six hours) or fairly long (thirty-five hours or more) (Kurtz *et al.*, 1985). A cursory scrutiny of those in the health professions suggests that the average length is probably somewhere around twenty hours. It has been our experience that little can be accomplished in less than, say, fifteen hours, unless it is intended to concentrate upon a single skill area or situation with minimal practice and feedback. It must be remembered that, in most cases, trainees have to be introduced to experiential techniques such as roleplay and video-recording, and that sufficient practice opportunities must be provided to encourage the transfer of training.

Temporal location of programme in course

Remarkably little agreement exists as to the stage of training at which students profit most from CST. This is evidenced by the fact that in the basic training curriculum of most professions, programmes of this type can be found from first through to final year (Kahn *et al.*, 1979a; Hargie and Morrow, 1986a). The majority though would seem to be located in first year (Kurtz *et al.*, 1985) and, at least in medicine, prior to clinical experience (Kahn *et al.*, 1979a). This is completely consonant with the underlying conceptualization of this form of training as a means of bridging theory and practice thus providing a more systematic preparation for practical involvement in the field (Ivey and Authier, 1978).

There may be disadvantages though, identified by Dickson and Maxwell (1987), in placing CST too early in the course. While it introduces students to the communicative dimension of the job, they typically embark upon it without any real appreciation of what that job entails. Not only do they lack practical experiences to draw upon during the programme, they may even fail to appreciate the relevance of this input to their training. Compared with the cognitive and technical skills of the profession, communication skills may appear, at first sight, commonplace and unproblematic. Under these circumstances the trainer is well advised, perhaps through some experiential exercise, to begin by impressing the need for effective communication and the many problems of this type which can beset the neophyte when dealing with patients, staff and the public.

An additional pitfall in scheduling the programme at the beginning of training is that students, through lack of professional knowledge and experience, may feel ill-prepared to take part in professionally oriented practical activities. If, on the other hand, the programme isn't explicitly oriented towards their profession if often loses face validity. Students cannot see the relevance of what they are doing – even accepting that communication plays a part in their chosen profession.

Difficulties which can arise through instituting CST towards the end of a course may be just as testing. Foremost amongst these is a possible lack of integration with other aspects of professional training. Additionally students, having most likely taken part in lengthy periods of placement, can feel that there is little to be gained from a college-based procedure of this nature which could be seen as artificial. To overcome such resistance it may be necessary to adopt the sort of approach which seems to work best with practising professionals. Thus experience (albeit limited) is acknowledged and built into training; felt needs are taken into account; content of training can target more complex skills, strategies or problematic situations; emphasis may be on *in vivo* practice or developmental roleplays; and a purposefully less directive style implemented during feedback, than with the first-year counterpart.

An alternative to having CST at some particular juncture is to organize it on a recurrent basis throughout the duration of the course. Such was the sequence described by Dickson and Maxwell (1985), for undergraduate physiotherapy students. Here students were involved in CST across the four years of their study amounting to five hours of instruction per week during a four-week module for each year group. In this way training is matched to students' development in professional knowledge and practical experience so as to more fully meet their requirements as the course unfolds. There is a danger, nevertheless, that, with relatively short isolated sequences, the total programme may become extremely fragmented.

Disposition of sessions

This has to do with two central considerations. The first is the issue of whether sessions should be concentrated in time or spaced out with intervening periods when trainees are doing other things. The second, the extent to which separate sessions should be given over to isolated constituent elements of performance.

Massed versus spaced practice

By tradition, CST has been structured in keeping with the principles of spaced practice. According to Pawlak *et al.* (1982, p.367), '... training is best delivered incrementally, in a series of sessions; marathon sessions may result in limited trainer learning'. The period of time between sessions has typically been a week in accordance, no doubt, with common timetabling habits. With the massed alternative, instruction is condensed so that skills and opportunities to practise them are introduced in quick succession. The rapid build-up of fatigue and decline in motivation which can result are weaknesses of massed practice which may become particularly evident with the less mature, experienced and committed student. Again there is little opportunity for students to supplement class activities through readings or homework assignments.

The consensus of opinion, therefore, would appear to favour spaced practice although there is little hard evidence in substantiation. Indeed instances of programmes where sessions are scheduled in a decidedly more massed fashion can be found. These tend to be of the all-day workshop variety, often involving practitioners, and the organizing principle is invariably logistical rather than andragogical. A considerable amount of material can be covered in a short period with trainees who would find it inconvenient to attend on a number of occasions. While learning does undoubtedly take place, Morton and Kurtz (1982) have questioned the extent to which it is retained or generalized to the place of work.

Spaced practice has also hidden dangers which should be recognized. If the interval of time between sessions is too long forgetting can occur to the detriment of cumulative learning effects. The optimum length of interval is not known and most likely varies depending upon such features as the group, homework assignments, concurrent placement experiences, etc. In some cases it could even be that a week, while convenient from a time-tabling point of view, is too long!

Whole versus part practice

The founding of CST upon a reductionist philosophy permitting the analysis of complex interactive processes into simpler elements, has already been established. Practising these constituent elements separately is the hallmark of the 'part' approach. The 'whole' method of learning involves, in comparison, going through the complete activity on each practice session until mastery is achieved. But 'part' and 'whole' are relative terms. While it would be unimaginably cumbersome to accept 'health professional communication' as the undifferentiated content of training, programmes can be located which operate at a more holistic level than that of basic skills such as questioning, listening, etc. In the instructional procedure detailed by Maguire (1984b), for example, it would seem that medical students who took part practised, from the beginning, taking a complete medical history.

Several factors are relevant when deciding upon which approach to employ. Perhaps the most important is the nature of the task. Those that are highly complex yet capable of being broken down into a number of simpler but meaningful constituent parts lend themselves to part practice. Characteristics of the trainees including ability, motivation, experience and learning style are also salient. The less able student with little prior experience, who already possesses few of the skills, may be easily discouraged and should therefore benefit from concentrating initially upon molecular aspects rather than advanced processes such as interviewing or counselling. Being accustomed to learning in accordance with the part strategy will also by an advantage.

A further determining factor in choosing which method to implement is the total time available for training. Focusing upon single skills per session is time-consuming. With more able students it is often possible to combine two or even three skills which complement each other and can readily be practised in the same practical e.g. paraphrasing and reflection of feeling. Morton and Kurtz (1982), however, caution against being too ambitious in this respect. Trying to include too much in a session can prevent over-learning taking place and hence inhibit generalization of outcomes.

A hybrid which goes some way to achieving a compromise between the 'whole' and 'part' options is the *progressive-part* technique. This involves concentrating initially upon the first and second content elements in isolation before practising both together. The third skill is likewise introduced on its own and then combined with the first two. A session is afterwards devoted to the fourth skill, and so on. The module reported by Tittmar *et al.* (1978) for use with health visiting students was organized along these lines. Scheduling sessions in this manner is also a highly effective way of achieving the integration of training content.

Integration of content

If CST operates on the principle that skilled communication is capable of being analysed to reveal a number of simpler elements each of which can, in isolation, be targeted during instruction, then, at some point, thought must be given to issues of synthesis. One of the potential shortcomings of the 'part' method of training is that students, at the end of the sequence, may be highly accomplished in the performance of isolated components but unable to integrate them in carrying out the complete task. To claim success the CST procedure must incorporate mechanisms whereby the original communicative process can be reconstituted. In many cases the final session of the programme is set aside for this purpose. The rationale would appear to be that the various bits and pieces can be readily and properly combined as the culmination to the sequence. But this may prove inadequate; integration of content should be an ongoing activity throughout the length of the programme.

A variant of the CST protocol was developed by Hargie *et al.* (1978) with this in mind and termed 'mini-teaching'. It incorporates a progressive-part format together with a systematic lengthening of skill practice episodes as training continues (See Fig. 12.2 for an illustration of this mode). This principle of progressively and systematically approximating the realities of the work setting was further refined by Dickson (1981) who produced evidence to suggest that it may lead to greater levels of skill retention and generalization.

Aspects of the integration of content to do with organization and choice of practical activity will be mentioned under these respective sub-headings.

Identification of content

A variety of techniques for determining the aspects of communication forming the content of training were presented in Chapter 7. The trainer who institutes the *intuitive* approach relies, it will be recalled, upon hunches and notions grounded most probably in personal experience, to generate the apposite skills and strategies for neophytes to acquire. The *analytical* approach derives training content on the basis of reasoned argument. Given what is known about the roles and sub-roles of the practitioner, the sorts of interpersonal transactions engaged in, together with a theoretical appreciation of germane communicative processes, an anthology of relevant

Session	Activity	Length of practice
1	Introduction and familiarization	–
2	Introduction to video	5 mins
3	Nonverbal communication	5 mins
4	Questioning	5 mins
5	Integration of NVC + Questioning	10 mins
6	Reflecting	10 mins
7	Integration of NVC + Questioning + Reflecting	15 mins
8	Explaining	15 mins
9	Integration of NVC + Questioning + Reflecting + Explaining	20 mins
10	Opening	20 mins
11	Closing	20 mins
12	Integration of all skills	25 mins
13	In-depth history interview	30 mins

Fig. 12.2 Outline of the practical element of a mini-teaching programme.

skills can be deduced. The *empirical* approach is distinct in that systematic observation, analysis and categorization are employed in the quest to improve trainees' communicative competence. Specific techniques which may be used include task analysis, the Delphi technique, critical incident analysis, constitutive ethnography, and the behavioural event interview.

The procedure followed by any particular trainer faced with the task of designing a programme and identifying the most relevant facets of communication for a specific group to consider will largely be determined by the broad objectives of the programme, the time available and the resources which can be utilized. While empirical procedures are more 'scientifically' respectable and arguably furnish a more valid set of skills specifically tailored to the needs of a certain group, they are time-consuming and draw heavily upon the resources available including hardware and software but particularly financial and personnel. Many of the techniques require a certain level of expertise to operate successfully.

It is true to say that in the majority of reported CST programmes, the skills featured have been established on the basis of intuition and analysis. A trainer with a straitened budget may not feel unduly disadvantaged if forced to adopt these approaches when planning modules on generic communication skills for basic level trainees. There may be less complacency, though, at the prospect of preparing, in the same way, to offer a CST programme in some more specialized area of the clinician's job. In this case there is a greater need to make use of some of the more sophisticated empirical procedures in order to identify the nuances of effective performance. Saunders and Caves (1986), for instance, unearthed subtle differences in speech therapists' perceptions of the appropriateness of skills depending upon whether therapy was conducted with an adult or child patient. Additionally, certain skills were utilized in distinct ways for particular purposes with different clinical types of patient.

Organization of content

Having identified material legitimately forming the content of training, decisions have to be taken in respect of its sequential organization over the length of the programme. Contrasting models for structuring the content of the curriculum in a coherent and meaningful way were sketched by Cork (1987). Chronological, structural logic and problem-centred sequences would seem to be three which are most evidently represented in the construction of different CST modules.

Chronological sequence

Here skills are presented in the temporal order in which they naturally occur in the commission of the interactive task. As discussed in Chapter 3 many social enounters follow a predictable course. According to Byrne and Long (1976), it will be recalled, the typical GP – patient consultation comprises six episodes, namely, relating to patient, discussing reasons for attendance, examining, considering patient's condition, detailing treatment or further investigation and finally terminating the interaction. This progression suggests that skills should be introduced in the order of opening skills, questioning (and perhaps reflecting), explaining and closure.

Although this is an uncommon approach to programme design it has been used to teach social work students interviewing techniques (Gibson *et al.*, 1981).

Structural logic

Without doubt, the vast majority of CST programmes have been planned in accordance with this method. Here the determining factor is conceptual relationship and level of complexity. If one facet of a subject depends upon the prior understanding of another, the latter should precede the former in the intructional sequence. Such programmes often begin with a consideration of the key features of skilled interaction.

It will be appreciated that the skills introduced in Chapters 4 and 5 differ in complexity. Some can be readily thought of as sub-skills of others e.g. listening subsumes reflecting. Processes such as interviewing and counselling are located at a still higher level. Thus effective counselling involves successful listening together with a variety of other skills. The potential afforded by this differentiation in the arrangement of training was recognized by French (1983) as follows: 'By identifying skill levels according to increasing complexity and interrelationships between skills, one can generate a hierarchy of social skills which can serve as a heuristic tool or "rule of thumb guide" to social skill learning . . .' (p.257).

While many specific examples of modules organized in keeping with the principles of this approach to CST design could be cited, one of the most recently significant has been that initiated as part of the Communication in Nurse Education project (CINE, 1986). (An abridged version of this sequence is given in Fig. 12.3.) The planned progression, following the two initial introductory sessions, from basic skills to more advanced skills and processes, finally culminating in their application in a range of nursing contexts, is clearly recognizable.

Constructing a programme in keeping with the philosophy of structured logic has a number of advantages. Since earlier inputs are systematically extended and elaborated as instruction continues it inevitably promotes the integration of content. Cork (1987) indicated that it is particularly suited to groups having little background knowledge of the subject to draw upon. We would concur with this view. This approach works particularly well with students who have just commenced their professional training with

Session	Activity
1	Communication in nursing
2	Elements of communication
3	Questioning skills
4	Listening and attending skills
5	Reinforcing and encouraging skills
6	Information-giving skills
7	Initiating and terminating interactions
8	Comfort and reassurance
9	Combining micro skills: the nursing process
10	Communicating with other members of the health-care team
11	Cancer and dying
12	Preparing a patient for discharge
13	Communicating with geriatric and stroke patients
14	Communicating with patients before and after surgery

Fig. 12.3 A programme organized according to the principles of structural logic. (Example drawn from the CINE project, 1986).

little or no knowledge of the discipline of communication or practical professional experience. Presenting material in this way also establishes a firm base on which to build further inputs, if required, at some subsequent stage.

Problem-centred sequence

Evidence of this approach having been utilized in reported programmes also exists. Here the key organizing feature is a problem with which students are confronted. It may be generated by the trainer or drawn from students' own experiences perhaps by means of a critical incidents procedure. The substance of training is introduced in an attempt to illuminate this concern and formulate solutions to it. In the case of the input on communication skills for dental students provided by Eigenbrode (1983), the problem situations addressed included dealing with fearful patients, patients in pain, emergency patients, pseudo-knowledgeable patients and patients who prescribe their own treatment.

Morton and Kurtz (1982) have argued strongly in support of the problem-centred approach in CST on the basis that '. . . Adult learner commitment and involvement is heightened when learners perceive its relevance to their work concerns. For example, a family assistance worker may not be especially interested in the skill of immediacy, but if the skill is taught in the context of how to deal with a hostile client, the worker may be more likely to perceive its value and concentrate on learning it' (p.413). We have found the problem-centred approach an especially apt way of establishing a framework for training mature, sophisticated and professionally experienced groups. The situations selected should reflect the experienced needs of members. As a result they can readily relate, from the beginning of the programme, to what takes place and accept its relevance.

Problem-centred planning is sometimes operationalized within a more inductive instructional framework involving a readjustment to the structure and function of the three phases of training, namely sensitization, practice and feedback. Thus trainees may deal with a problem situation without prior sensitization to any specific tactics or strategies for coping. It is during feedback that these are established together with more general principles relating to the nature of skilled interaction.

Practical activities

A further area which requires decisions to be taken at the planning stage is the practical one of types of experiential technique to incorporate, bearing in mind that learning communication skills should be very much a 'doing' enterprise. Various exercises which can be considered have, of course, been included throughout the book. In terms of procedures for providing skill practice opportunities the possibilities outlined in Chapter 9 include covert rehearsal; behaviour rehearsal; structured, semi-structured and unstructured roleplay together with multiple roleplay, fish-bowl, role-rotation and role-reversal variants; simulation exercises and games; and *in vivo* practice. Those selected inevitably depend upon one or more of the constraining factors mentioned in the first part of the chapter. Decisions taken with regard to temporal location of the module in the course, together with the organization and integration of content, will also play a part. Perhaps the most central considerations, though, concern the characteristics of the group and the objectives established for the programme.

While there are few hard and fast rules which must be adhered to, we have found that less mature, confident or experienced trainees do not cope as well with techniques such as covert rehearsal, unstructured or developmental roleplay and, of course, *in vivo* practice. The relationship between group characteristics, needs and programme objectives has already been established. If the trainer is principally intent upon developing proficiency in the performance of relatively basic skills, structured or method-centred roleplay and, perhaps, simulation exercises are suitable. Behaviour rehearsal may also be considered depending partly upon the skill content. It is also an effective way of providing initial practice of more complex skills. At more advanced levels, though, incorporating interactive strategies and situations, developmental roleplay is often the preferred alternative.

When the objective is essentially to increase awareness of certain difficult issues or to gain insights into the operation of some procedure, the fish-bowl variant of developmental roleplay, as well as simulation exercises and games, are typically implemented. A particularly useful approach to changing attitudes and increasing self-awareness and sensitivity, on the other hand, is through procedures such as role-reversal.

The appropriateness of these techniques will also depend upon the stage of the programme at which they are introduced. With less sophisticated and confident students it may be best to begin with simulation games and exercises, which are usually viewed as less threatening, before moving on to roleplay. Indeed, under these circumstances, Miles (1987) advocates concentrating largely upon didactic instruction at the start before gradually including experiential exercises as the programme unfolds.

The point at which particular practical activities are utilized becomes more significant when the sequence is organized in keeping with the principles of structural logic. In this case, after the introductory exercises, it is common to progress from the method-centred roleplay of simpler skills to developmental roleplay and, finally perhaps, *in vivo* practice. The latter two also promote the integration of earlier content and serve an important function in this respect.

Constitution of sub-groups

The practice and feedback stages of training are, in most cases, undertaken in sub-groups. Some thought should be given to their number and composition as part of planning. Decisions taken will be strongly determined by the size of the initial group together with the resources available.

Suggestions vary as to the optimal size of sub-group. Barnes (1983) proposed that twelve should be regarded as a maximum. For MacLeod Clark and Faulkner (1987) this upper limit is twelve to fourteen with eight members regarded as ideal. We would advocate slightly smaller groups. If at all possible they should contain no more than ten members with six being a figure to aim for. While teaching groups of this size is andragogically sound, it does pose logistical difficulties. It may mean having to teach a higher number of hours and doing so in a less efficient manner in terms of staff-student ratios if a tutor is assigned to each sub-group. It can, in addition, pose considerable resource problems.

Two further points about the constitution of sub-groups are worth making. In the view of Barnes (1983), once formulated, sub-groups should remain unchanged for the duration of the programme. This enables members to become familiar and comfortable with each other so that greater levels of trust can be attained thus promoting increased openness. Members should be dissuaded, though, from constantly practising with the same partner since this may serve to limit the generalizability of training outcomes. One advantage of changing sub-groups, on the other hand, is that it usually offers each trainee a broader range of practice experiences and feedback opportunities.

The second issue concerns the homogeneity of sub-group composition. We tend to favour having a broad cross-section of the overall group represented in each sub-group. Differences in age, sex, experience, etc. often lead to a richer flux of views and opinions during feedback. Again transfer of training may be improved in this way. If, however, members differ in some important respect which has implications for how skills content would normally be implemented or the types of situations encountered, then more selective groupings can be made. Thus in the module described by Morrow and Hargie (1985a), hospital pharmacists were grouped together as were their community colleagues.

Utilization of resources

Resources available frequently place a frustrating restriction upon the form which the programme takes. Here video-recording equipment and staffing considerations immediately come to the fore. Being confronted with a large group of students and having only a single video unit to call upon can pose obvious problems. These are compounded if the trainer is adamant that the central objective of the module is essentially performance-oriented requiring students to participate in practical activities designed to improve some aspect of their communicative repertoire. Nevertheless, much can be accomplished even under these circumstances.

Strategies to be considered include timetabling sub-sections of the cohort for practicals at different times. Morrow and Hargie (1985a) for example, have catered for groups of sixteen in sub-groups of four by scheduling their use of a single video-recording unit on a rota basis. While one sub-group was recording, others were variously preparing their roleplay for practice, engaging in post-practice analysis or having a staggered coffee break. Afterwards sub-groups took it in turn to show and comment on their recordings to the large group as part of feedback.

It may, alternatively, be necessary to operate larger sub-groups of say ten members when resources are limited. One of the disadvantages though, is the impracticability of permitting each member to practise each skill during each practice session – especially if it is intended to provide feedback as well. As a compromise, it might be acceptable to have only half the sub-group practice per session with the rest having their turn on the next occasion. Those not actually practising can take part as roleplay partners and contribute fully during feedback.

Even so, it may not be possible to allocate a tutor to each sub-group. It has already been pointed out (Chapter 10) that trainees prefer to have their group led by a tutor although it is uncertain if this is associated with improved training outcomes. The effects of tutor presence are likely to be mediated by what the tutor does together with other features of the programme (Ellis and Whittington, 1981). Operating a flexible system whereby one tutor oversees several sub-groups can, therefore, be contemplated. This can work particularly successfully with the more mature trainee. It is desirable, though, that:

(a) sub-groups be thoroughly briefed prior to practice
(b) one member of the sub-group be appointed as co-ordinator
(c) a specific and clearly defined task be set
(d) sub-groups should combine for a plenary session.

Allocation of time

The allocation of the total hours available to the different phases of the training process and the different elements of content is a feature of many of the constraining influences already mentioned. As such it is extremely difficult to be other than tentative as to how this should best be accomplished. With largely inexperienced, pre-service groups, operating in sub-groups of say six members, however, we would recommend that from three to six hours per week be set aside for CST. This time should be mainly devoted to a single skill although with those skills that are quite basic it may be possible to combine two together as already indicated. On the other hand dealing with more complex processes or situations frequently requires much longer, perhaps taking place over several weekly sessions. Nevertheless, the notion of three to six hours per week is a useful starting point.

Assuming that programme objectives are to directly improve performance in addition to increasing knowledge, sensitivity, self-awareness, etc. about a quarter of this time should be given over to skill sensitization, roughly the same to practice and the remainder to feedback. These proportions may vary of course. For example, as the length of skill practice interactions increases during the course of the programme so too will the amount of time required to complete this phase. Again, if a problem-solving rather than a structural logic approach to curriculum design is followed, proportionately more time may be taken up with practice but especially with feedback.

The temporal relationship between the phases of training is also relevant. We have found it beneficial to leave at least a day between sensitization and practice. This gives students time to assimilate the skill content and undertake any additional readings or homework exercises suggested. If possible, however, feedback should follow practice within the same session. Indeed where video or audio feedback modalities are not available this is imperative.

In concluding this sub-section, it should again be appreciated that there is little hard evidence favouring any particular allocation of training time. One important consideration, however, is that sufficient time should be allowed for full and detailed feedback to be given (van Ments, 1983).

Integration within the curriculum

Integrating the content of CST has already been discussed. When it forms part of a broader curriculum, the relationship of CST to other course elements must, in addition, be addressed. It would seem that, in practice, trainers are often negligent in this respect. This is borne out by the results of the survey by Hargie and Morrow (1986a) which identified three models of CST implementation. The *interspersed model* characterized training which was distributed throughout the curriculum. It was often poorly co-ordinated and arranged on an *ad hoc* basis. The *isolated model* was so called for several reasons. Communication studies tended to be taught by a social or behavioural scientist as an academic subject in a separate, self-contained unit. With no explicit attempt made to relate these concepts to health-care practice this, in as much as it did take place, was left entirely to the perspicuity of individual students.

The *integrated model* rectified many of these shortcomings. Here the organizing principle was identified as the application of communication issues to the interpersonal dimension of the health professions. The successful operationalization of this resolve was accomplished through a team-teaching strategy involving a behavioural scientist (mostly a psychologist) together with a health practitioner tutor. The unfortunate fact that much instruction appeared to reflect the first two rather than the third model led Hargie and Morrow (1986a, p.174) to conclude, '. . . that there was a need for more guidance and direction about how to organize and implement CST'.

The need for CST to form part of a fully integrated course of professional preparation has also been vigorously argued by Ellis and Whittington (1981). Furthermore, a *modus operandi* is articulated in what they call the *action focus* curriculum. The action which is the object of focus is that of the competent practitioner. Effective interpersonal performance is, of course, of central import. The curriculum can be visualized as forming a series of concentric circles with *skill acquisition*, including communication skills, at the nucleus. This process draws upon *related theory* which informs and critically evaluates professional competence and is, therefore, directly and immediately applicable. Such theory is frequently presented under titles such as 'Professional principles and practice'. Related theory can, in turn, be located in the wider setting of *contextual studies* drawn, for example, from disciplines such as psychology, sociology, anthropology, social policy, social philosophy, etc. These address much wider issues of possible professional activity.

A curriculum devised in this way places major emphasis upon practical work and experience enabling professional skills to be nurtured. The relationship between inputs which are college-based and field-based, warrants special attention. If properly sequenced to complement each other, students can gain an invaluable learning opportunity. Having a period of placement following on from a CST programme organized in keeping with the principles of structural logic, for instance, provides opportunities for the integration of earlier content to take place through *in vivo* practice. Subsequent college-based work can, in turn, incorporate and build upon these experiences. In the procedure reported by Bamford and Hargie (1981), with social work students, the initial basic skills sequence was extended, following placement, by adopting a thematic approach in which topics like interprofessional conflict, child abuse and confidentiality were introduced. The successful operation of this approach depends upon careful scheduling of inputs to enable students to make use of relevant material from other parts of the course.

When CST is taught as part of a course, it must link with the other elements to form a coherent and unified whole if a worthwhile outcome is to be achieved. Ellis and Whittington (1981, p.176) encapsulate the sentiment admirably in the following succinct statement: 'At best [CST] is an integral part of an organism of which it is a microcosm: at worst it is a cosmetic graft soon rejected or isolated by the host'.

Evaluation

Establishing the most suitable strategies for evaluating the instructional intervention should also feature as part of the process of programme planning. Such evaluation may be conducted with different purposes in mind as was indicated in Chapter 11. The major aim, in certain cases, is to assess students' level of performance to enable judgements to be made about their competence as they proceed through training. Upon its completion decisions have to be taken as to whether professional accreditation is merited. The procedure may alternatively be conducted with the primary intention of improving the quality of the programme itself. Subsequent inputs can be modified in accordance with feedback obtained in this way.

A range of evaluation techniques from which choices can be made were outlined in the preceding chapter and categorized as direct or indirect. In deciding which to adopt, the trainer should be aware of why he wants to evaluate, what he wants to evaluate and the resources which can be called upon to enable him to evaluate.

If the undertaking is essentially formative, with the aim of promoting the success of training, an obvious starting point is with the predetermined objectives of the programme. When these stipulate changes in, for instance, knowledge, cognitive processes or attitudes, indirect methods such as paper and pencil tests and questionnaires may be quite adequate assessment techniques. Perceptual sensitivity and awareness can be judged by means of tests requiring trainees to respond to videotaped presentations of interpersonal behaviour. However, CST is typically designed to influence what trainees actually do – it is targeted on performance. Here indirect methods, while relatively convenient, are less satisfactory. Direct observation of behaviour enables a more valid evaluation to be conducted. The ultimate test, of course, is live 'real' practice with the trainee being assessed during actual patient encounters. But direct observation procedures are usually more demanding of resources. They tend to be time-consuming and the trainer, intent only upon monitoring the success of a programme in order to make improvements, may be content to settle for less stringent alternatives.

Comparing learning outcomes to predetermined objectives permits global estimates of success or failure to be arrived at. This may be all that is required to base decisions upon whether the continuation of the programme is justified. But such procedures don't reveal particular strengths and weaknesses and will consequently be of limited utility to the trainer intent upon improving the efficiency of instruction. Asking participants to complete questionnaires of the type suggested in Exercise 11.2 and Table 11.2 is a useful way of generating feedback on their CST experience. Modifications can then be contemplated as part of subsequent planning in accordance with the model of CST outlined in the introduction to Part Three.

When it comes to assessing students' competence in order to make decisions about them rather than the instructional sequence, somewhat different criteria and standards pertain. Indirect methods may be employed but most likely as adjuncts to more direct techniques, especially at advanced stages of professional preparation. Being assessed while involved with a patient is the ultimate test and many charged with the responsibility of bestowing professional accreditation may feel that this form of evaluation is essential if the checks and safeguards protecting not only that profession but the public are to be properly exercised.

12.4 OVERVIEW

This chapter has addressed a range of organizational and logistical issues pertinent to the planning and implementation of CST programmes. In so doing it extends the cross-sectional focus on the training procedure taken in preceding chapters.

Trainers must formulate programmes to meet the requirements of particular groups and within the realities of specific settings and sets of circumstances. CST is most effective when approached in this way. There is no template of the 'model programme' which can be immutably worked through on each and every occasion. In consequence, the focus in this chapter has very much been upon the process of devising a training sequence. This was discussed within a framework of decisions taken with regard to a range of features of the programme. These are determined by a set of immediate influencing factors including the needs and characteristics of the group, the objectives of the programme, resources available, size of group and time available for training. The fact that the formulation of certain programme characteristics could place constraints on choices available in respect of others was also acknowledged. Features discussed included the duration of the programme, temporal location in course, utilization of resources, disposition of sessions, organization of content, allocation of time, choice of practical activities, constitution of sub-groups, integration of content and of the programme within the curriculum, and the selection of evaluation procedures.

13

Concluding comments

The ability to communicate effectively is now regarded, by those who have written on the topic, as central to the provision of quality health care. Without it the establishment of facilitative relationships within which changes can take place in values, attitudes, feelings, knowledge, beliefs and ultimately habits and practices, is impossible. There is evidence to suggest that patients who are related to by staff in an interpersonally skilled fashion can benefit physiologically, psychologically and behaviourally (Gerrard *et al.*, 1980; Davis, 1985).

There is, unfortunately, also evidence that patients frequently express dissatisfaction at the lack of proper communication engaged in by health workers (Ley, 1983). Badenoch (1986) suggests societal changes accompanied by raised expectations on the part of the public may account for these findings. A less clearly differentiated class structure, the lowering of class barriers with corresponding adjustments to established norms now means that the individual is more insistent that his rights be acknowledged and respected and less willing to unquestioningly acquiesce in the face of authority. Consequently the, 'old doctor-patient relationship – half-father/ half-child, half-master/half-servant – has already given way to a consultation where the doctor offers guidance and seeks the cooperation of the patient . . .' (Badenoch, 1986, p.565).

Again, better education and increased knowledge of, and interest in, health matters have meant that many patients now insist on being fully informed of their medical condition and its treatment and are better able to understand such information when given. Failure to comply is no longer justified on the grounds that engaging in such dialogue is pointless since patients or their families won't grasp the complexities of diagnosis, therapeutic procedures or prognosis, even if carefully explained.

These trends in society are likely to continue. When combined with the role implications of a growing emphasis, in many quarters, upon health promotion and preventive care, they represent an increasing challenge to the interpersonal competence of the health professional. MacLeod Clark and

Faulkner (1987, p.203), for instance, anticipate that, 'Society's expectations of nurses in the year 2000 will make even greater demands on their communication skills . . .'.

But practitioners in the past have been poorly prepared in such interpersonal procedures as interviewing, counselling, informing intelligibly, gaining compliance, etc. Until quite recently this social dimension of the job was largely ignored in training, being relegated to the 'hidden curriculum'. General views prevailed that expertise would be gradually acquired through increased contact with patients or even that intelligent individuals should, almost by definition, already possess these skills. Maguire (1981, 1986) among others, has argued convincingly against the complacency of such notions and the need for the formal curriculum to encompass explicit instruction in interpersonal communication is being increasingly accepted (e.g. General Nursing Council, 1977; General Medical Council, 1980; Pharmaceutical Society of Great Britain, 1984; Department of Health and Social Security, 1986).

It would seem, however, that recommendations for innovation in this area have, in many instances, found those with an executive responsibility decidedly ill-prepared. While readily agreeing in principle with the legitimacy of such an endeavour, MacLeod Clark and Faulkner (1987) discovered that less than 5% of nurse tutors surveyed in schools and colleges of nursing throughout the UK felt that they were ready to offer such teaching. This disquiet was further reflected in the expressed need for suitable training in how to teach communication skills. This book has been written to meet the requirement, by trainers, for information on, and guidance in, apposite techniques for promoting students' interpersonal proficiency in professional contexts.

The CST process elaborated encompasses preparation, training and evaluation phases. The training phase, in turn, incorporates sensitization, practice and feedback components and is in keeping with our underlying conceptualizations of communicative competence and skill. Throughout, however, we have been at pains to dispel the illusion of CST as a fixed and immutable regime which must be inflexibly adhered to in all circumstances. Rather we have striven to encourage tutors, within the resource constraints imposed upon them, to mould and adapt the basic model, in accordance with guidelines provided to accommodate the needs of student groups. Indeed one of the advantages of the system is its tolerance of variability in terms of skill content, institutional setting, and trainee population. Having affirmed the efficacy of this orientation to training, Authier and Gustafson (1982) go on to state that the trainer is only limited by his or her ability to define the skills component of the communicative process targeted for intervention and, 'by his or her ability to modify the structural format to accommodate the needs and demands of the trainee' (p.122).

In addition to being flexible, there is merit in the tutor adopting an open approach to CST by monitoring the effectiveness of the programme, in accordance with the techniques discussed in Chapter 11, and being prepared to utilize such feedback to make further modifications and refinements in an attempt to ensure that the aims of training are fully met.

The thesis of this text has been that by establishing communication as a valid component of the curriculum and by offering structured and systematic instruction in clearly identified aspects of it, the competence of practitioners, in this dimension of their work, can be improved. The effectiveness of CST, in this respect, will depend, nevertheless, upon a range of broader contextual factors associated not only with the education and training of health workers but the organization and administration of health care provision. These factors include:

1. The traditional adherence to an essentially medical model of the patient, derived from the natural sciences. Referring specifically to the medical profession, Täkhä (1984), acknowledges that the doctor's frame of reference in approaching the patient is typically derived from the natural rather than the behavioural sciences. The upshot has been a predisposition to characterize the patient as a purely biological entity comprised of complex of physical and chemical systems and sub-systems, within which pathology can be defined and treated, rather than as a fellow human being with a personal dignity and needs which may be psychosocial as well as physical. Attitudes of medical staff which result, 'may be manifested as a tendency to see the patient as a thing or to concentrate upon the parts rather than the whole' (Täkhä, 1984, p.3). Under these circumstances the necessity for skilled communication is unlikely to be fully appreciated. This was found to be the case by Sanson-Fisher and Poole (1980) who attributed the ready acceptance of inappropriate patient behaviour, in a psychiatric unit, to the operationalization by staff of a primarily medical model of mental illness. If this condition is believed to be essentially a neurological or biochemical abnormality receptive only to physical interventions in the form of drugs, surgery, ECT, etc. then therapeutically it matters little how the patient is related to at an interpersonal level.

   When the medical model pervades the curriculum it is unlikely that an input on communication skills training will be readily accommodated. A broader conceptualization of human well-being is required incorporating contributions from the behavioural sciences. Faulkner (1985) regards this paradigm shift as crucial in nurse training if interpersonal communication is to be accepted as a core element of the curriculum contributing to all other aspects of care.

2. Senior staff as role models. It is improbable that college-based teaching in communication will have a lasting influence on students' health-care practices if it is at variance with what is experienced by them during

clinical placement. If the general ethos of the ward is such that a low priority seems to be given to relating interpersonally to patients, students will not doubt behave accordingly. Indeed Helfer (1970) reported that the interpersonal skills of medical students may actually deteriorate over the course of their medical training.

Senior staff have considerable responsibility in this respect. Poor practice on their part or the belief that they place low value on adequate communication will influence students adversely. Such impressions can be insidious and transmitted in subtle ways. Lillie (1985) draws attention to how the use of language by staff can serve to dehumanize as in the labelling of patients e.g. 'the hysterectomy in bed 2', or 'the asthmatic in 6', etc.

College-based teaching in communication skills must be complemented and extended by experiences provided during clinical placement.

3. Organizational and administrative influences. Pracitioners, when challenged, frequently account for poor communication in terms of insufficient time to devote to the individual patient. In some instances this may be no more than a convenient excuse, in others it is undoubtedly a reality reflecting the shortcomings of the system within which the clinician operates (Badenoch, 1986). Reductions in funding for the health service leading to shortages in personnel inevitably increase the pressures which staff work under. Clearly this has implications for the quality of interpersonal relationships formed not only with patients, but also colleagues (McIntee and Firth, 1984). Faced with an ever increasing case-load and the necessity to prioritize, it is likely that the physical rather than psychosocial needs of patients will be tended to. Turton and Faulkner (1983) intimate that district nursing management may place a higher premium on figures denoting the number of injections or bed-baths given than with visits to patients experiencing emotional problems. A regression to old attitudes and ways of thinking typified by accusations of 'skiving' which were levelled at nurses caught taking time to talk to patients, must be guarded against.

In-service training directed at improving the interpersonal competence of practitioners in certain areas is also unlikely to be given a high priority in a climate of straitened budgets and shortfalls in staffing levels.

While accepting the difficulty of the task under present difficult economic circumstances, policy makers, planners and administrators must be made to acknowledge the value of effective interpersonal communication with patients (even if only on the hard economic basis of less stressed patients making quicker recoveries and being discharged from hospital sooner) and be prepared to take steps to promote it.

4. Lack of adequate psychoemotional support for staff. In a way this point relates to the previous one. Staff who are experiencing heightened levels of stress are unlikely to be prepared to risk close emotional contact with

patients. Indeed Marshfield (1985) proposed that the avoidance of all but the most superficial communication by nurses when dealing with patients may not be due to a lack of skill as such. Rather it may be a defensive strategy operating in the interests of emotional self-protection. This is most probable in areas of health care which are potentially more distressing, such as working with the terminally ill or the bereaved.

Concomitant psychoemotional demands placed upon practitoners must not be overlooked in advocating an increased supportive role. In keeping with sentiments expressed by Altschul (1983), Banister and Kagan (1985) state that, 'support systems will be essential if the profession is seriously interested in encouraging and facilitating more meaningful and therapeutic forms of communication between nurses and patients' (p.48).

5. Inappropriate relationships and inadequate contact between those providing care. The internal social structure of the NHS has a clearly identifiable status hierachy extending from consultants down through doctors and paramedics to nurses and ancillary staff (Burton, 1985). The direction of power and influence follows. This structure militates against full and open discussion between strata taking place on the basis of equality, for the good of the patient. It also causes dilemmas for some who may avoid getting involved in conversations with patients about their diagnosis or prognosis lest they incur the wrath of a higher-status colleague whose policy is not to divulge such information. Faulkner (1985, p.69) chronicles the response of a ward sister on a communication course, thus: 'It's all right for you to talk of improving communication with patients. You should meet my consultant – he won't let me tell them a bloody thing!' Faulkner continues by asserting that, 'The relationship between doctors and nurses needs further exploration if the organization of patient care is to be improved, especially in the area of interpersonal skills' (p.71).

Clearly these contextual realities of CST must be acknowledged. It would be naïve to believe that CST can, single-handedly, reverse the impression, all too frequently formed, of health professionals as poor communicators. We are convinced, however, that it has an invaluable contribution to make as part of a wider movement which recognizes the centrality of this facet of professional competence and is pledged to improving it.

References

Adams, J. (1987) Historical review and appraisal of research on the learning, retention, and transfer of human motor skills, *Psychol. Bull.*, **101**, 41–74.

Adler, M. (1983) *How to Speak, How to Listen*, Macmillan, New York.

Albert, S. and Kessler, S. (1976) Processes for ending social encounters, *J. of Theory of Soc. Behav.*, **6**, 147–70.

Allen, D. and Ryan, K. (1969) *Microteaching*, Addison-Wesley, Reading, Mass.

Altman (1977) The communication of interpersonal attitudes: an ecological approach in *Foundations of Interpersonal Attraction* (ed. T.L. Houston), Academic Press, London.

Altschul, A. (1983) The consumer's voice: nursing implications, *J. of Ad. Nurs.*, **8**, 175–83.

Alssid, L. and Hutchinson, W. (1977) Comparison of modeling techniques in counselor training, *Counselor Education and Supervision*, **17**, 36–42.

American Dental Association (1977) *Dental Education in the United States 1976*, American Dental Association, Chicago.

Annett, J. (1969) *Feedback and Human Behaviour*, Penguin, Harmondsworth.

Annett, J. (ed.) (1974) *Human Information Processing, Part 1*, Open University Press, Milton Keynes.

Antaki, C. and Lewis, A. (ed.) (1986) *Mental Mirrors: Metacognition in Social Knowledge and Communication*, Sage, London.

Archer, J. and Lloyd, B. (1986) *Sex and Gender* (2nd edn), Cambridge University Press, Cambridge.

Archer, R. (1979) Role of personality and the social situation in *Self-disclosure* (ed. G. Chelune), Jossey-Bass, San Francisco.

Argyle, M. (1975) *Bodily Communication*, Methuen, London.

Argyle, M. (1981) The nature of social skill in *Social Skills and Health* (ed. M. Argyle), Methuen, London.

Argyle, M. (1983) *The Psychology of Interpersonal Behaviour*, Penguin, Hammondsworth, England.

Argyle, M., Furnham, A. and Graham, J. (1981) *Social Situations*, Cambridge University Press, Cambridge.

Argyle, M. and Kendon, A. (1967) The experimental analysis of social performance in *Advances in Experimental Social Psychology: Vol. 3* (ed. L. Berkowitz), Academic Press, New York.

Arkowitz, H. (1981) The assessment of social skills in *Behavioral Assessment. A Practical Handbook* (eds M. Hersen and A. Bellack), Pergamon Press, New York.

Armstrong, P. (1982) The 'needs meeting' ideology in liberal adult education, *International Journal of Lifelong Education*, **1**, 330–34.

Arvey, R. and Campion, J. (1984) Person perception in the employment interview in *Issues in Person Perception* (ed. M. Cook), Methuen, London.

Authier, J. (1986) Showing warmth and empathy in *A Handbook of Communication Skills* (ed. O. Hargie), Croom Helm, London.

Authier, J. and Gustafson, K. (1982) Microtraining: focusing on specific skills in *Interpersonal Helping Skills* (ed. E. Marshall *et al.*), Jossey-Bass, San Francisco.

Averill, J. (1975) A semantic atlas of emotional concepts, *JSAS Catalogue of Selected Documents in Psychology*, **5**, 330.

Backlund, P. (1977) *Issues in Communication Competence Theory*, paper presented at the meeting of the Speech Communication Association, Washington, DC.

Badenoch, J. (1986) Communication skills in medicine: the role of communication in medical practice, *J. of the Roy. Soc. of Med.*, **79**, 565–67.

Bader, J. (ed.) (1983) Proceedings of the National Conference on Applied Behavioral Science. Case Western Reserve University, Cleveland, Ohio, October 5–6, 1981, *J. of Dent. Ed.*, **47**, (2) Special issue.

Bailey, C. and Butcher, D. (1983) Interpersonal skills training II: the trainer's role, *Management Education and Development*, **14**, 106–12.

Baker, S., Johnson, E., Kopala, M. and Strout, N. (1985) Test interpretation competence: a comparison of microskills and mental practice training, *Counsellor Education and Supervision*, **25**, 31–43.

Baker, S., Johnson, E. and Strout, N *et al.* (1986) Effects of separate and combined overt and covert practice modes on counselling trainee competence and motivation, *J. of Couns. Psychol.*, **33**, 469–70.

Baldwin, J. and Baldwin, J. (1981) *Behavior Principles in Everyday Life*, Prentice-Hall, Englewood Cliffs, New Jersey.

Bamford, D. and Hargie, O. (1981) Teaching social work students: a model for integrating skills and social work concepts, *Social Work Education*, **1**, 15–18.

Bandura, A. (1977a) *Social Learning Theory*, Prentice-Hall, Englewood Cliffs, New Jersey.

Bandura, A. (1977b) Self-efficacy: toward a unifying theory of behavioural change, *Psychol. Rev.*, **84**, 191–215.

Banister, P. and Kagan, C. (1985) The need for research into interpersonal skills in nursing in *Interpersonal Skills in Nursing: Research and Applications* (ed. C. Kagan), Croom Helm, London.

Barnes, D. (1983) Teaching communication skills to student nurses – an experience, *Nurse Education Today*, **3**, 45–8.

Bartlett, F. (1948) The measurement of human skill, *Occupational Psychology*, **22**, 83–91.

Beattie, A. (1987) Making a curriculum work in *The Curriculum in Nursing Education* (eds P. Allan and M. Jolley), Croom Helm, London.

Beck, K. and Frankel, A. (1981) A conceptualization of threat communication and protective health behavior, *Soc. Psychol. Quart.*, **3**, 204–17.

Becker, M., Drachman, R. and Kirscht, J. (1972) Motivations as predictors of health behavior, *Health Services Reports*, **87**, 852–61.

Becker, M. and Maiman, L. (1975) Sociobehavioral determinants of compliance with health and medical care recommendations, *Medical Care*, **13**, 10–24.

Becker, M. and Maiman, L. (1980) Strategies for enhancing patient compliance, *J. of Comm. Health*, **6**, 113–35.

Becker, M. and Rosenstock, I. (1984) Compliance with medical advice in *Health Care and Human Behaviour* (eds A. Steptoe and A. Mathews), Academic Press, London.

Beggs, D. and Lewis, E. (1975) *Measurement and Evaluation in the Schools*, Houghton-Mifflin Company, Boston.

Bellack, A. (1979) A critical appraisal of strategies for assessing social skill, *Behavioral Assessment*, **1**, 157–76.

Berger, M. (ed.) (1978) *Videotape Techniques in Psychiatric Training and Treatment*, Brunner/Mazel, New York.

Bernstein, D. and Borkovec, T. (1973) *Progressive Relaxation Training: A Manual for the Helping Professions*, Research Press, Champaign, Illinois.

Bernstein, L. and Bernstein, R. (1980) *Interviewing: A Guide for Health Professionals* (3rd edn), Appleton-Century-Crofts, New York.

Bilodeau, E. and Bilodeau, I. (1961) Motor-skills learning, *Annual Review of Psychology*, **12**, 243–80.

Bligh, D. (1971) *What's the Use of Lectures*, D.A. and B. Bligh, Briar House, Exeter.

Block, M., Schaffner, K. and Coulehan, J. (1985) Ethical problems of recording physician – patient interactions in family practice settings, *J. of Fam. Pract.*, **21**, 467–72.

Blondis, M. and Jackson, B. (1982) *Nonverbal Communication with Patients*, Wiley, New York.

Bochner, A. and Yerby, J. (1977) Factors affecting instruction in interpersonal competence, *Communication Education*, **26**, 91–103.

Boice, R. (1983) Observational skills, *Psychol. Bull.*, **93**, 3–29.

Boster, F. and Mongeau, P. (1984) Fear-arousing persuasive messages in *Communication Yearbook: 8* (eds B. Bostrom and B. Westley), Sage, Beverly Hills, California.

Boulton, M., Griffiths, J. and Hall, D. *et al.* (1984) Improving communication: a practical programme for teaching trainees about communication issues in the general practice consultation, *Medical Education*, **18**, 269–74.

Bradburn, N. and Sudman, S. (1980) *Improving Interview Method and Questionnaire Design: Response Effects to Threatening Questions in Survey Research*, Aldine, Chicago.

Bradley, J. and Edinberg, M. (1982) *Communication in the Nursing Context*, Appleton-Century-Crofts, Connecticut.

Bradshaw, J. (1977) The concept of social need in *Welfare in Action* (eds M. Fitzgerald, P. Halmos, J. Murcie and D. Zoldin), Routledge and Kegan Paul, London.

Bradshaw, P., Ley, P., Kincey, J. and Bradshaw, J. (1975) Recall of medical advice: comprehensibility and specificity, *Brit. J. of Soc. and Clin. Psychol.*, **14**, 55–62.

Brenner, M. (1981) Skills in the research interview in *Social Skills and Work* (ed. M. Argyle), Methuen, London.

Briggs, K. (1986) Assertiveness: speak your mind, *Nursing Times*, **82**, 24–6.

Brigham, J. (1986) *Social Psychology*, Little, Brown & Co, Boston.

Brook, C. (1985) Providing feedback: the research on effective oral and written feedback strategies, *Central States Speech Journal'*, **36**, 14–23.

Brooks, W. and Heath, R. (1985) *Speech Communication*, W.C. Brown, Dubuque, Iowa.

Brown, G. (1985) How to make and use video in teaching, *Medical Teacher*, **7**, 139–49.

Brown, G. (1986) Explaining in *A Handbook of Communication Skills* (ed. O. Hargie), Croom Helm, London.

Brown, J. and Elmore, R. Jr. (1982) Interpersonal skills training for dental students, *Psychol. Rep.*, **50**, 390.

Brown, M. (1983) *Developing Skills in Helping Relationships* (Videotape Package), Tavistock Publications, London.

Bruner, J. and Tagiuri, R. (1954) The perception of people in *Handbook of Social Psychology* (ed. G. Lindzey), Addison-Wesley, Reading, Massachusetts.

Bull, P. (1983) *Body Movement and Interpersonal Communication*, Wiley, Chichester.

Burley-Allen, M. (1982) *Listening: The Forgotten Skill*, Wiley, New York.

Burton, M. (1985) The environment, good interactions and interpersonal skills in nursing in *Interpersonal Skills in Nursing: Research and Applications* (ed. C. Kagan), Croom Helm, London.

Byrne, P. and Long, B. (1976) *Doctors Talking to Patients*, HMSO, London.

Cairns, L. (1986) Reinforcement in *A Handbook of Communication Skills* (ed. O. Hargie), Croom Helm, London.

Caney, D. (1983) The physiotherapist in *The Study of Real Skills, Vol. 4* (ed. W. Singleton), MTP Press, Lancaster.

Carkhuff, R. (1969) *Helping and Human Relations: a Primer for Lay and Professional Helpers*, Holt, Rinehart and Winston, New York.

Carlson, R. (1984) *The Nurse's Guide to Better Communication*, Scott, Foresman & Co, Glenview, Illinois.

Carroll, J. (1980) Analysing decision behavior: the magician's audience in *Cognitive Processes in Choice and Decision Behavior* (ed. T. Wallsten), Lawrence Erlbaum Associates, Hillsdale.

Carroll, J. and Monroe, J. (1979) Teaching medical interviewing: a critique of educational research and practice, *J. of Med. Ed.*, **54**, 498–500.

Carroll, J. and Monroe, J. (1980) Teaching clinical interviewing in the health professions: a review of empirical research, *Evaluation and the Health Professions*, **3**, 21–45.

Cartledge, G. and Milburn, J. (eds) (1986) *Teaching Social Skills to Children*, Pergamon, New York.

Cartwright, A. (1964) *Human Relations and Hospital Care*, Routledge and Kegan Paul, London.

Cartwright, A. and Anderson, R. (1981) *General Practice Revisited*, Tavistock, London.

Cartwright, A., Hockey, L. and Anderson, J. (1973) *Life Before Death*, Routledge and Kegan Paul, London.

Cartwright, S. (1986) *Training with Video*, Knowledge Industry Publications, White Plains, New York.

Cassata, D. (1978) Health communication theory and research: an overview of the communication specialist interface in *Communication Yearbook 2* (ed. B. Ruben), International Communication Association, Transaction Books, New Jersey.

Cattell, R. (1970) *Sixteen Personality Factor Questionnaire*, Institute of Personality and Ability Testing, Champaign, Illinois.

Chaikin, S. (1979) Communicator physical attractiveness and persuasion, *J. of Pers. and Soc. Psychol.*, **37**, 1387–97.

Chalmers, R. (1983) Chair report of the study committee on preparation of students for the realities of contemporary pharmacy practice, *Amer. J. of Pharmac. Ed.*, **47**, 393–401.

Chambers, D. (1970) Managing the anxieties of young dental patients, *J. of Dentistry in Children*, **37**, 363–7, 370–3.

Chomsky, N. (1965) *Aspects of the Theory of Syntax*, MIT Press, Cambridge, Massachusetts.

Cialdini, R. (1985) *Influence: Science and Practice*, Scott, Foresman & Co, Glenview, Illinois.

CINE (1986) *Report of the Communication in Nursing Education Curriculum Development Project (Phase 1)*, Health Education Council, London.

Clark, C. (1978) *Classroom Skills for Nurse Educators*, Springer, New York.

Clark, R. (1984) *Persuasive messages*, Harper & Row, New York.

Conine, N. (1976) Listening in the helping relationship, *Physical Therapy*, **56**, 159–62.

Cooley, R. and Roach, D. (1984) A conceptual framework in *Competence in Communication: A Multidisciplinary Approach* (ed. R. Bostrom), Sage, Beverly Hills, California.

Cooper, C. (1981) *Improving Interpersonal Relations*, Gower, Aldershot.

Cork, N. (1987) Approaches to curriculum planning in *Nursing Education: Research and Developments* (ed. B. Davis), Croom Helm, London.

Cormier, W. and Cormier, L. (1979) *Interviewing Strategies for Helpers. A Guide to Assessment, Treatment and Evaluation*, Brooks/Cole Pub. Co., Monterey.

Crichton, E., Smith, D. and Demanuele, F. (1978) Patient recall of medication information, *Drug Intelligence and Clinical Pharmacy*, **12**, 591–99.

Crisp, A. (1986) Undergraduate training for communications in medical practice, *J. of the Roy. Soc. of Med.*, **79**, 568–74.

Crossman, E. (1960) *Automation and Skill. DSIR Problems of Progress in Industry*, No. 9, HMSO, London.

Crow, B. (1983) Topic shifts in couple's conversations in *Conversational Coherence: Form, Structure and Strategy* (eds B. Craig and K. Tracy), Sage, Beverly Hills, California.

Crute, V. (1986) Microtraining in health visitor education: an intensive examination of training outcomes, feedback processes and individual differences. Unpublished PhD thesis, University of Ulster, Jordanstown.

Daly, J. and McCroskey, J. (eds) (1984) *Avoiding Communication: Shyness, Reticence, and Communication Apprehension*, Sage, Beverly Hills, California.

Danish, S., D'Augelli, A. and Brock, G. (1976) An evaluation of helping skills training: effects of helper's verbal responses, *J. of Counsel. Psychol.*, **23**, 259–66.

Davies, I. (1976) *Objectives in Curriculum Design*, McGraw-Hill, New York.

Davis, B. (1981) Social skills in nursing in *Social Skills and Health* (ed. M. Argyle), Methuen, London.

Davis, B. (1985) The clinical effect of interpersonal skills: the implementation of pre-operative information giving in *Interpersonal Skills in Nursing* (ed. C. Kagan), Croom Helm, London.

Davis, B. and Ternuff-Nyhlin, K. (1982) Social skills training. The assessment of training in social skills in nursing, with particular reference to the patient profile interview, *Nursing Times*, **78**, 1765–8.

Davis, M.S. (1968) Physiologic, psychological and demographic factors in patients' compliance with doctors' orders, *Medical Care*, **6**, 115–22.

Davitz, J.R. (1964) *The Communication of Emotional Meaning*, McGraw-Hill, New York.

Decker, P. (1983) The effects of rehearsal group size and video feedback in behaviour modeling training, *Personnel Psychology*, **36**, 763–73.

Deets, C. and Blume, D. (1977) Evaluating the effectiveness of selected continuing education offerings, *J. of Cont. Ed. in Nurs.*, **8**, 63–71.

Department of Health and Social Security (1986) *Primary Health Care: An Agenda for Discussion*, HMSO, London.

Derlega, V. and Chaikin, A. (1975) *Sharing Intimacy: What We Reveal to Others and Why*, Prentice-Hall, Englewood Cliffs, New Jersey.

Derlega, V. and Grzelak, J. (1979) Appropriateness of self-disclosure in *Self-disclosure* (ed. G. Chelune), Jossey-Bass, San Francisco.

DeVito, J. (1986) *The Interpersonal Communication Book*, Harper and Row, New York.

Dichter Institute for Motivational Research Inc. (1973) *Communicating the Value of Comprehensive Pharmaceutical Services to the Consumer*, American Pharmaceutical Association, Washington DC.

Dickson, D. (1981) *Microcounselling: An Evaluative Study of a Programme*, Unpublished PhD Thesis, Ulster Polytechnic.

Dickson, D. (1986) Reflecting in *A Handbook of Communication Skills* (ed. O. Hargie), Croom Helm, London.

Dickson, D. and Maxwell, M. (1985) The interpersonal dimension of physiotherapy: implications for training, *Physiotherapy*, **71**, 306–10.

Dickson, D. and Maxwell, M. (1987) A comparative study of physiotherapy students' attitudes to social skills training undertaken before and after clinical placement, *Physiotherapy*, **73**, 60–4.

Dickson, D., Tittmar, H. and Hargie, O. (1984) Social skills training in the preparation of the counsellor of the alcoholic in *Advanced Concepts in Alcoholism* (ed. H. Tittmar), Pergamon, Oxford.

Dillon, J. (1986) Questioning in *A Handbook of Communication Skills* (ed. O. Hargie), Croom Helm, London.

Di Matteo, M. and Di Nicola, D. (1982) *Achieving Patient Compliance: The Psychology of the Medical Practitioner's Role*, Pergamon, New York.

Dimbleby, R. and Burton, G. (1985) *More than Words: An Introduction to Communication*, Methuen, London.

Dohrenwend, B. and Richardson, S. (1964) A use for leading questions in research interviewing, *Human Organization*, **3**, 76–7.

Drachman, D., De Carufel, A. and Insko, C.A. (1978) The extra credit effect in interpersonal attraction, *J. of Exp. Soc. Psychol.*, **14**, 458–67.

Dukes, R. and Seidner, C. (1978) *Learning with Simulations and Games*, Sage, Beverly Hills, California.

Dunn, W. and Hamilton, D. (1984) Continuing pharmaceutical education and the competence based approach – a discussion, *J. of Soc. and Admin. Pharm.*, **2**, 136–43.

Dworkin, S. (1981) Behavioral sciences in dental education: past, present and future, *J. of Dent. Ed.*, **45**, 692–8.

Eastwood, C. (1985) Nurse-patient communication skills in Northern Ireland – the educational problems, *Internat. J. of Nurs. Stud.*, **22**, 99–104.

Edwards, B. and Brilhart, J. (1981) *Communication in Nursing Practice*, C.V. Mosby, St Louis.

Edwards, C. (1974) Personality correlates of a microteaching programme: a function of instructional strategy, *Illinois School Research*, **11**, 1–13.

Egan, G. (1986) *The Skilled Helper* (3rd edn), Brooks/Cole, California.

Eigenbrode, C. (1983) Interpersonal skills training in a dental setting: a group inter-action approach, *J. of Dent. Ed.*, **47**, 86–90.

Eijkman, M., Karsdorp, N., Boeke, B. and Karsdorp-Bimmerman, E. (1977) Experiences with a training course in patient counseling, *J. of Dent. Ed.*, **41**, 623–25.

Eisler, R. and Frederiksen, L. (1980) *Perfecting Social Skills*, Plenum, New York.

Ekman, P. and Friesen, W. (1982) Measuring facial movement with the facial action coding system in *Emotion in the Human Face* (ed. P. Ekman) (2nd edn), Cambridge University Press, Cambridge.

Elliot, J. (1980) Introduction in *Interviewing: A Guide for Health Professionals* (L. Bernstein and R. Bernstein), Appleton-Century-Crofts, New York.

Ellis, A. (1962) *Reason and Emotion in Psychotherapy*, Lyle Stuart, New York.

Ellis, A. and Beattie, G. (1986) *The Psychology of Language and Communication*, Weidenfeld and Nicolson, London.

Ellis, R. and Whittington, D. (1981) *A Guide to Social Skill Training*, Croom Helm, London.

Evens, S. and Curtis, P. (1983) Using patient simulators to teach telephone communication skills to health professionals, *J. of Med. Ed.*, **58**, 894–98.

Ewles, L. and Simnett, I. (1985) *Promoting Health: A Practical Guide to Health Education*, John Wiley & Sons, Chichester.

Falloon, I., Lindley, P., McDonald, R. and Marles, I. (1977) Social skills training of out-patient groups: a controlled study of rehearsal and homework, *Brit. J. of Psych.*, **131**, 599–609.

Faulkner, A. (1980) *The Student Nurse's Role in Giving Information to Patients*, M. Litt. Thesis, University of Aberdeen.

Faulkner, A. (ed.) (1984) *Recent Advances in Nursing, 7, Communication*, Churchill Livingstone, Edinburgh.

Faulkner, A. (1985) Evaluation of teaching interpersonal skills in *Interpersonal Skills in Nursing: Research and Applications* (ed. C. Kagan), Croom Helm, London.

Faulkner, A. (1986) Human interest, *Nursing Times*, **82**, 33–4.

Faulkner, A., Bridge, W. and Macleod-Clark, J. (1983) Teaching communication in schools of nursing: a survey of directors of nurse education, paper given at RCN conference, Brighton.

Faulkner, A. and Maguire, P. (1984) Teaching assessment skills in *Recent Advances in Nursing, 7, Communication* (ed. A. Faulkner), Churchill Livingstone, Edinburgh.

Fehrenbach, P., Miller, D. and Thelen, M. (1979) The importance of consistency of modeling behavior upon imitation. A comparison of single and multiple models, *J. of Pers. and Soc. Psych.*, **37**, 1412–17.

Feldman, R. (1985) *Social Psychology: Theories, Research and Applications*, McGraw-Hill, New York.

Fichten, C. and Wright, J. (1983) Videotape and verbal feedback in behavioural couple therapy: a review, *J. of Clin. Psychol.*, 39, 216–21.

Field, S., Draper, J., Kerr, M. and Hare, M. (1982) A consumer view of the health visiting service, *Health Visitor*, 55, 299–301.

Fillmore, C. (1979) On fluency in *Individual Differences in Language Ability and Language Behaviour* (eds C. Fillmore, D. Kemper and W. Wang), Academic Press, New York.

Fishbein, M. (1982) Social psychological analysis of smoking behaviors in *Social Psychology and Behavioral Medicine* (ed. J. Eiser), Wiley, Chichester.

Fisher, J., Rytting, M. and Heslin, R. (1976) Hands touching hands: affective and evaluative effects of an interpersonal touch, *Sociometry*, 39, 416–21.

Fiske, J. (1982) *Introduction to Communication Studies*, Methuen, London.

Fitts, P. (1962) Factors in complex skill training in *Training Research and Education* (ed. R. Glaser), University of Pittsburgh, Pittsburgh.

Fitts, P. (1964) Perceptual-motor skill training in *Categories of Human Learning* (ed. A. Melton), Academic Press, New York.

Fitts, P. and Posner, M. (1973) *Human Performance*, Prentice-Hall, London.

Fletcher, C. (1979) Towards better practice and teaching of communication between doctors and patients in *Mixed Communications* (ed. G. McLachlan), Nuffield Provincial Hospitals Trust, London.

Flowers, J. and Booraem, C. (1980) Simulation and role playing methods in *Helping People Change* (eds F. Kanfer and A. Goldstein), Pergamon, New York.

Floyd, J. (1985) *Listening: A Practical Approach*, Foresman, Glenview, Illinois.

Follette, W. and Cummings, N. (1967) Psychiatric services and medical utilization in a prepaid health plan setting, *Medical Care*, 5, 25–35.

Forgas, J. (1983) What is social about social cognition? *Brit. J. of Soc. Psychol.*, 22, 129–44.

Forgas, J. (1985) *Interpersonal Behaviour*, Pergamon, Oxford.

Foxman, R., Moss, P., Boland, G. and Owen, C. (1982) A consumer view of the health visitor at six weeks post practicum, *Health Visitor*, 55, 302–8.

French, P. (1983) *Social Skills for Nursing Practice*, Croom Helm, London.

Freund, H. (1969) Listening with any ear at all, *Amer. J. of Nurs.*, 69, 1650.

Friedman, H. (1982) Nonverbal communication in medical interaction in *Interpersonal Issues in Health Care* (eds H. Friedman and M. Di Matteo), Academic Press, New York.

Friedrich, R., Lively, S. and Schacht, E. (1985) Teaching communication skills in an integrated curriculum, *J. of Nurs. Ed.*, 24, 164–6.

Fritz, P., Russell, C., Wilcox, E. and Shirk, F. (1984) *Interpersonal Communication in Nursing*, Appleton-Century-Crofts, Norwalk, Connecticut.

Froehle, T., Robinson, S. and Kurpius, D. (1983) Enhancing the effects of modelling through role-play practice, *Counsellor Education and Supervision*, 22, 197–206.

Froelich, R. and Bishop, F. (1977) *Clinical Interviewing Skills*, C.V. Mosby, St Louis.

Fuller, F. and Manning, B. (1973) Self-confrontation reviewed: a conceptualisation for video playback in teacher education, *Rev. of Ed. Res.*, 43, 469–528.

Fuqua, D. and Gade, E. (1982) A critical re-examination of the practice component in counsellor training, *Counsellor Education and Supervision*, **21**, 282–95.

Furnham, A. (1979) Assertiveness in three cultures: multidimensionality and cultural differences, *J. of Clin. Psychol.*, **35**, 522–27.

Furnham, A. (1983a) Social skills and dentistry, *Brit. Dent. J.*, **154**, 404–8.

Furnham, A. (1983b) Situational determinants of social skill in *New Directions in Social Skill Training* (eds R. Ellis and D. Whittington), Croom Helm, London.

Furnham, A., King, J. and Pendleton, D. (1980) Establishing rapport: interaction skills and occupational therapy, *Brit. J. of Occup. Therapy*, **43**, 322–5.

Gahagan, J. (1984) *Social Interaction and its Management*, Methuen, London.

Gallagher, M. (1987) The microskills approach to counsellor training: a study of counsellor personality, attitudes and skills, Unpublished D. Phil. Thesis, University of Ulster at Jordanstown, N. Ireland.

Gallego, A. (1987) Evaluation in nursing education in *Nursing Education: Research and Developments* (ed. B. Davis), Croom Helm, London.

Gambrill, E. and Richey, C. (1975) An assertion inventory for use in assessment and research, *Behavior Therapy*, **6**, 550–61.

Gardner, M. and Burpeau-DiGregorio, M. (1985) Objective assessment of pharmacy students' interviewing skills, *Amer. J. of Pharmac. Ed.*, **49**, 137–44.

Gellatly, A. (ed.) (1986) *The Skilful Mind*, Open University Press, Milton Keynes.

General Medical Council (1977) *Basic Medical Education in the British Isles: Report of the G.M.C. Survey*, Nuffield Provincial Hospital Trust.

General Medical Council (1980) *Recommendations as to Basic Medical Education*, General Medical Council, London.

General Nursing Council (1977) *Syllabus of Training for the Register*, G.N.C., London.

Gergen, K. and Gergen, M. (1981) *Social Psychology*, Harcourt Brace Jovanovich, New York.

Gerrard, B., Boniface, W. and Love, B. (1980) *Interpersonal Skills for Health Professionals*, Reston Publishing Company, Reston.

Gershen, J. (1983) Use of experiential techniques in interpersonal skill training, *J. of Dent. Ed.*, **47**, 72–5.

Gibson, F., Lewis, J., Loughrey, J. and Lount, M. (1981) Developments in the teaching of social work skills, *Social Work Education*, **1**, 8–14.

Gill, C. (1973) Types of interview in general practice: the flash in *Six Minutes for the Patient: Interactions in General Practice Consultation* (eds E. Balint and J. Norell), Tavistock, London.

Goffman, E. (1961) *Asylums*, Anchor Books, New York.

Goldberg, D., Smith, C., Steele, J. and Spivey, L. (1980) Training family doctors to recognise psychiatric illness with increased accuracy, *Lancet* ii, 521–3.

Goldfried, M. and Goldfried, A. (1980) Cognitive change methods in *Helping People Change* (eds F. Kanfer and A. Goldstein), Pergamon, New York.

Goldstein, A. and Sorcher, M. (1974) *Changing Supervisor Behavior*, Pergamon, New York.

Gorden, R. (1980) *Interviewing: Strategy, Techniques and Tactics* (3rd edn), The Dorsey Press, Homewood, Illinois.

Gott, M. (1984) *Learning Nursing*, Royal College of Nursing, London.

Graham, J. and Heywood, S. (1975) The effects of elimination of hand gestures and of verbal codability on speech performance, *Europ. J. of Soc. Psychol.*, **5**,

189–95.

Greenspoon, J. (1955) The reinforcing effect of two spoken sounds on the frequency of two responses, *Amer. J. of Psychol.*, **68**, 409–16.

Gregg, V. (1986) *Introduction to Human Memory*, Routledge and Kegan Paul, London.

Griffiths, R. (1974) The contribution of feedback to microteaching technique in *Microteaching Conference Papers* (ed. A. Trott), APLET Occasional Publications, No. 3.

Griffiths, R. (1976) The preparation of models for use in microteaching programmes, *Educational Media*, **1**, 25–31.

Gronlund, N. (1976) *Measurement and Evaluation in Teaching* (3rd edn), Macmillan, New York.

Guilbert, J. (1981) *Educational Handbook for Health Personnel*, World Health Organization, Geneva.

Hall, E. (1959) *The Silent Language*, Doubleday, New York.

Hanson, A. (1981) Use of standards of practice in the design and evaluation of a continuing education programme, *Amer. J. of Pharm. Ed.*, **45**, 56–60.

Hargie, O. (1986) From teaching to counselling: an evaluation of the role of micro-counselling in the training of school counsellors. Invited address to the First International Meeting on Psychological Teacher Education, University of Minho, Braga, Portugal.

Hargie, O., Dickson, D. and Tittmar, H. (1978) Mini-teaching: an extension of the microteaching format, *Brit. J. of Teacher Ed.*, **4**, 1–6.

Hargie, O. and Marshall, P. (1986) Interpersonal communication: a theoretical framework in *A Handbook of Communication Skills* (ed. O. Hargie), Croom Helm, London.

Hargie, O. and McCartan, P. (1986) *Social Skills Training and Psychiatric Nursing*, Croom Helm, London.

Hargie, O. and Morrow, N. (1986a) A survey of interpersonal skills teaching in pharmacy schools in the United Kingdom and Ireland, *Amer. J. of Pharm. Ed.*, **50**, 172–4.

Hargie, O. and Morrow, N. (1986b) Analytical and practical considerations of illustrative model videotapes, *J. of Audiovisual Media in Medicine*, **9**, 65–8.

Hargie, O. and Morrow, N. (1986c) Using videotape in communication skills training: a critical evaluation of the process of self-viewing, *Medical Teacher*, **8**, 359–64.

Hargie, O. and Morrow, N. (1987a) Introducing interpersonal skills training into the pharmaceutical curriculum, *Inter. Pharm. J.*, **1**, 175–78.

Hargie, O. and Morrow, N. (1987b) Interpersonal communication in pharmacy: the counselling approach, *Pharmacy Update*, **3**, 417–21.

Hargie, O. and Morrow, N. (1987c) Interpersonal communication: the sales approach, *Pharmacy Update*, **3**, 320–24.

Hargie, O. and Morrow, N. (1988) Interpersonal communication in pharmacy: the skill of self-disclosure, *Pharmacy Update* (in press).

Hargie, O. and Saunders, C. (1983a) Training professional skills in *Using Video: Psychological and Social Applications* (eds P. Dowrick and S. Biggs), Wiley, Chichester.

Hargie, O. and Saunders, C. (1983b) Individual differences and SST in *New Direc-*

tions in Social Skill Training (eds R. Ellis and D. Whittington), Croom Helm, London.

Hargie, O., Saunders, C. and Dickson, D. (1987) *Social Skills in Interpersonal Communication* (2nd edn), Croom Helm, London.

Hart, A. (1984) Some implications of audiovisual recordings of patients, *J. of Audiovisual Media in Medicine*, **7**, 48–50.

Hasler, J. (1983) The consultation and postgraduate general practice training in *Doctor–Patient Communication* (eds D. Pendleton and J. Hasler), Academic Press, London.

Hazler, R. and Hipple, T. (1981) The effects of mental practice on counselling behaviours, *Counsellor Education and Supervision*, **20**, 211–18.

Heath, C. (1986) *Body Movement and Speech in Medical Interaction*, Cambridge University Press, Cambridge.

Hein, E. (1973) *Communication in Nursing Practice*, Little, Brown & Co., Boston.

Helfer, R. (1970) An objective comparison of the paediatric interviewing skills of freshmen and senior medical students, *Paediatrics*, **45**, 623–27.

Henley, N. (1977) *Body Politics*, Prentice-Hall, Englewood Cliffs, New Jersey.

Herzmark, G. (1985) Rections of patients to video recording of consultations in general practice, *B. M. J.*, **291**, 315–7.

Hewitt, C. (1984) Training in social skills in *Occupational Therapy in Short-Term Psychiatry* (ed. M. Willson), Churchill Livingstone, Edinburgh.

Higgins, M., McCabe, D. and Vanetzian, E. (1984) Integration of communication theory in an accelerated nursing curriculum, *J. of Nurs. Ed.*, **23**, 262–4.

Hirsh, H. and Freed, H. (1978) Pattern sensitisation in psychotherapy supervision by means of videotape recording in *Videotape Technique in Psychiatric Training and Treatment* (ed. M. Berger), Brunner/Mazel, New York.

HMSO (1978) *Health Services Commissioner – Annual Report of Session 1977–1978*, HMSO, London.

Hodges, A. (1977) *Psychosocial Counseling in General Medical Practice*, D.C. Heath & Co., Lexington, Massachusetts.

Hofling, C., Brotzman, E. and Dalrymple, S. *et al.* (1966) An experimental study in nurse-physician relationships, *J. of Nerv. and Ment. Dis.*, **143**, 171–80.

Hogstel, M. (1987) Teaching students observational skills, *Nursing Outlook*, **35**, 89–91.

Holding, D. (1965) *Principles of Training*, Pergamon, Oxford.

Hopson, B. (1981) Counselling and helping in *Psychology And Medicine* (ed. D. Griffiths), MacMillan, London.

Hornsby, J., Deneen, L. and Heid, D. (1975) Interpersonal communication skills development: a model for dentistry, *J. of Dent. Ed.*, **39**, 728–32.

Hosford, R. (1981) Self-as-a-model: a cognitive social learning technique, *The Counselling Psychologist*, **9**, 45–61.

Hung, J. and Rosenthal, T. (1978) Therapeutic videotaped playback: a critical review, *Adv. in Behav. Res. and Therapy*, **1**, 103–35.

Hymes, D. (1972) On communicative competence in *Sociolinguistics: Selected Readings* (eds J. Pride and J. Holmes), Penguin, Baltimore.

Inskipp, F., Johns, H. and Heaviside, P. (1978) *Principles of Counselling*, BBC Further Education Publication, London.

Irwin, W. and Bamber, J. (1984) An evaluation of medical student behaviours in communication, *Medical Education*, **18**, 90–5.

Ivey, A. (1976) *Basic Attending Skills* (Videotape Package), Microtraining Associates Inc., North Amherst, Massachusetts.

Ivey, A. and Authier, J. (1978) *Microcounselling: Innovations in Interviewing, Counselling, Psychotherapy and Psychoeducation*, C.C. Thomas, Springfield, Illinois.

Ivey, A. and Gluckstern, N. (1974) *Basic Attending Skills: Participant Manual*, Microtraining Associates Inc., North Amherst, Massachusetts.

Ivey, A. and Gluckstern, N. (1976) *Basic Influencing Skills: Leader and Participant Manual*, Microtraining Associates Inc., Massachusetts.

Ivey, A., Ivey, M. and Simek-Dowling, L. (1987) *Counseling and Psychotherapy: Integrating Skills, Theory and Practice* (2nd edn), Prentice Hall, Englewood Cliffs, New Jersey.

Izard, C. (1977) *Human Emotions*, Plenum Press, New York.

Jackson, E. (1978) Convergent evidence for the effectiveness of interpersonal skill training for dental students, *J. of Dent. Ed.*, **42**, 517–23.

Jackson, E. and Katz, J. (1983) Implementation of interpersonal skill training in dental schools, *J. of Den. Ed.*, **47**, 66–71.

Jarvis, P. (1983) *Professional Education*, Croom Helm, London.

Jarvis, P. and Gibson, S. (1985) *The Teacher Practitioner in Nursing, Midwifery and Health Visiting*, Croom Helm, London.

Jessop, A. (1979) *Nurse-Patient Communication: A Skills Approach*, Microtraining Associates, North Amherst, Massachusetts.

Joint Committee on Postgraduate Training for General Practice (1982) *Training for General Practice*, London.

Jones, C. (1984) Process recording for communication with psychiatric patients – techniques for improving skills of communication in *Recent Advances in Nursing, 7, Communication* (ed. A. Faulkner), Churchill Livingstone, Edinburgh.

Jones, J. (1973) Helping relationship inventory in *The Annual Handbook for Group Facilitators* (eds W. Pfeiffer and J. Jones), University Associates, San Diego, California.

Jones, K. (1985) *Designing Your Own Simulations*, Methuen, London.

Kagan, C. (ed.) (1985) *Interpersonal Skills in Nursing: Research and Applications*, Croom Helm, London.

Kagan, C., Evans, J. and Kay, B. (1986) *A Manual of Interpersonal Skills for Nurses: An Experiential Approach*, Harper & Row, London.

Kagan, N. (1980) Influencing human interaction: eighteen years with IPR in *Psychotherapy Supervision: Theory, Research and Practice* (ed. A. Hess), Wiley, New York.

Kahn, G., Cohen, B. and Jason, H. (1979a) The teaching of interpersonal skills in US medical schools, *J. of Med. Ed.*, **54**, 29–35.

Kahn, G., Cohen, B. and Jason, H. (1979b) Teaching interpersonal skills in family practice: results of a national survey, *J. of Fam. Prac.*, **8**, 309–16.

Kahn, R. and Cannell, C. (1957) *The Dynamics of Interviewing*, Wiley, New York.

Kasch, C. (1986) Toward a theory of nursing action: skills and competency in nurse-patient interaction, *Nursing Research*, **35**, 226–30.

Kasteler, J., Kane, R., Olsen, D. and Thetford, C. (1976) Issues underlying prevalence of "doctor shopping" behavior, *J. of Health and Soc. Beh.*, **17**, 328–39.

Kauss, D., Robbins, A. and Abrass, I. *et al.* (1980) The long-term effectiveness of interpersonal skills training in medical schools, *J. of Med. Ed.*, **55**, 595–601.

Kelley, H. (1971) *Attribution in Social Interaction*, General Learning Press, Morristown.

Kelly, L. (1984) Social skills training as a mode of treatment for social communication problems in *Avoiding Communication: Shyness, Reticence and Communication Apprehension* (eds J. Daly and J. McCroskey), Sage, Beverly Hills, California.

Kent, G., Clarke, P. and Dalrymple-Smith, D. (1981) The patient is the expert: a technique for teaching interviewing skills, *Medical Education*, **15**, 38–42.

Kerr, D. (1986) Teaching communication skills in postgraduate medical education, *J. of the Roy. Soc. of Med.*, **79**, 575–80.

Kimberlin, C. (1985) Characteristics desired in tests: validity, *Amer. J. of Pharmac. Ed.*, **49**, 73–6.

Kincey, J., Bradshaw, P. and Ley, P. (1975) Patients satisfaction and reported acceptance of advice in general practice, *J. of the Roy. Coll. of Gen. Pract.*, **25**, 558–66.

Kipper, D. and Ginot, E. (1979) Accuracy of evaluating videotape feedback and defense mechanisms, *J. of Consulting and Clinical Psychol.*, **47**, 493–99.

Kitching, J. (1986) Communication and the community pharmacist, *The Pharmac. J.*, **10**, 449–52.

Kleinke, C. (1986) *Meeting and Understanding People*, Freeman, New York.

Klinzing, D. and Klinzing, D. (1985) *Communication for Allied Health Professionals*, W.C. Brown, Dubuque, Iowa.

Knowles, M. (1980) *The Modern Practice of Adult Education*, Association Press, New York.

Knox, J. and Bouchier, I. (1985) Communication skills teaching, learning and assessment, *Medi. Ed.*, **19**, 285–89.

Kolotkin, R., Wielkiewicz, R., Judd, B. and Weisler, S. (1983) Behavioral components of assertion: comparison of univariate and multivariate assessment strategies, *Behavioral Assessment*, **6**, 61–78.

Kopp, C. and Krakow, J. (1982) *The Child: Development in a Social Context*, Addison-Wesley, Reading, Massachusetts.

Korsch, B., Gozzi, E. and Francis, V. (1968) Gaps in doctor-patient communication: doctor-patient interaction and patient satisfaction, *Paediatrics*, **42**, 855–71.

Kratz, C. (1978) *Care of the Long Term Sick in the Community*, Churchill Livingstone, Edinburgh.

Kurtz, P. and Marshall, E. (1982) Evolution of interpersonal skills training in *Interpersonal Helping Skills* (eds E. Marshall *et al.*), Jossey-Bass, San Francisco.

Kurtz, P., Marshall, E. and Banspach, S. (1985) Interpersonal skill-training research: a 12–year review and analysis, *Counsellor Education and Supervision*, **24**, 249–63.

Larsen, K. and Smith, C. (1981) Assessment of nonverbal communication in the patient-physician interview, *J. of Fam. Prac.*, **12**, 481–88.

Lawson, K. (1975) *Philosophical Concepts and Values in Adult Education*, University of Nottingham, Department of Education.

Leigh, H. and Reiser, M. (1980) *The Patient: Biological, Psychological, and Social Dimensions of Medical Practice*, Plenum, New York.

Leventhal, H. (1970) Findings and theory in the study of fear communications in

Advances in Experimental Social Psychology: Vol. 5 (ed. L. Berkowitz), Academic Press, New York.

Ley, P. (1977a) Psychological studies of doctor-patient communication in *Contributions to Medical Psychology* (ed. S. Rachman), Pergamon Press, Oxford.

Ley, P. (1977b) Communicating with the patient in *Introductory Psychology* (ed. J. Coleman), Routledge and Kegan Paul, London.

Ley, P. (1982a) Satisfaction, compliance and communication, *Brit. J. of Clin. Psychol.*, **21**, 241–54.

Ley, P. (1982b) Giving information to patients in *Social Psychology and Behavioral Medicine* (ed. J.R. Eiser), Wiley, New York.

Ley, P. (1983) Patients' understanding and recall in clinical communication failure in *Doctor-Patient Communication* (eds D. Pendleton and J. Hasler), Academic Press, London.

Ley, P. (1988) *Communicating with Patients*, Chapman and Hall, London.

Ley, P., Bradshaw, P., Eaves, D. and Walker, C. (1973) A method for increasing patients' recall of information presented by doctors, *Psychological Medicine*, **3**, 217–20.

Ley, P., Goldman, M., Bradshaw, P., Kincey, J. and Walker, C. (1972) The comprehensibility of some X-ray leaflets, *J. of the Inst. of Health Ed.*, **10**, 47–53.

Lezberg, A. and Fedo, D. (1980) Communication skills and pharmacy education: a case study, *Amer. J. of Pharmac. Ed.*, **44**, 257–59.

Lillie, F. (1985) The wider social context of interpersonal skills in nursing in *Interpersonal Skills in Nursing: Research and Applications* (ed. C. Kagan), Croom Helm, London.

Linehan, M. and Egan, K. (1979) Assertion training for women in *Research and Practice in Social Skills Training* (eds A. Bellack and M. Hersen), Plenum, New York.

Linstone, H. and Turoff, M. (1975) *The Delphi Method: Techniques and Applications*, Addison-Wesley Publishing Company, Reading, Massachusetts.

Livesey, P. (1986) *Partners in Care: The Consultation in General Practice*, Heinemann, London.

Loftus, E. (1975) Leading questions and the eyewitness report, *Cogn. Psychol.*, **7**, 560–72.

Long, H. (1983) *Adult Learning*, Cambridge Book Co., New York.

Long, L., Paradise, L. and Long, J. (1981) *Questioning: Skills for The Helping Process*, Brooks-Cole, Monterey, California.

Lott, D. and Sommer, R. (1967) Seating arrangements and status *J. of Per. and Soc. Psychol.*, **7**, 90–5.

Love, D., Weise, H. and Parker, C. (1978) Continuing education in factors affecting communication: a novel approach, *Amer. J. of Pharm. Ed.*, **42**, 304–7.

MacLeod, G. (1977) The effects of videotape and skill-related feedback on students' perceptions of their microteaching performance in *Investigations of Microteaching* (eds D. McIntyre, G. MacLeod and R. Griffiths), Croom Helm, London.

MacLeod Clark, J. (1981) Nurse-patient communication, *Nursing Times*, **77**, 12–18.

MacLeod Clark, J. (1982) Nurse-patient verbal interaction: an analysis of recorded conversations from selected surgical wards, Unpublished PhD thesis, University of London.

MacLeod Clark, J. (1984) Verbal communication in nursing in *Recent Advances in*

Nursing, 7, Communication (ed. A. Faulkner), Churchill Livingstone, Edinburgh.

MacLeod Clark, J. (1985) The development of research in interpersonal skills in nursing in *Interpersonal Skills in Nursing: Research and Applications* (ed. C. Kagan), Croom Helm, London.

MacLeod Clark, J. and Faulkner, A. (1987) Communication skills teaching in nurse education in *Nursing Education: Research and Developments* (ed. B. Davis), Croom Helm, London.

Mader, P. (1974) Differential effects of immediate and delayed feedback in role-playing counselling sessions, *Dissertation Abstracts International*, **34**, 3878A.

Maguire, G. and Rutter, D. (1976) History taking for medical students *Lancet* ii, 556–58.

Maguire, P. (1981) Doctor-patient skills in *Social Skills and Health* (ed. M. Argyle), Methuen, London.

Maguire, P. (1984a) Communication skills and patient care in *Health Care and Human Behaviour* (eds A. Steptoe and A. Mathews), Academic Press, London.

Maguire, P. (1984b) How we teach interviewing skills, *Med. Teacher*, **6**, 128–33.

Maguire, P. (1985) Deficiencies in key interpersonal skills in *Interpersonal Skills in Nursing* (ed. C. Kagan), Croom Helm, London.

Maguire, P. (1986) Social skills training for health professionals in *Handbook of Social Skills Training, Vol. 2* (eds C. Hollin and P. Trower), Pergamon, Oxford.

Maguire, P., Fairbairn, S. and Fletcher, C. (1986) Consultation skills of young doctors, *B. M. J.*, **292**, 1573–78.

Maguire, P., Roe, P., and Goldberg, D. *et al.* (1978) The value of feedback in teaching interviewing skills to medical students, *Psychol. Med.*, **8**, 695–704.

Maguire, P., Tait, A., Brooke, M. and Sellwood, R. (1980a) Emotional aspects of mastectomy: a conspiracy of pretence, *Nursing Mirror*, January **10**, 17–19.

Maguire, P., Tait, A., Brooke, M., and Thomas, C. *et al.* (1980b) The effect of counselling on the psychiatric morbidity associated with mastectomy, *B. M. J.*, **2**, 1454–6.

Mahoney, M. (1974) *Cognitive and Behaviour Modification*, Ballinger, Cambridge, Massachusetts.

Marquis, K. (1970) Effects of social reinforcement on health reporting in the household interview, *Sociometry*, **33**, 203–15.

Marshall, E., Kurtz, P. and Associates (eds) (1982) *Interpersonal Helping Skills*, Jossey-Bass, San Francisco.

Marshfied, G. (1985) Issues arising from teaching interpersonal skills in general nurse training in *Interpersonal Skills in Nursing: Research and Applications* (ed. C. Kagan), Croom Helm, London.

Marson, S. (1985) *Communication Skills – A Trainer's Guide*, National Health Service, Learning Resources Unit, Sheffield.

Marteniuk, R. (1976) *Information Processing in Motor Skills*, Holt, Rinehart and Winston, New York.

Martin, E. and Martin, P. (1984) The reactions of patients to a video camera in the consulting room, *J. of the Roy. Coll. of G. P.*, **34**, 607–11.

Marwell, G. and Schmitt, D. (1967a) Compliance-gaining behavior: a synthesis and model, *Sociol. Quart.*, **8**, 317–28.

Marwell, G. and Schmitt, D. (1967b) Dimensions of compliance-gaining behavior: an empirical analysis, *Sociometry*, **30**, 350–64.

Maslow, A. (1954) *Motivation and Personality*, Harper and Row, New York.

Mason, H. and Svarstad, B. (1984) Medication counseling behaviors and attitudes of rural community pharmacists, *Drug Intelligence and Clincial Pharmacy*, **18**, 409–14.

Mayo, C. and Henley, N. (eds.) (1981) *Gender and Nonverbal Behavior*, Springer-Verlag, New York.

McCroskey, J. (1977) Oral communication apprehension: a survey of recent theory and research, *Hum. Com. Res.*, **4**, 78–96.

McCroskey, J. (1984) Communication competence: the elusive construct in *Competence in Communication: A Multidisciplinary Approach* (ed. R. Bostrom), Sage, Beverly Hills, California.

McGarvey, B. and Swallow, D. (1986) *Microteaching in Teacher Education and Training*, Croom Helm, London.

McGhee, A. (1961) *The Patient's Attitude to Nursing Care*, Livingstone, London.

McGuire, W. (1968) The nature of attitudes and attitude change in *Handbook of Social Psychology: Vol. 3* (eds G. Lindzey and E. Aronson), Addison-Wesley, Reading, Massachusetts.

McIntee, J. and Firth, H. (1984) How to beat the burnout, *Health and Soc. Serv. J.*, February **9**, 166–68.

McIntyre, D. (1983) Social skills training for teaching in *New Directions in Social Skill Training* (eds R. Ellis and D. Whittington), Croom Helm, London.

McIntyre, T., Jeffrey, D. and McIntyre, S. (1984) Assertion training: the effectiveness of a contemporary cognitive-behavioral treatment package with professional nurses, *Behav. Res. and Ther.*, **22**, 311–18.

McKenny, J., Slining, J. and Henderson, H. *et al.* (1973) The effect of clinical pharmacy services on patients with essential hypertension, *Circulation*, **48**, 1104–11.

McKinlay, J. (1972) Some approaches and problems in the study of the use of services: an overview, *J. of Health and Soc. Beh.*, **13**, 115–52.

McPherson, C., Sachs, L., Knapp, W. and Wolf, F. (1984) The doctor-patient relationship: systematic training in effective communication skills, *The J. of Psychiat. Ed.*, **8**, 87–92.

McQuellon, R. (1982) Interpersonal process recall in *Interpersonal Helping Skills* (eds E. Marshall, P. Kurtz *et al.*), Jossey-Bass, San Francisco.

McSweeney, P. (1986) Sight and sound – any use for video found? Part 2: a potential still untapped, *Nurse Education Today*, **6**, 223–27.

Menikheim, M. and Ryden, M. (1985) Designing learning to increase competency in interpersonal communication skills, *J. of Nurs. Ed.*, **24**, 216–8.

Miles, R. (1987) Experiential learning in the curriculum in *The Curriculum in Nursing Education* (eds P. Allan and M. Jolley), Croom Helm, London.

Miller, G., Boster, F., Roloff, M. and Seibold, D. (1987) MBRS rekindled: some thoughts on compliance gaining in interpersonal settings in *Interpersonal Processes: New Directions in Communication Research* (eds M. Roloff and G. Miller), Sage, Beverly Hills, California.

Millis, J. (1975) *Pharmacistis for the Future: The Report of the Study Commission on Pharmacy*, Health Administration Press, Ann Arbor, Michigan.

Milroy, E. (1982) *Role-Play: A Practical Guide*, Aberdeen University Press, Aberdeen.

Montagu, A. (1978) *Touching*, Harper & Row, New York.

Moreno, J. (1953) *Who Shall Survive*, Beacon House, Beacon, New York.

Morris, R. (1980) Fear reduction methods in *Helping People Change* (eds F. Kanfer and A. Goldstein), Pergamon, New York.

Morrow, N. (1986) *Communication as a Focus in Pharmacy Education and Practice*, PhD Thesis, The Queen's University of Belfast, Northern Ireland.

Morrow, N. and Hargie, O. (1985a) Improving interpersonal communication in pharmacy practice, *The Pharmac. J.*, **235**, 23–5.

Morrow, N. and Hargie, O. (1985b) Interpersonal communication: questioning skills, *Pharmacy Update*, **1**, 255–57.

Morrow, N. and Hargie, O. (1986) Communication as a focus in the continuing education of pharmacists, *Studies in Higher Education*, **11**, 279–88.

Morrow, N. and Hargie, O. (1987a) Effectiveness of a communication skills training course in continuing pharmaceutical education in Northern Ireland: a longitudinal study, *Amer. J. of Pharm. Ed.*, **51**, 148–52.

Morrow, N. and Hargie, O. (1987b) An investigation of critical incidents in interpersonal communication in pharmacy practice, *J. of Soc. and Admin. Pharmacy*, **4**, 112–18.

Mortensen, C. (1972) *Communication: The Study of Human Interaction*, McGraw-Hill, New York.

Morton, T. and Kurtz, P. (1982) Conditions affecting skills learning in *Interpersonal Helping Skills* (eds E. Marshall *et al.*), Jossey-Bass, San Francisco.

Mulac, A. (1974) Effects of three feedback conditions employing videotape and audiotape on acquired speech skill, *Speech Monographs*, **41**, 205–14.

Mullan, T. (1986) *Generalization in SST*, Unpublished M. Phil. Thesis, University of Ulster, Jordanstown.

Murdock, B. (1962) The serial position effect in free recall, *J. of Exper. Psychol.*, **64**, 482–88.

Myers, G. and Myers, M. (1985) *The Dynamics of Human Communication*, McGraw-Hill, New York.

National Board for Nursing, Midwifery and Health Visiting for Northern Ireland (1983), *General Nursing Syllabus for Part 1 of the Register of Nurses, Midwives and Health Visitors*.

Neisser, U. (1967) *Cognitive Psychology*, Appleton-Century-Crofts, New York.

Nelson, A., Gold, B., Hutchinson, R. and Benezra, E. (1975) Drug default among schizophrenic patients, *Amer. J. of Hosp. Pharm.*, **32**, 1237–42.

Nelson-Jones, R. (1983) *Practical Counselling Skills*, Holt, Rinehart & Winston, London.

Niland, T., Duling, J., Allen, V. and Panther, E. (1971) Student counsellors' perceptions of videotaping, *Counsellor Education and Supervision*, **10**, 97–101.

Norris, J. (1986) Teaching communication skills: effects of two methods of instruction and selected learner characteristics, *J. of Nurs. Ed.*, **25**, 102–6.

Northouse, P. and Northouse, L. (1985) *Health Communication: A Handbook for Health Professionals*, Prentice-Hall, Englewood Cliffs, New Jersey.

Nuffield Committee of Inquiry (1986) *Pharmacy. The Report of the Committee of Inquiry Appointed by the Nuffield Foundation*, The Nuffield Foundation, London.

Nurse, G. (1977) *The Professional Helping Relationship and its Relevance for Nurse*

Education, Dip Ed Thesis, Institute of Education, University of London.

Nurse, G. (1980) *Counselling and the Nurse*, HM&M Publishers, Aylesbury, England.

Nyquist, J. and Wulff, D. (1982) The use of simultaneous feedback to alter teaching behaviours to university instructors, *J. of Classroom Interaction*, **18**, 11.

Oetting, E. (1976) Evaluative research and orthodox science *Personal and Guidance Journal*, **55**, 11–15.

Oland, L. (1978) The need for territoriality in *Human Needs and The Nursing Process* (eds A. Yura and M. Walsh), Appleton-Century-Crofts, New York.

Olson, J. and Iwasiw, C. (1987) Effects of a training model on active listening skills of post-RN students, *J. of Nurs. Ed.*, **26**, 104–7.

Omololu, C. (1984) Communication behaviours of undergraduate medical students before and after training, *Brit. J. of Med. Psychol.*, **57**, 97–100.

Oppenheim, A. (1966) *Questionnaire Design and Attitude Measurement*, Heinemann, London.

Owen, G. (ed.) (1983) *Health Visiting*, Ballière Tindall, London.

Page, G. and Fielding, D. (1985) Appraising Tests, *Amer. J. of Pharm. Ed.*, **49**, 80–5.

Patterson, M. (1983) *Nonverbal Behavior: A Functional Perspective*, Springer-Verlag, New York.

Pavlov, I. (1927) *Conditioned Reflex*, Dover Reprint, New York.

Pawlak, E., Way, I. and Thompson, D. (1982) Assessing factors that influence skills training in organizations in *Interpersonal Helping Skills* (eds E. Marshall *et al.*), Jossey-Bass, San Francisco.

Pendleton, D. (1981) Learning communication skills, *Update*, **22**, 1708–14.

Pendleton, D. and Bochner, S. (1980) The communication of information in general practice consultations as a function of patients' social class, *Soc. Sci. and Med.*, **14**, 669–73.

Pendleton, D., Schofield, T., Tate, P. and Havelock, P. (1984) *The Consultation: An Approach to Learning and Teaching*, Oxford University Press, Oxford.

Pennington, D. (1986) *Essential Social Psychology*, Edward Arnold, London.

Perry, M. and Furukawa, M. (1986) Modeling methods in *Helping People Change* (eds F. Kanfer and A. Goldstein), Pergamon, New York.

Peters, G., Cormier, L. and Cormier, W. (1978) Effects of modelling, rehearsal, feedback and remediation on acquisition of a counselling strategy, *J. of Couns. Psychol.*, **25**, 231–37.

Pettegrew, L. (1982) Some boundaries and assumptions in health communication in *Straight Talk: Explorations in Provider and Patient Interaction* (eds L. Pettegrew, P. Arntson, D. Bush and K. Zoppi), Humana, Louisville, Kentucky.

Pfeiffer, J. and Jones, J. (1970) *A Handbook of Structured Experiences for Human Relations Training*, University Associates Press, Iowa.

Pharmaceutical Society of Great Britain (1984) First report of the Working Party on pharmaceutical education and training, *Pharm. J.*, **232**, 495–508.

Phillips, E. (1978) *The Social Skills Basis of Psychotherapy: Alternative to Abnormal Psychology and Psychiatry*, Grune and Statton, New York.

Phillips, K. and Fraser, T. (1982) *The Management of Interpersonal Skills Training*, Gower, Aldershot.

Pietrofesa, J., Hoffman, A., Splete, H. and Pinto, D. (1978) *Counseling: Theory,*

Research and Practice, Rand McNally, Chicago.

Pillow, W. and Schlegel, J. (1981) Training future communicators, *American Pharmacy*, **NS21**, 43–5.

Plat, F. and McMath, J. (1979) Clinical hypocompetence: the interview, *Annals of Internal Medicine*, **91**, 898–902.

Podell, K. (1975) *Physician Guide to Compliance in Hypertension*, Merck, Rahway, New Jersey.

Poole, D. and Sanson-Fisher, R. (1981) Long-term effects of empathy training on the interview skills of medical students, *J. of Patient Counseling and Health Ed.*, **2**, 125–9.

Pope, B. (1986) *Social Skills Training for Psychiatric Nurses*, Harper and Row, London.

Porritt, L. (1984) *Communication: Choices for Nurses*, Churchill Livingstone, Edinburgh.

Pringle, M., Robins, S. and Brown, G. (1984) Assessing the consultation: methods of observing trainees in general practice, *B. Med. J.*, **288**, 1659–60.

Purtilo, R. (1984) *Health Professional/Patient Interaction*, W.B. Saunders and Co., Philadelphia.

Rackham, N. and Morgan, T. (1977) *Behaviour Analysis in Training*, McGraw-Hill, London.

Rae, L. (1985) *The Skills of Human Relations Training*, Gower, Aldershot.

Rakos, R. (1986) Asserting and confronting in *A Handbook of Communication Skills* (ed. O. Hargie), Croom Helm, London.

Rand, C. (1981) Communication of affect between patient and physician, *J. of Health and Soc. Beh.*, **22**, 18–30.

Rapport, H. (1983) A Methodology for the identification and assessment of health planning goals: application to pharmacy services, *J. of Soc. and Admin. Pharm.*, 1, 161–71.

Rasmuson, T. (1987) The effects of pausing and listening ability on retention of a spoken message, *J. of the International Listening Society*, 1, 114–28.

Raven, B. and Haley, R. (1982) Social influence and compliance of hospital nurses with infection control policies in *Social Psychology and Behavioral Medicine* (ed. J. Eiser), Wiley, Chichester.

Raven, B. and Rubin, J. (1983) *Social Psychology* (2nd edn), Wiley, New York.

Reich, C. and Meisner, A. (1976) A comparison of colour and black and white television as instructional media, *Brit. J. of Educ. Tech.*, 7, 24–34.

Renne, C., Dowrick, P. and Wasek, G. (1983) Considerations of the participant in video recording in *Using Video: Psychological and Social Applications* (eds P. Dowrick and S. Biggs), Wiley, Chichester.

Richardson, S., Dohrenwend, N. and Klein, D. (1965) *Interviewing: Its Forms and Functions*, Basic Books, New York.

Rimm, D. and Masters, J. (1979) *Behavior Therapy: Techniques and Empirical Findings* (2nd edn), Academic Press, New York.

Robinson, J. (1982) *An Evaluation of Health Visiting*, C.E.T.H.V., London.

Rodenhauser, P. and Sayer, J. (1987) A workshop to increase communication competence in medical students, *J. of Med. Ed.*, **62**, 141–42.

Rogers, C. (1951) *Client-Centred Therapy*, Houghton Mifflin, Boston.

Rogers, C. (1975) Empathic: an unappreciated way of being, *The Counseling*

Psychologist, **5**, 2–10.

Rogers, R. (1984) Changing health-related attitudes and behavior: the role of preventive health psychology in *Social Perception in Clinical and Counseling Psychology: Vol. 2* (eds J. Harvey, J. Maddux, R. McGlynn, and D. Stoltenberg), Texas Tech. University Press, Lubbock, Texas.

Roloff, M. and Kellermann, K. (1984) Judgements of interpersonal competency: how you know, what you know, and who you know in *Competence in Communication: A Multidisciplinary Approach* (ed. R. Bostrom), Sage, Beverly Hills, California.

Roloff, M. and Miller, G. (eds) (1980) *Persuasion: New Directions in Theory and Research*, Sage, Beverly Hills, California.

Rose, Y. and Tryon, W. (1979) Judgements of assertion behavior as a function of speech, loudness, latency, content, gestures, inflection and sex, *Behavior Modification*, **3**, 112–23.

Rosenberg, M.; Nelson, C. and Vivekananthan, P. (1968) A multidimensional approach to the structure of personality impression, *J. of Pers. and Soc. Psychol.*, **9**, 283–94.

Rosenblatt, P. (1977) Cross-cultural perspective on attraction in *Foundations of Interpersonal Attraction* (ed. T. Houston), Academic Press, London.

Rosenfeld, H. and Hancks, M. (1980) The nonverbal context of verbal listener responses in *The Relationship of Verbal and Nonverbal Communication* (ed. M. Kay), Mouton, The Hague.

Rosser, J. and Maguire, P. (1982) Dilemmas in general practice: the care of the cancer patient, *Social Science and Medicine*, **16**, 315–22.

Roter, D. (1977) Patient participation in the patient-provider interaction: the effects of patient question asking on the quality of interaction satisfaction and compliance, *Health Education Monographs*, Winter, 281–315.

Royal College of General Practitioners Working Party (1972) *The Future General Practitioner*, Royal College of General Practitioners, London.

Rozelle, R., Druckman, D. and Baxter, J. (1986) Nonverbal communication in *A Handbook of Communication Skills* (ed. O. Hargie), Croom Helm, London.

Ruffner, M. and Burgoon, M. (1981) *Interpersonal Communication*, Holt, Rinehart and Winston, New York.

Runyon, H. and Cohen, L. (1979) The effects of systematic human relations training on freshman dental students, *J. of the Amer. Dent. Assoc.*, **98**, 196–201.

Ryan, M. (1978) Planning, development, and evaluation of continuing education programme in *Pharmacy in Health Care and Institutional Systems* (eds P. Lecca and C. Tharp), C.V. Mosby Company, St Louis.

Salmoni, A., Schmidt, R. and Walter, C. (1984) Knowledge of results and motor learning: a review and critical reappraisal, *Psychological Bulletin*, **95**, 355–86.

Salvendy, J. (1984) Improving interviewing techniques through the bug-in-the-ear, *Canadian J. of Psychiatry*, **29**, 302–5.

Sanders, M. (1982) The effects of instructions, feedback and cueing procedures in behavioural parent training, *Austral. J. of Psychol.*, **34**, 53–69.

Sanson-Fisher, R. and Poole, A. (1980) The content of interactions: naturally occurring contingencies within a short-stay psychiatric unit, *Advances in Behaviour Research and Therapy*, **2**, 145–57.

Saunders, C. (1986) Opening and closing in *A Handbook of Communication Skills* (ed. O. Hargie), Croom Helm, London.

Saunders, C. and Caves, R. (1986) An empirical approach to the identification of communication skills with reference to speech therapy, *J. of Further and Higher Ed.*, **10**, 29–44.

Sause, R., Carlstedt, B. and Peterson, C. (1976) Pharmacist-patient interactions in terms of 'appropriate behaviours', *Amer. J. of Pharm. Ed.*, **40**, 261–65.

Scherer, K. (1972) Judging personality from voice: a cross-cultural approach to an old issue in person perception, *J. of Pers.*, **40**, 191–210.

Schofield, T. (1983) The application of the study of communication skills to training for general practice in *Doctor-Patient Communication* (eds D. Pendleton and J. Hasler), Academic Press, London.

Servant, J. and Matheson, J. (1986) Video recording in general practice: the patients do mind, *J. of the Roy. Coll. of G. P.*, **36**, 555–6.

Shannon, C. and Weaver, W. (1949) *The Mathematical Theory of Communication*, University of Illinois Press, Illinois.

Shaw, B. (1979) The theoretical and experimental foundations of a cognitive model for depression in *Advances in the Study of Communication and Affect: Volume 5* (eds P. Pliner, K. Blankstein and I. Spigel), Plenum Press, New York.

Sheppe, W. and Stevenson, I. (1963) Techniques of interviewing in *The Psychological Basis of Medical Practice* (eds H. Lief, F. Lief and N. Lief), Hoeber, New York.

Shienwold, A., Asken, M. and Cincotta, J. (1979) Family practice residents' perceptions of behavioural science training, relevance and needs, *J. of Fam. Prac.*, **8**, 97.

Shorter, E. (1985) *Bedside Manners*, Viking Penguin, New York.

Shuy, R. (1983) Three types of interference to an effective exchange of information in the medical interview in *Social Organisation of Doctor–Patient Communication* (eds S. Fisher and A. Todd), Center for Applied Linguistics, Washington DC.

Siegman, A. and Feldstein, S. (eds) (1987) *Nonverbal Behavior and Communication* (2nd edn), Lawrence Erlbaum Associates, Hillsdale, New Jersey.

Simms, M. and Smith, C. (1984) Teenage mothers: some views on health visitors, *Health Visitor*, **57**, 269–70.

Skinner, B. (1953) *Science and Human Behaviour*, Collier Macmillan, London.

Skinner, B. (1969) *Contingencies of Reinforcement*, Appleton-Century-Crofts, New York.

Skinner, B. (1971) How to teach animals in *Contemporary Psychology* (ed. R. Atkinson), Freeman, San Francisco.

Skinner, B. (1976) *About Behaviourism*, Vintage Books, New York.

Smith, P. (1983) Teaching and learning to communicate, *Nursing Times*, **79**, 51–3.

Smith, V. (1986) Listening in *A Handbook of Communication Skills* (ed. O. Hargie), Croom Helm, London.

Smith, V. and Bass, T. (1982) *Communication for the Health Care Team*, Harper & Row, London.

Snyder, M. (1974) The self-monitoring of expressive behavior, *J. of Person. and Soc. Psychol.*, **30**, 526–37.

Snyder, M. (1987) *Public Appearances, Private Realities*, Freeman, New York.

Sorenson, R. and Pickett, T. (1986) A test of two teaching strategies designed to improve interview effectiveness: rating behaviour and videotape feedback, *Com-*

munication Education, **35**, 13–22.

Sparks, S., Vitalo, P., Cohen, B. and Kahn, G. (1980) Teaching of interpersonal skills to nurse practitioner students, *J. of Cont. Ed. in Nursing*, **11**, 5–16.

Speas, C. (1979) A comparison of the effectiveness of model exposure and role-playing with videotape feedback, and no treatment for training prison inmates in job-seeking interview skills, *Dis. Abs. Internat.*, **39**, 6552A.

Speedie, S. (1985) Reliability: the accuracy of a test, *Amer. J. of Pharmac. Ed.*, **49**, 76–9.

Spencer, L. (1979) *Identifying, Measuring and Training 'Soft Skill' Competencies which Predict Performance in Professional Mangerial and Human Service Jobs.* Paper presented at the Soft Skill Analysis Symposium, Department of the Army Training Development Institute, Fort Monroe, Virginia.

Spitzberg, B. and Cupach, W. (1984) *Interpersonal Communication Competence*, Sage, Beverly Hills, California.

Stammers, R. and Patrick, J. (1975) *The Psychology of Training*, Methuen, London.

Steil, L., Barker, L. and Watson, K. (1983) *Effective Listening: Key to Your Success*, Addison-Wesley, Reading, Massachusetts.

Stevens, R. (1975) *Interpersonal Communication*, Open University Press, Milton Keynes.

Stewart, L. and Ting-Toomey, S. (eds) (1987) *Communication, Gender and Sex Roles in Diverse Interaction Contexts*, Guildford Press, Hove, England.

Stewart, W. (1983) *Counselling in Nursing: A Problem Solving Approach*, Harper & Row, London.

Stimson, G. and Webb, B. (1975) *Going to the Doctor*, Routledge and Kegan Paul, London.

Stokes, T. and Baer, D. (1977) An implicit technology of generalization, *J. of Appl. Behav. Analy.*, **10**, 349–67.

Stuart, G. and Sundeen, S. (1983) *Principles and Practice of Psychiatric Nursing* (2nd edn), C.V. Mosby, St Louis.

Sudman, S. and Bradburn, N. (1982) *Asking Questions*, Jossey-Bass, San Francisco.

Sundeen, S., Stuart, G., Rankin, E. and Cohen, S. (1985) *Nurse–Client Interaction*, C.V. Mosby, St Louis.

Sutton, S. (1982) Fear-arousing communications: a critical examination of theory and research in *Social Psychology and Behavioral Medicine* (ed. J. Eiser), Wiley, Chichester.

Taba, H. (1962) *Curriculum Developments: Theory and Practice*, Harcourt, Brace and World, New York.

Tähkä, V. (1984) *The Patient-Doctor Relationship*, ADIS Health Science Press, Sydney.

Taylor, D. (1979) Motivational bases in *Self-disclosure* (ed. G. Chelune), Jossey-Bass, San Francisco.

Tedeschi, J. (ed.) (1972) *The Social Influence Processes*, Aldine, Chicago.

Ter Horst, G., Leeds, J. and Hoogstraten, J. (1984) Effectiveness of communication skills training for dental students, *Psychol. Rep.*, **55**, 7–11.

Thibaut, J. and Kelley, H. (1959) *The Social Psychology of Groups*, Wiley, New York.

Thompson, J. and Anderson, J. (1982) Patient preferences and the bedside manner, *Med. Ed.*, **16**, 17–21.

Thompson, T.L. (1986) *Communication for Health Professionals*, Harper & Row, New York.

Thorndike, D. (1927) The law of effect, *Amer. J. of Psychol.*, **39**, 212–22.

Tindal, W., Beardsley, R. and Curtis, F. (eds) (1984) *Communication in Pharmacy Practice*, Lea and Febiger, Philadelphia.

Tittmar, H., Hargie, O. and Dickson, D. (1978) The moulding of health visitors: the evolved role played by mini-training, *Health Visitor J.*, **51**, 130–6.

Tomlinson, A. (1985) The use of experiential methods in teaching interpersonal skills to nurses in *Interpersonal Skills in Nursing: Research and Application* (ed. C. Kagan), Croom Helm, London.

Trower, P. (ed.) (1984) *Radical Approaches to Social Skills Training*, Croom Helm, London.

Trower, P., Bryant, B. and Argyle, M. (1978) *Social Skills and Mental Health*, Methuen, London.

Trower, P. and Kiely, B. (1983) Video feedback: help or hindrance? A review and analysis in *Using Video: Psychological and Social Applications* (eds P. Dowrick and S. Biggs), Wiley, Chichester.

Truax, C. (1966) Reinforcement and non-reinforcement in Rogerian psychotherapy, *J. of Abn. Psychol.*, **71**, 1–9.

Tuckett, D., Boulton, M. and Olson, C. *et al.* (1985) *Meetings Between Experts: A Study of Medical Consultations*, Tavistock, London.

Turock, A. (1980) Trainer feedback: a method for teaching interpersonal skills, *Counsellor Education and Supervision*, **19**, 216–22.

Turton, P. and Faulkner, A. (1983) Carer and educator, *J. of Dist. Nurs.*, **2**, 20–2.

Twentyman, C. and Zimering, R. (1979) Behavioural training of social skills: a critical review in *Progress in Behaviour Modification, Vol. 7* (eds M. Hersen, R. Eisler and P. Miller), Academic Press, New York.

van Ments, M. (1983) *The Effective Use of Role-Play: A Handbook for Teachers and Trainers*, Kogan Page, London.

Verby, J., Holden, P. and Davis, R. (1979) Peer review of consultations in primary care: the use of audiovisual recordings, *B. M. J.*, **1**, 1686–8.

Wainwright, G. (1985) *Body Language*, Hodder & Stoughton, London.

Waitzkin, H. (1984) Doctor-patient communication. Clinical implications of social scientific research, *J. of the Amer. Med. Assoc.*, **252**, 2441–6.

Wakeford, R. (1983) Communication skills training in United Kingdom medical schools in *Doctor-Patient Communication* (eds D. Pendleton and J. Hasler), Academic Press, London.

Wallace, G., Marx, R. and Martin, J. (1981) Training psychiatric nursing staff in social approval skills, *Canad. J. of Behav. Sci.*, **13**, 171–180.

Wallace, W., Horan, J., Baker, S. and Hudson, R. (1975) Incremental effects of modeling and performance feedback in teaching decision-making counselling, *J. of Counsel. Psychol.*, **22**, 570–2.

Wallbott, H. (1983) The instrument in *Using Video: Psychological and Social Applications* (eds P. Dowrick and S. Biggs), Wiley, Chichester.

Wallen, J., Waitzkin, H. and Stoeckle, J. (1979) Physicians' stereotypes about female health and illness: a study of patients' sex and the information process during medical interviews, *Women and Health*, **4**, 135–146.

Walsh, P. and Green, J. (1982) Pathways to impact evaluation in continuing education in the health professions, *J. of All. Health*, **11**, 115–23.

Walton, L. and MacLeod Clark, J. (1986) Making contact, *Nursing Times*, **82**, 28–32.

Watson, K. and Barker, L. (1984) Listening behavior: definition and measurement in *Communication Yearbook: 8* (eds R. Bostrom and B. Westley), Sage, Beverly Hills, California.

Watzlawick, P., Beavin, J. and Jackson, D. (1967), *Pragmatics of Human Communication*, W.W. Norton, New York.

Waxer, P. (1974) Nonverbal cues for depression, *J. of Abn. Psychol.*, **83**, 319–22.

Waxer, P. (1977) Nonverbal cues for anxiety: an examination of emotional leakage, *J. of Abn. Psychol.*, **86**, 306–14.

Weiner, M. (1980) Personal openness with patients: help or hindrance, *Texas Medicine*, **76**, 60–2.

Weinman, J. (1984) A modified essay question evaluation of pre-clinical teaching of communication skills, *Med. Ed.*, **18**, 164–7.

Weinstein, P. and Getz, T. (1978) Preclinical laboratory course in dental behavioral science: changing human behavior, *J. of Dent. Ed.*, **42**, 147–9.

Wessler, R. (1984) Cognitive – social psychological theories and social skills: a review in *Radical Approaches to Social Skills Training* (ed. P. Trower), Croom Helm, London.

West, C. (1983) Ask me no questions . . . an analysis of questions and replies in *The Social Organization of Doctor-Patient Communication* (eds S. Fisher and A. Todd), Center for Applied Linguistics, Washington DC.

Whitcher, S. and Fisher, J. (1979) Multi-dimensional reactions to therapeutic touch in a hospital setting, *J. of Pers. and Soc. Psychol.*, **37**, 87–96.

White, R. and Clemens, D. (1971) Trainee reaction to videotape as a feedback technique in a counselling practicum, *Can. Counsel.*, **5**, 225–30.

Whyte, B. (1980) Commentary on 'listening to patients', *Nursing Times*, September 9, 1784.

Wiemann, J. (1977) Explication and test of a model of communicative competence, *Human Commun. Res.*, **3**, 195–213.

Williams, L. (1978) Patient role-play by learners, *Nursing Times*, **74**, 1402–6.

Willis, F. and Hamm, H. (1980) The use of interpersonal touch in securing compliance, *J. of Nonverb. Behav.*, **5**, 49–55.

Wilmot, W. (1979) *Dyadic Communication: A Transactional Perspective*, Addison-Wesley, Reading, Massachusetts.

Winefield, H. (1982) Subjective and objective outcomes of communication skills training in first year, *Med. Ed.*, **16**, 192–6.

Wishner, J. (1960) Reanalysis of 'Impressions of Personality', *Psychol. Rev.*, **67**, 96–112.

Wohlking, W. and Gill, P. (1980) *Role Playing*, Educational Technology Publications, Englewood Cliffs, New Jersey.

Wolff, F., Marsnik, N., Tacey, W. and Nichols, R. (1983) *Perceptive Listening*, Holt, Rinehart and Winston, New York.

Wolinsky, J. (1983) Research crumbles stereotypes of age, *APA Monitor*, **14**, 26–8.

Wolpe, J. (1973) *The Practice of Behaviour Therapy*, Pergamon, Oxford.

Wolvin, A. and Coakley, C. (1982) *Listening*, W.C. Brown, Dubuque, Iowa.

Working Party Report on pharmaceutical education and training (1984) *Pharm. J.*, **232**, 495–508.

Yager, G. and Beck, T. (1985) Beginning practicum: it only hurt until I laughed, *Counselor Education and Supervision*, **25**, 149–56.

Young, L. and Willie, R. (1984) Effectiveness of continuing education for health professionals: a literature review, *J. of All. Health*, **13**, 112–23.

Zanna, M., Olson, J. and Herman, C. (eds) (1987) *Social Influence: The Ontario Symposium, Vol. 5*, Lawrence Elbaum Associates, Hillsdale, New Jersey.

Author index

Subject index